Vertebral Osteoporotic Compression Fractures

Vertebral Osteoporotic Compression Fractures

Editors

Marek Szpalski, M.D.
Senior Consultant and Associate Professor
Hôpitaux Iris Sud-Molière Longchamp
Université Libre de Bruxelles
Bruxelles, Belgium

Robert Gunzburg, M.D., Ph.D.
Senior Consultant
Department of Orthopedics
Centenary Clinic
Antwerp, Belgium

LIPPINCOTT WILLIAMS & WILKINS
A **Wolters Kluwer** Company
Philadelphia • Baltimore • New York • London
Buenos Aires • Hong Kong • Sydney • Tokyo

Acquisitions Editor: Robert Hurley
Developmental Editor: Kerry Barrett
Supervising Editor: Mary Ann McLaughlin
Production Service: Bermedica Production, Ltd.
Manufacturing Manager: Colin Warnock
Cover Designer: Patricia Gast
Compositor: Lippincott Williams & Wilkins Desktop Division
Printer: Maple Press

530 Walnut Street
Philadelphia, PA 19106 USA
LWW.com

Printed in the USA

Library of Congress Cataloging-in-Publication Data
Vertebral osteoporotic compression fractures / [edited by] Marek Szpalski, Robert Gunzburg.
p. ; cm.
Includes bibliographical references and index.
ISBN 0-7817-4262-5
1. Spine—Fractures. 2. Spinal cord compression. 3. Osteoporosis—Complications. I. Szpalski, Marek. II. Gunzburg, Robert.
[DNLM: 1. Spinal Cord Compression—therapy. 2. Spinal Fractures—therapy. 3. Osteoporosis—complications. 4. Spinal Cord Compression—etiology. 5. Spinal Fractures—etiology. WE 175 V567 2002]
RD768.V45 2002
617.1′51—dc21 2002030192

---

10 9 8 7 6 5 4 3 2 1

Contents

Contributing Authors

Federico Balagué, M.D. *Adjunct Associate Professor, Department of Orthopedic Surgery, New York University School of Medicine, New York, New York; Médecin-chef adjoint, Service de Rhumatologie, Médecine physique et Rééducation, Hôpital cantonal, Fribourg, Switzerland*

Michel Benoist, M.D. *Consultant Rheumatologist of Paris Hospitals, University of Paris VII, Paris, France; Consultant in Rheumatology, Department of Orthopedic Surgery, Hôpital Beaujon, Clichy, France*

Jérôme Berge, M.D. *Service de Neuroradiologie diagnostique et therapeutique, Centre Hospitalier Pellegrin, Bordeaux, France*

Luc Vanden Berghe, M.D. *Orthopaedic Spine Surgeon, Department of Orthopaedic Surgery, Sint Lucas Hospitaal, Sint Lucas Laam, Brugge, Belgium*

Michael Bierschneider, M.D. *Resident, Department of Neurosurgery, Berufsgenossenschaftliche Unfallklinik Murnau, Murnau, Germany*

Bronek M. Boszczyk, M.D. *Resident, Department of Neurosurgery, Berufsgenossenschaftliche Unfallklinik Murnau, Murnau, Germany*

Helena Brisby, M.D., Ph.D. *Assistant Professor, Department of Orthopaedics, Sahlgrenska Academy, Göteborg University, Göteborg, Sweden; Assistant Professor, Department of Orthopaedics, Sahlgrenska University Hospital, Göteborg, Sweden*

Chris De Laet, M.D., Ph.D. *Senior Researcher, Department of Public Health, Erasmus University Medical Center, Rotterdam, The Netherlands*

Joel Delécrin, M.D., Ph.D. *Associate Professor, Department of Orthopedic Surgery, Nantes University, Nantes, France; Associate Professor, Department of Orthopedic Surgery, Hôtel Dieu Place Ricordeau, Nantes, France*

Hervé Deramond, M.D. *Professor, Service de Radiologie A, CHU Amiens-Hôpital Nord, Amiens, France*

Jean Dudler, M.D. *Maître d'enseignement et de recherche (MER), Service de Rhumatologie, Médecine physique et Rééducation, Université de Lausanne, Dorigny, Lausanne, Switzerland; Chef de Clinique, Service de Rhumatologie, Médecine physique et Rééducation, Centre hospitalier universitaire vaudois, Lausanne, Switzerland*

Stephen Eisenstein, Ph.D., F.R.C.S. (Edin) *Director, Centre for Spinal Studies, The Robert Jones and Agnes Hunt Orthopaedic Hospital, Oswestry, Shropshire, United Kingdom*

Afshin Gangi, M.D. *Professor, Hopitaux Universitaires de Strasbourg, Hospices Civiles, Strasbourg, France*

Philippe Gillet, M.D. *Professor of Orthopaedic Surgery and Anatomy, University of Liège, Liège, Belgium; Chief, Department of Orthopaedic Surgery, Liège, Belgium*

Robert Gunzburg, M.D., Ph.D. *Senior Consultant, Department of Orthopedics, Centenary Clinic, Antwerp, Belgium*

Michael Hadjiargyrou, Ph.D. *Assistant Professor, Department of Biomedical Engineering, State University of New York, Stony Brook, Stony Brook, New York*

Véronique Halkin, M.D. *Consultant, Unité d'Exploration du Métabolisme de l'Os et du Cartilage, Centre Hospitalier Universitaire de Liège, Liège, Belgium*

Tommy Hansson, M.D., Ph.D. *Professor and Vice Dean, Göteborg University, The Faculty of Medicine, Sahlgren Academy, Göteborg, Sweden; Department of Orthopaedics, Sahlgren University Hospital, Göteborg, Sweden*

Paul F. Heini, M.D. *Head, Spine Unit, Department for Orthopaedic Surgery, Inselspital, University of Berne, Berne, Switzerland*

G. Michael Hess, M.D. *Staff Surgeon, Spine Center, Orthopedic Hospital Munich–Harlaching, Munich, Germany*

Hans Jaksche, M.D. *Chief, Department of Neurosurgery, Berufsgenossenschaftliche Unfallklinik Murnau, Murnau, Germany*

Olof Johnell, M.D., Ph.D. *Professor, Department of Orthopaedics, Lund University, Malmö University Hospital, Malmö, Sweden*

John A. Kanis, M.D. *Professor, Centre for Metabolic Bone Diseases, University of Sheffield Medical School, Sheffield, United Kingdom*

Tony S. Keller, Ph.D. *Professor, Department of Mechanical Engineering, The University of Vermont, Burlington, Vermont; Professor, Department of Orthopaedics & Rehabilitation, The University of Vermont, Burlington, Vermont*

Bart W. Koes, Ph.D. *Professor, Department of General Practice, Erasmus MC, University Medical Centre Rotterdam, Rotterdam, The Netherlands*

Victor Kosmopoulos, M.S. *Department of Mechanical Engineering, The University of Vermont, Burlington, Vermont*

Stephen D. Kuslich, M.D. *Consultant in Spinal Surgery, St. Croix Orthopedics, Stillwater, Minnesota; Assistant Clinical Professor, University of Minnesota, Minneapolis, Minnesota*

Angelo A. Licata, M.D., Ph.D. *Clinical Assistant Professor of Medicine, Department of Endocrinology, Case Western Reserve School of Medicine, Cleveland, Ohio; Director of Research, Metabolic Bone Center of Endocrinology, The Cleveland Clinic Foundation, Cleveland, Ohio*

Isador H. Lieberman, M.D., F.R.C.S.(C) *Orthopaedic and Spine Surgeon, Departments of Orthopaedics and Neurosurgery, The Cleveland Clinic, Cleveland, Ohio*

Michael A. K. Liebschner, Ph.D. *Assistant Professor, Department of Bioengineering, Rice University, Houston, Texas*

Angela Maria Lis, P.T., M.A. *Instructor, Departments of Orthopaedic and Environmental Health Sciences, Graduate School of Arts and Science, New York University, New York, New York; Research Physical Therapist, Occupational and Industrial Orthopaedic Center (OIOC), Hospital for Joint Diseases, New York, New York*

H. Michael Mayer, M.D., Ph.D. *Privat Dozent und Chefarzt, Spine Center, Orthopadische Klinik Munchen-Harlachinger, Muchen, Germany*

Christian Mélot, M.D., Ph.D., M.Sci.Biostat., M.Sci.HealthManag. *Professor of Biostatistics, Faculty of Medicine, Free University of Brussels, Brussels, Belgium; Associate Professor of Medicine, Intensive Care Department, Erasme University Hospital, Brussels, Belgium*

Everard A. Munting, M.D., Ph.D. *Associate Professor, Department of Orthopaedic Surgery, Université Catholique de Louvain, Brussels, Belgium; Staff Member, Department of Orthopaedic Surgery, Clinique St. Pierre, Ottignies, Belgium*

Margareta Nordin, Dr.Sci. *Research Professor, Departments of Orthopaedics and Environmental Health Sciences, Graduate School of Arts and Science, New York University, New York, New York; Director, Occupational and Industrial Orthopaedic Center (OIOC), Hospital for Joint Diseases, New York, New York*

Anders Odén *Consulting Statistician, Göteborg, Sweden*

Jean Palussière, M.D. *Service de Radiologie, Institut Bergonié, Imagerie Médicale, cours de l'Argonne, Bordeaux, France*

Norbert Passuti, M.D., Ph.D. *Professor, Department of Orthopedic Surgery, Nantes University, Nantes, France; Chief, Department of Orthopedic Surgery, Hôtel Dieu Place Ricordeau, Nantes, France*

Charles E. Pither, M.B.B.S., F.R.C.A. *Consultant, Pain Management Department, and Medical Director, Input Pain Unit, St. Thomas's Hospital, London, United Kingdom*

Malcolm H. Pope, D.Sc. *Professor, Department of Occupational Medicine, University of Aberdeen, Aberdeen, Scotland, United Kingdom*

Jean-Yves Reginster, M.D., Ph.D. *Professor and Head, Unité d'Exploration du Métabolisme de l'Os et du Cartilage, Centre Hospitalier Universitaire de Liège, Liège, Belgium*

Björn Robert, M.D. *Consultant, Department of Neurosurgery, Berufsgenossenschaftliche Unfallklinik Murnau, Murnau, Germany*

Clinton T. Rubin, Ph.D. *Professor and Chairman, Department of Biomedical Engineering, State University of New York, Psychology-A, Stony Brook, New York*

Janet Rubin, M.D. *Professor, Department of Medicine, Emory University School of Medicine, Atlanta, Georgia; Staff Physician, Department of Medicine, Atlanta Veterans Affairs Medical Center, Decatur, Georgia*

Björn Rydevik, M.D., Ph.D. *Professor, Department of Orthopaedics, Sahlgrenska Academy, Göteborg University, Göteborg, Sweden; Professor, Department of Orthopaedics, Sahlgrenska University Hospital, Göteborg, Sweden*

Sieglinde Major Schumacher, M.D. *Médecin-assistante, Service de Rhumatologie, Médecine physique et Rééducation, Hôpital cantonal, Fribourg, Switzerland*

Dirk W. Sommerfeldt, M.D. *Assistant Professor, Department of Surgery, Hamburg University, Martinistr. Hamburg, Germany; Attending Surgeon, Department of Trauma and Reconstructive Surgery, Hamburg University Hospital, Hamburg, Germany*

Marek Szpalski, M.D. *Senior Consultant and Associate Professor, Hôpitaux Iris Sud-Molière Longchamp, Université Libre de Bruxelles, Bruxelles, Belgium*

Jan T. Wilmink, Prof.Dr. *Neuroradiologist, Department of Radiology, University Hospital, Maastricht, The Netherlands*

Paul I. J. M. Wuisman, M.D., Ph.D. *Professor, Department of Orthopedics, Vrije Universiteit, Amsterdam, The Netherlands*

Preface

Osteoporosis is a major health problem and, with the ageing of the population, the problems related to this condition will undoubtedly increase. Between 20 and 25% of postmenopausal women have radiological evidence of at least one vertebral fracture and in some countries the prevalence climbs to 39% over 65 years of age. It is not without reason that the World Health Organization launched the Bone and Joint Decade (2000 – 2010), with the endorsement of the United Nations, and gave osteoporosis problems an important place in it. Whereas prevention of osteoporosis remains one of the primary goals, we still have to offer state-of-the-art treatment for the secondary effects and complications resulting from this condition. Vertebral compression fractures are a major example of these. This book is devoted to a better understanding of their etiopathogenesis, diagnosis, treatment, and, of course, prevention of recurrence.

In the first section of this book, we present an overview of the normal and pathological metabolism of bone in relation to osteoporosis, as well as principles of biomechanics. Computer modelization techniques enable a better understanding of the bone ultrastructure and the mechanisms of calcium loss.

The second section takes us into the field of the etiopathogenesis of vertebral compression fractures and its clinical presentation. Risk factors, incidence, epidemiology, and natural history are in turn discussed, as well as the mechanisms of pain and the possible neurological complications.

Diagnostic algorithms and differential diagnostic challenges are detailed and illustrated in the light of state-of-the-art imaging techniques.

The main section of this volume deals with the treatment of osteoporotic vertebral compression fractures. The conservative treatment modalities include pharmacological approaches, mechanical support through orthoses, elective pain therapy, physical medicine, exercise, and revalidation. The use of a series of new and promising substances is presented.

The surgical treatment is divided in two sections: vertebral augmentation and open surgery.

Vertebral augmentation comprises vertebroplasty and kyphoplasty techniques. The use of these procedures has shown a spectacular increase over the last few years and has reached a "fashionable" status discussed in the greater public media. These relatively new techniques are described in detail, as are the devices and many different biomaterials they require. The possible serious risks and complications are discussed in the light of the emerging results.

The rare indications for open surgery are discussed. Proposed techniques range from open decompression and spondylodesis to pedicle screw augmentation and total vertebrectomy and vertebral replacement.

Special attention is given to the problem of recurring osteoporotic vertebral fractures. Prevention of these may comprise prophylactic vertebral augmentation besides medical and behavioral approaches.

Finally, economic considerations governing the management of osteoporotic vertebral compression fractures are analysed. This is a major issue for a pathology whose medical costs are estimated to be in excess of $14 billion yearly in the United States.

In sum, the editors believe that the readers will experience this book as state of the art in the field of osteoporotic vertebral compression fractures. To this end, it is addressed to both clinicians and researchers in this field.

Marek Szpalski
Robert Gunzburg

1

Clinical Implications of Recent Advances in the Biology and Physiology of Bone[1]

*Dirk W. Sommerfeldt, †Michael Hadjiargyrou, ‡Janet Rubin, and *†Clinton T. Rubin

**Musculoskeletal Research Laboratory, Department of Biomedical Engineering, State University of New York, Stony Brook, New York; †Center for Biotechnology, State University of New York, Stony Brook, New York; *†Division of Endocrinology, Department of Medicine, Emory University, Atlanta, Georgia*

Bone is a highly specialized form of connective tissue that provides an internal support system and facilitates locomotion. The skeleton also serves as a mineral reservoir that contains 99% of the body's total calcium, 85% of its phosphorus, and 66% of its magnesium, all of which are key elements for the function of the organism. These contrasting and yet interdependent responsibilities are met through bone's ability to augment its structure in response to increased functional demand, as well as its ability to remodel, to retain mineral homeostasis and repair itself. Metabolic challenges, such as aging, nutritional deficiencies, endocrinopathy, or menopause, however, disrupt and uncouple bone's resorptive and formative activity, potentiating the loss of bone to the point of structural failure, or osteoporosis. Indeed, many interventional strategies for preventing or reversing this skeletal loss are based on restoring the balance of bone formation and resorption (1).

The first vertebrates appeared in the Ordovician period, approximately 500 million years ago; their bone provided anchors and levers for musculature and thus made locomotory and masticatory activities more efficient and powerful. Since that time, bone has evolved to become a complex living tissue in which the mineralized extracellular matrix confers marked rigidity and strength to the skeleton while adjusting its degree of elasticity according to need. Phylogenetically, antlers of deer have adapted to elastically absorb the impact of intentional collision by increasing collagen content; the temporal bullae of the whale have maximized acoustic transmissibility by establishing a matrix almost devoid of collagen; and the tibiae of migrating cursors are capable of withstanding thousands, if not millions, of loading cycles without failure by optimizing a resilient collagen/mineral composite in such a way that there is the ability to resist loads and avoid fatigue failure (2,3).

Despite the remarkable attributes of bone tissue, skeletal injury concomitant with metabolic bone disease, particularly atraumatic fractures of the spine and hip as potentiated by osteoporosis, gravely compromise the lifestyle of millions around the world (4) and indicates that the tissue no longer serves as an optimized biological system. With the current pandemic of musculoskeletal conditions and the opportunities now available through

[1]This work has been kindly supported by grants from the German Research Foundation, the National Institutes of Health, the National Aeronautics and Space Administration, and the National Space Biomedical Research Institute.

genomic data to prevent and/or treat diseases and injuries to bone (5), it is critical that both physicians and scientists improve their understanding of the biology of bone and how its ability to form and resorb tissue ultimately results in the success of the skeleton.

THE CELLS OF BONE

Bone is a composite material composed of a mineralized matrix interspersed with an organic scaffold that consists primarily of collagen. There are three different cell types in the bone tissue: osteoblasts, which forms osteoid—the unmineralized matrix—of bone; osteocytes, which account for well over 95% of all cells in the adult skeleton; and osteoclasts, which are multinucleated giant cells responsible for the resorption of bone. The osteoblast and osteocyte in the postcranial skeleton derive from pluripotent mesenchymal stem cells (6), whereas the osteoclast is of hematopoietic origin and its precursors are located in the monocytic fraction of the bone marrow (7).

Osteoblasts

Morphologically, osteoblasts are cuboidal in shape and located at the bone surface, along with their precursors and their less active form, bone-lining cells. The tight canopy of the lining cells enables the selective isolation of the mineralized surface from the extracellular milieu, which is critical for the site-specific control of mineralization or resorption. Osteoblasts are highly anchorage-dependent and rely on extensive cell-matrix and cell-cell contacts through a variety of transmembranous proteins (integrins, connexins, cadherins) and specific receptors (for cytokines, hormones, growth factors) to maintain cellular function and responsiveness to metabolic and mechanical stimuli (8,9).

The osteoblast's principal function is to form bone, first with secretion of the osteoid and then by nucleation and mineralization of the osteoid matrix. Osteoid can be functionally described by a panel of secretory proteins, including type I collagen and several noncollagenous proteins and proteoglycans that are critical to the appropriate orchestration of the remodeling response. Many of the proteins secreted or displayed by the osteoblasts have signaling roles in bone *resorption,* such as the suggested role of osteocalcin to recruit osteoclasts (10); the plasminogen activator, which initiates the cascade of collagen breakdown (11); or receptor activator of nuclear factor κB (NF-κB) ligand (RANKL), which is critical for osteoclastogenesis (12). Others, such as osteopontin and bone sialoprotein, strongly bind ionic calcium and may serve as cell attachment factors (13).

Study of the molecular mechanisms involved in osteoblast maturation has uncovered a specific nuclear factor critical for entry of the pluripotent mesenchymal stem cell into the osteoblast lineage. This helix-loop-helix factor, termed CBFA1, is reminiscent of other nuclear factors that designate differentiation of the mesenchymal stem cell in other directions, such as the induction of myotubule formation by MyoD. In the case of CBFA1, expression of osteoblastic characteristics and bone development requires its presence *in vitro* (14). Heterozygous loss of CBFA1 in several human kindreds causes cleidocranial dysplasia, a condition in which short stature and hypoplasia of the clavicles (15) was predictive of a similar phenotype generated by targeted disruption of the CBFA1 gene in mice (16).

Wnt-mediated signaling has been established as critical to osteoblast function. The autosomal recessive disorder osteoporosis-pseudoglioma syndrome, distinguished by reduced bone mass, has been shown to arise from mutations in the low-density lipoprotein (LDL) receptor—related protein 5 (LRP5) (17). These investigators have shown that LRP5 is expressed by osteoblasts and is involved in transducing *Wnt* signaling. A mutant form of soluble LRP5 apparently can reduce bone thickness in mouse calvarial cultures. Work is being done to establish that reduced LRP5 expression is associated with reduced bone mass, and it is possible that inherited alterations in bone mass may be traced to polymorphisms in the LRP5 gene as well as to other components of the *Wnt* pathway in osteoblasts.

The life span of an osteoblast ranges from 3 days in young rabbits up to 8 weeks in humans, during which it lays down 0.5 to 1.5 μm of osteoid per day (18,19). At a rate of 0.5 to 1.5 μm per day, an active human osteoblast produces a seam of osteoid about 15 μm thick before mineralization ensues, which suggests that the average osteoblast life in humans is 15 days. While seams have been reported to exceed 70 mm, such a seam width can also indicate a disruption or flaw in the mineralization process (e.g., rickets [20] and osteomalacia [21]). As mineralization proceeds, the osteoblast may become engulfed in its own calcifying osteoid matrix. Osteoblasts remaining behind in small lacunae retain connections with other similarly disposed cells, creating the osteocyte network.

Osteocytes

Derived from osteoblasts and yet distinctly different in morphology and function, osteocytes are the most abundant cells in bone. As terminally differentiated osteoblasts, the osteocytes have relatively reduced their cell organelles, such as ribosomes and endoplasmic reticula, and have an increased ratio of nucleus to cytoplasm. These cells continue to produce, obviously to a lesser extent, matrix-modulating proteins (MMP; e.g., collagen, MMP-1), which may offer a means for modifying the architecture of their lacunae, and thus can self-regulate their mechanical environment (22). A complex of cell processes, or filopodia, from the osteocyte body extend through canaliculae to neighboring osteocytes and surface-residing bone-lining cells, creating an extensive network of intercellular communication (Fig. 1.1). This three-dimensional syncytium is ideally placed to sense subtle changes in the mechanical and/or hormonal milieu (23), including a means of guiding the repair and replacement of damaged matrix or apoptotic osteocytes (24–26). Considering that the osteocyte is the principal constituent of adult bone and that neither the osteoclast or osteoblast is evident in any significant numbers in the relatively quiescent adult skeleton, it is reasonable to presume that the osteocyte is responsible for orchestrating the spatial and temporal recruitment of the cells that form and resorb bone (27,28).

Osteoclasts

The main feature of the osteoclast is its ability to resorb fully mineralized bone at sites called Howship's lacunae. Both macrophages and osteoclasts are derived from hematopoietic stem cells, and, like macrophages, osteoclasts are highly migratory, multinucleated, and polarized cells that carry an arsenal of lysosomal enzymes (29). They have to be highly specialized to fulfill their task and possess several unique ultrastructural characteristics, such as pleomorphic mitochondria, vacuoles, and lysosomes (30). Probably the most intriguing feature is the apical membrane, which is able to form a tight seal with the calcified matrix (Fig. 1.2). A resorption bay into which the lytic enzymes are secreted is formed underneath the cell. In addition, proton pumps lower the pH in this subosteoclastic space to values between 2 and 4, activating the secreted enzymes such as tartrate-resistant acid phosphatase (31) and cathepsin K (32). An activated osteoclast is able to resorb 200,000 μm^3 per day, an amount of bone formed by seven to ten generations of osteoblasts with an average life span of 15 to 20 days (33).

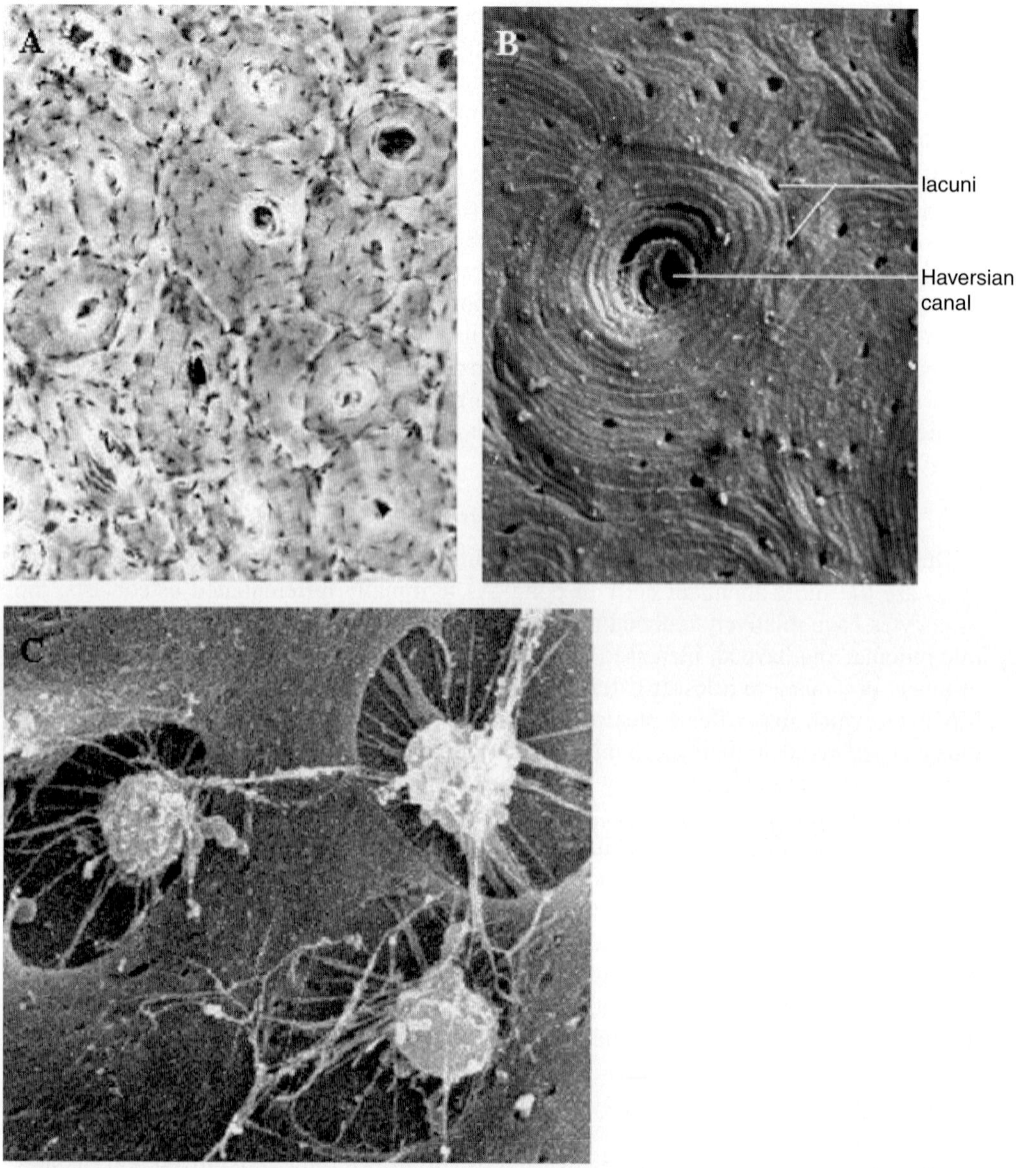

FIG. 1.1. Ultrastructure of bone. **A:** Light microscopic image (350× magnification) of a ground section of compact bone. Osteons or haversian systems can be seen. The central dark circle is the haversian canal, which contains a nutrient artery *in vivo*. It is surrounded by concentric lamellae of calcified bone matrix. The dark spots visible within the compacta are the lacunae, in which osteocytes become entrapped. **B:** Scanning electron micrograph (SEM; 800× magnification) of a haversian system. **C:** SEM at higher magnification (1600×) reveals individual osteocytes with cellular processes reaching out toward the lacunar wall and interconnecting cells in an intricate network. (Reproduced with permission from the Department of Functional Anatomy, University of Glasgow, Glasgow, Scotland, http://www.anatomy.gla.ac.uk/fab/).

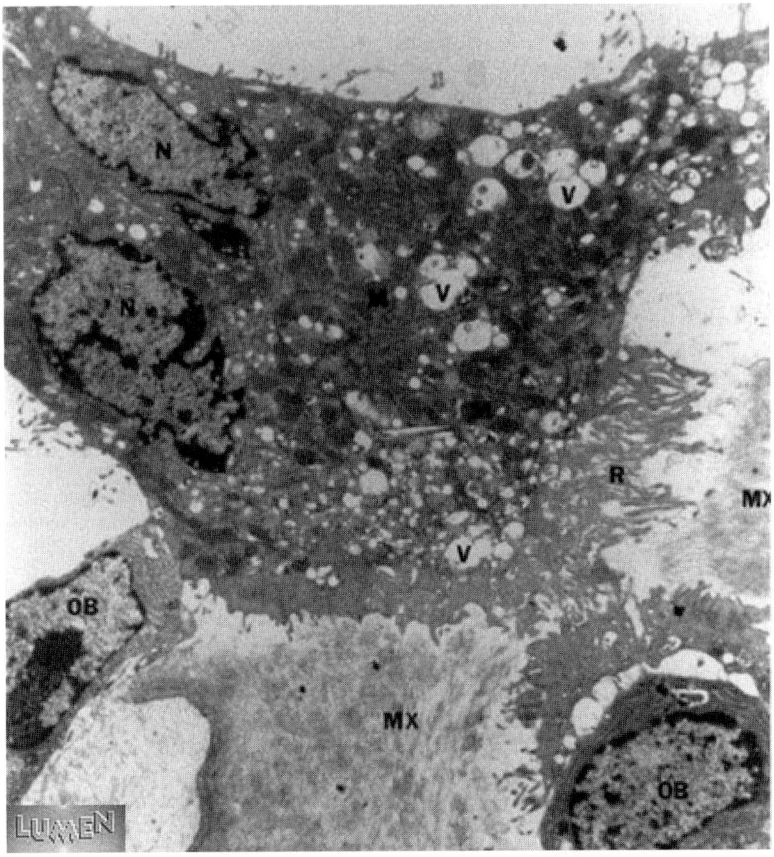

FIG. 1.2. Electron microscopy (1500× magnification) of an active osteoclast adjacent to two osteoblasts (OB). Its ruffled border (R) is visible next to the area where bony matrix (MX) is being resorbed. Note the high number of vacuoles (V) containing lysosomal enzymes and the multinucleated (N) nature of this cell derived from hematopoetic stem cells. (Reproduced with permission from LUMEN, Loyola University Medical Network, http://www.lumen.luc.edu/lumen).

The processes controlling osteoclast differentiation have been the subjects of intense scrutiny, allowing the process to be reduced, at least in tissue culture, to three basic elements: the osteoclast precursor cell, which arises out of the macrophage lineage of hematopoietic stem cells; macrophage colony stimulating factor (MCSF), which is necessary for the differentiation, proliferation and survival of cells of macrophage lineage; and RANKL (variably referred to as osteoprotegerin ligand, TRANCE, or osteoclast differentiation factor [ODF]) (12,34). The most important factor promoting entry of hematopoietic stem cells into the macrophage lineage is MCSF. Loss of MCSF action engenders deficiencies of both osteoclasts and macrophages: the osteopetrotic *op/op* mouse, which secretes an ineffective MCSF, is characterized by a prematurely terminated MCSF protein molecule, which results in absence of both macrophages and osteoclasts (35). Interestingly, when *op/op* mice are "rescued" with MCSF infusions early in life, they no longer require MCSF for normal bone remodeling (36). The reason for this late sufficiency remains uncertain, but it was reported that the *op/op* mouse could also be rescued by vascular endothelial growth factor (VEGF), which suggests that VEGF may be able to substitute for MCSF under certain conditions (37).

Coupling of Osteoblast to Osteoclast Activity

Although it had been suggested for many years that communication between osteoblasts and osteoclasts must exist to coordinate processes of bone formation and resorption, it was not until 1997 that a molecular basis for this paradigm was discovered in the form of osteoprotegerin (OPG) (38), and shortly after, its cognate ligand, RANKL, a transmembranous protein expressed on osteoblasts and immune cells (39). RANKL can bind to RANK (receptor activator of NF-κB), a transmembranous receptor expressed on osteoclast precursor cells. Interaction between RANKL and RANK initiates a signaling and gene expression cascade, resulting in the promotion of osteoclast formation from the precursor pool. In this setting, OPG, which is secreted by osteoblasts but is also expressed in many other tissues, acts as a soluble competitive binding partner for RANKL, which inhibits osteoclast formation and, consequentially, bone resorption (40) (Fig. 1.3). Inter-

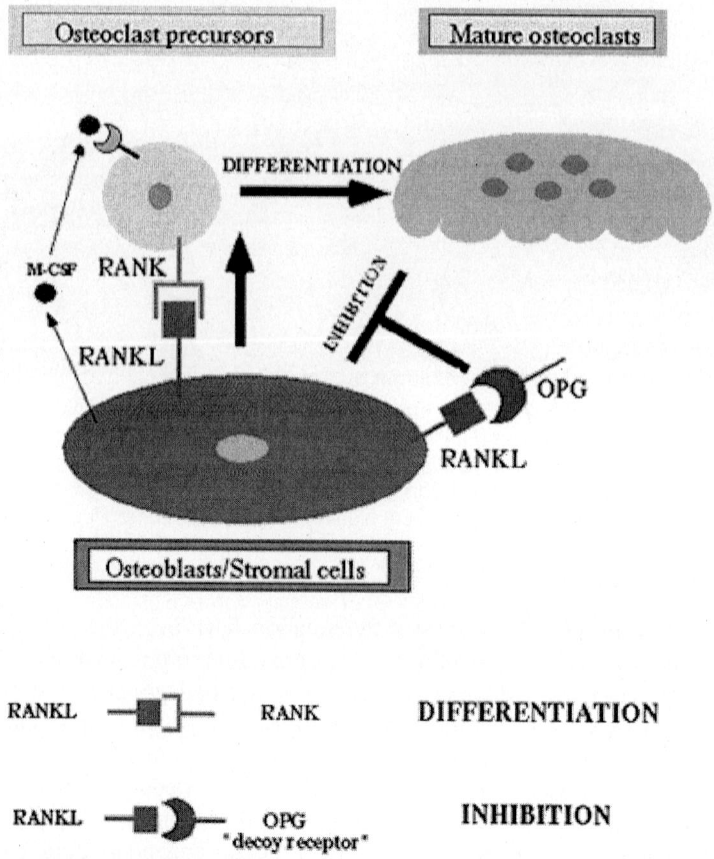

FIG. 1.3. Schematic of osteoblast: osteoclast interaction via receptor activator of nuclear factor κB (RANK)-RANK ligand (RANKL) and osteoprotegerin (OPG). RANKL, a transmembranous receptor on the surface of mature osteoblasts, interacts with the transmembranous RANK receptor on osteoblast precursor cells. This interaction induces proliferation and differentiation of osteoclasts in the presence of the permissive factor M-CSF and can be inhibited by the soluble protein OPG. (Reproduced with permission from Aubin JE, Bonnelye E. Osteoprotegerin and its ligand: a new paradigm for regulation of osteoclastogenesis and bone resorption. *Medscape Womens Health* 2000;5[2]:5.)

estingly, the RANKL-RANK-OPG system is being recognized as a modulator of both cancer metastasis and hypercalcemia. For instance, prostate carcinoma that has metastasized to bone expresses soluble RANKL, and OPG prevents bone metastasis (41). The hypercalcemia associated with multiple myeloma appears to involve a disrupted RANKL-OPG axis (42). This communication mechanism also appears to be an end point for the action of several calciotropic hormones and cytokines, such as 1,25-$(OH)_2D_3$, parathormone (PTH), estrogen, prostaglandin E_2 (PGE_2), interleukins, and tumor necrosis factor α (TNF-α). As a result of these findings, and a mere 3 years after its discovery, OPG entered clinical trials as a promising therapeutic agent for osteoporosis (43,44).

EXTRACELLULAR MATRIX

Calcified bone contains about 25% of organic matrix, including cells (2% to 5%), water (5%), and inorganic mineral (e.g., hydroxyapatite) (70%). Osteoid, which is the freshly synthesized matrix before its mineralization, consists primarily (94%) of collagen. Other proteins, some of them unique to bone, such as osteocalcin, are embedded in the extracellular matrix (ECM) and can have important signaling functions (bone morphogenetic proteins [BMPs], growth factors, cytokines, adhesion molecules) or play a role during the mineralization process (osteopontin, osteonectin, matrix Gla protein) either during the early stages of modeling or when released during the resorptive phase of remodeling to ensure coupling of formative activity (45). Studies of knockout mice lacking the ability to synthesize these proteins have shed light on the individual functions of some of these proteins. Osteocalcin-deficient mice, for example, display increased bone formation (14), whereas mice lacking osteonectin are osteopenic because of reduced bone remodeling (46).

The majority of the noncollagenous proteins in bone consist of proteoglycans, the function of which was regarded until the mid 1990s as structural. Studies of transgenic mouse models, however, showed that at least some of these molecules, such as perlecan and biglycan, in addition to their role in defining the spatial organization of the ECM, can also have unique functions at a biochemical level. In the case of perlecan, for example, synthesis of the proteoglycan is essential for survival of these animals, possibly because of roles in facilitating cellular signaling and/or interactions with growth factors during development (47).

Ten to 15 days after the organic matrix has been laid down, it begins to mineralize. During this period, the mineral content increases suddenly to 70% of its final amount; deposition of the final 30%, in contrast, takes several months (recall that unusually wide osteoid seams do not necessarily indicate overly active osteoblasts; they may also signify dysfunctional mineralization, such as with osteomalacia). Although the actual process of mineralization remains poorly understood, several investigators believe that the initiators of this process are small, round, extracellular lipid-bilaminar organelles, which bud from hypertrophic chondrocytes or osteoblasts. These matrices contain phosphatases, phospholipids, and calcium ions (48). At a point of supersaturation, mineral crystalization begins, and as the matrix vesicles disintegrate, the mineral is exposed to the matrix, in which the process of mineralization proceeds in a self-perpetuating manner. During this process, collagen fibrils, fibronectin, and some glycoproteins, such as osteonectin and osteopontin, determine the orientation and organization of the bone mineral crystal (49). Other glycoproteins, such as matrix Gla protein and glycosaminoglycans, appear to play a role in the inhibition of excessive mineralization (50).

Bone mineral is generically referred to as hydroxyapatite $[Ca_{10}(PO_4)_6(OH)_2]$, a platelike crystal 20 to 80 nm in length and 2 to 5 nm thick. Because it is 4X smaller than naturally occurring apatites and less perfect in structure, it is more reactive and soluble and facilitates chemical turnover (51). In other words, it would be more difficult for a more "perfect" crystal to be resorbed, and thus repair of the matrix would be hindered. Typically, the degree of mineralization of bone, or bone mineral density (BMD), is estimated in the clinic by dual energy x-ray absorptiometry (DXA) or quantitative computed tomography (qCT) and is the principal diagnostic measure for osteoporosis (52).

BONE DEVELOPMENT

The vertebrate skeleton is the product of a complex, coordinated, and synergistic interaction among three distinctly different cell lineages: Cells derived from the neural crest are responsible for the development of the branchial arches and, ultimately, the craniofacial skeleton; sclerotome cells, a subdivision of the somites and of mesodermal origin, give rise to the axial skeleton; and the lateral plate mesoderm is the starting point for limb bud formation and long bone development (53).

There are two possible mechanisms of bone formation during morphogenesis. According to one, mesenchymal cells differentiate directly into osteoblasts, which then proceed to form bone. This membranous or intramembranous bone formation is found during skull development and in maxilla and mandibula morphogenesis. If differentiation of mesenchymal cells proceeds through chondrocytes, which then form cartilaginous templates, or anlagen, of the future bones, the process is termed *endochondral ossification*. The cartilage anlagen develop by interstitial and appositional growth and are at some point replaced by invading osteoblasts, which replace the hypertrophic cartilage and allow ossification of the structure (54). Although there are obvious genomic influences on anlagen morphology, it has been proposed that the stresses and strains encountered even during fetal development are critical determinants of the architecture of the element, including trabecular patterns (55).

Development of the axial skeleton in the human starts during the fourth week post gestation, when cells from the paraxial mesoderm condense to form somites and, subsequently, sclerotomes. After differentiating into chondrocytes and migrating ventrally, dorsally, and laterally of the neural tube, the cartilage anlagen for the vertebral body, neural arches, and ribs or transverse processes, respectively, are formed.

A key aspect during development of the vertebral column is to create a flexible enclosure to allow continuous growth of the neural components, which develop slower and at a later time. During the precartilaginous stage (weeks 4 to 6) the vertebral anlage is formed by the sclerotomal mesenchyme surrounding the notochord. Each sclerotome has two components, whose cranial loose cells fuse with the next segment, whereas the caudal dense cells form the annulus fibrosus of the intervertebral disk and surrounding the notochord, which eventually forms the nucleus pulposus. The most caudal cells then fuse with the cranial cells from the next segment, and so on (Fig. 1.4). During the cartilaginous stage, the mesenchy-

→

FIG. 1.4. Development of the vertebral column. Somatogenesis begins during gestational week 4 with condensation in the paraxial mesoderm **(A)**. Cells within the somites further differentiate, and the cells surrounding the notochord then proceed to form the sclerotome **(B)**. Sclerotome cells then differentiate into chondrocytes that form the anlagen of vertebral bodies **(C)**. Somite formation is clearly visible in a human embryo at day 22.5 **(D, E)**. (Images courtesy of Professor Kohei Shiota, Congenital Anomaly Research Center, Kyoto University Faculty of Medicine, Kyoto, Japan.) In **F**, a section through the cartilaginous anlage of vertebral body Th1 in a human embryo at day 55, the ventral sclerotome (vS) forming the vertebral body and the two dorsal sclerotomes (dS) forming the vertebral arches, which will fuse after birth, are clearly visible. dL, dorsal lamina; sG, spinal ganglion. (Courtesy of Dr. Mark Hill, Cell Biology Lab, School of Anatomy, University of New South Wales, Sydney, Australia.)

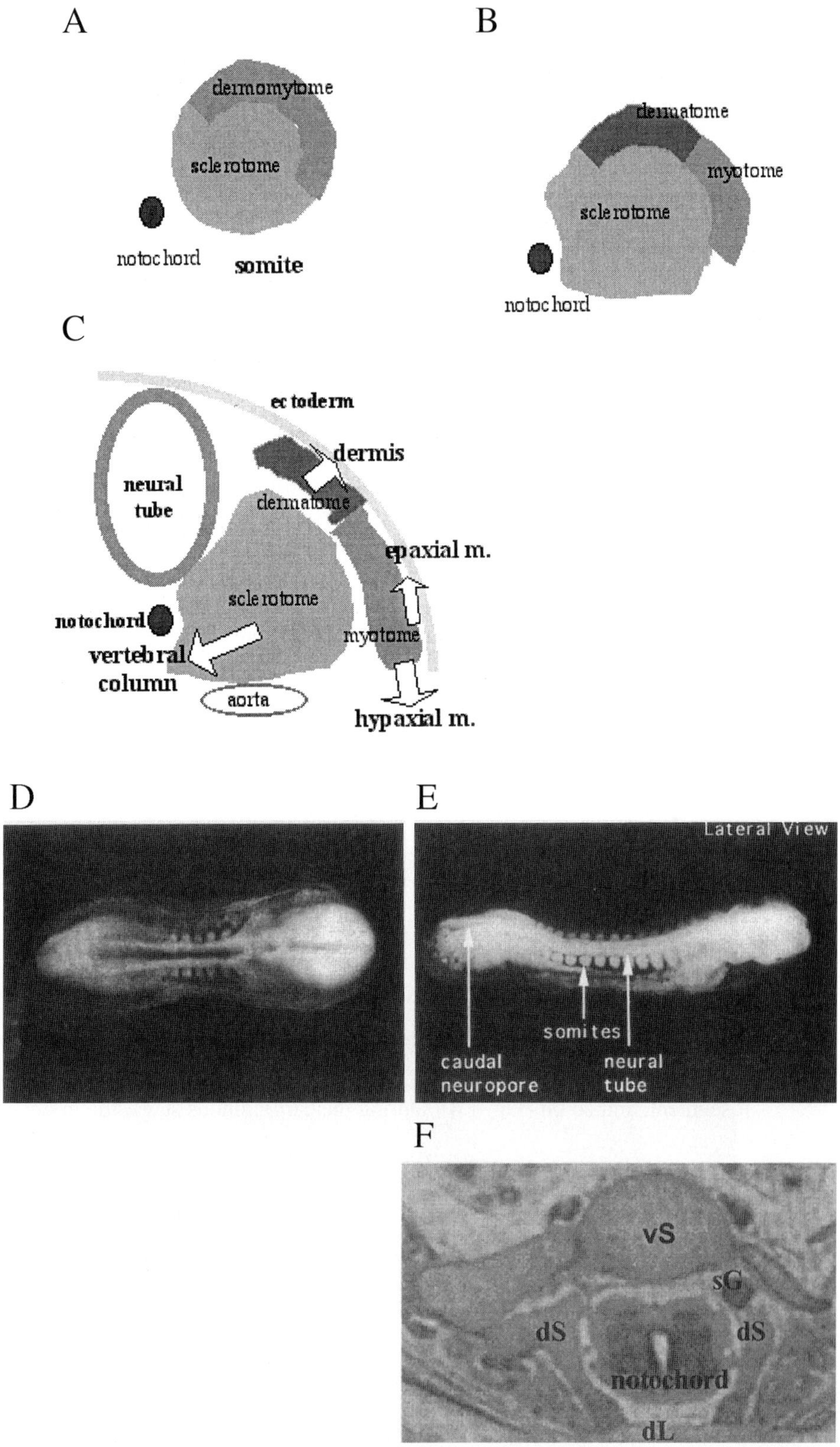
A
dermomyotome
sclerotome
notochord
somite
B
dermatome
myotome
sclerotome
notochord
C
ectoderm
dermis
neural tube
dermatome
epaxial m.
sclerotome
notochord
vertebral column
myotome
aorta
hypaxial m.
D
E
Lateral View
somites
caudal neuropore
neural tube
F
vS
sG
dS
dS
notochord
dL

mal anlagen are replaced by cartilage (week 7) and finally, during the bony stage of vertebral development (week 7 to age 25 years), by three primary ossification centers from within the cartilaginous vertebrae. The two dorsal centers form the two vertebral arches, which do not fuse until the age of 3 to 5 years. The central and more ventral ossification center forms the vertebral body. Vertebral development is not completed until puberty, as the secondary ossification centers on the vertebral body and facets are constituted.

This lengthy process of spine development is under tight and complex genetic control and regulation. For example, a master gene for development of the vertebral column is the secreted cytokine *sonic hedgehog.* Mice carrying inactivated alleles of this gene do not form a spine and are lacking the posterior parts of their ribs (56). *Sonic hedgehog* and a number of highly conserved homeobox transcription factors, which have been under intense investigation since the mid-1990s, are equally important during limb formation, for which they control dorsal-ventral, proximal-distal, and posterior-anterior patterning (57).

BONE MORPHOLOGY

Bones are exceptionally well suited for their structural demands. At the gross morphological level, as hollow tubes they provide great strength and durability in response to axial compression forces while at the same time minimizing weight to accomplish this response efficiently. The ultimate tensile strength of bone approaches that of cast iron, and its capacity to absorb and release energy is twice that of oak; however, the weight of bone is only one third that of steel (58). At the next level, the integrated architecture of the dense cortical shell and the intricate cancellous scaffolding that together, can accommodate the complex array of stresses and strains that arise during functional load bearing. The trabecular cascades of the proximal femur, for example, readily distribute the forces and moments to the cortical shell of the diaphysis. The loss of trabeculae within this proximal region is not only a sign of osteopenia but also an indication of an increased

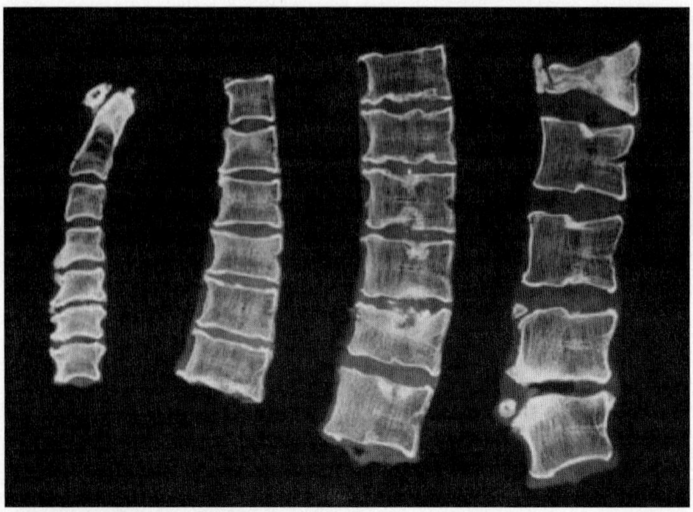

FIG. 1.5. Contact radiograph of a cervical, thoracic, and lumbar human spine. The trabecular architecture within the vertebral body is shown, as is the orientation of trabeculi, preferably in the direction of axial loading. Note the multiple degenerative changes, such as C1/C2 fusion with the formation of osteophytes and the osteoporotic compression fracture of L1. (Image courtesy of Dr. M. Amling, Department of Trauma and Reconstructive Surgery, University of Hamburg, Hamburg, Germany.)

risk of femoral neck fracture. The vertebral body distributes axial compressive forces throughout a tightly woven network of trabecular bone, thus minimizing fracture risk even under extreme conditions of flexion and extension of the spine under load (Fig. 1.5). Indeed, it is exactly the deterioration of this trabecular network that allows the catastrophic collapse of the vertebral body.

Microscopically, bone is made up of two distinct phenotypes: woven and lamellar. As mentioned earlier, woven bone is characteristic of embryonic and fetal development, but it is also found in the healthy adult skeleton at ligament and tendon insertions as well as under pathological conditions, such as osteogenic tumor and metastasis formation or in the temporary callus of a healing fracture, where it is typically remodeled into lamellar bone within a few weeks of deposition. Architecturally, it has an irregular, disorganized pattern of collagen fiber orientation and osteocyte distribution. Mechanical stimulation can cause rapid production of woven bone, which ultimately remodels into dense, lamellar bone (59); this indicates that the woven bone response is a strategic means of rapidly responding to changes in functional activity.

Lamellar, or mature, bone is found in cortical as well as trabecular bone. The structural subunits, the lamellae, run parallel to the trabeculae or, as is the case in cortical bone, are arranged in osteons, which are composed of up to 20 concentric lamellar plates that form a cylinder with a diameter of 200 to 300 μm. A central capillary runs through the osteon, and up to seven concentric rings of osteocytes are incorporated into its wall. It is possible to identify primary osteons, which form *de novo* (e.g., during woven bone consolidation) and secondary osteons or haversian systems, which form through resorption of preexisting bone and account for most of the adult human bone tissue (33).

SYSTEMIC REGULATION OF BONE REMODELING

Modeling is the process in which bone is laid down onto surfaces without necessarily being preceded by resorption. Examples of this are the appositional increases to the periosteal or endosteal surface. In the case of remodeling, osteoclastic resorption of bone leaves pockets that are subsequently filled by osteoblast activity. This cyclic sequence of turnover is also called the activation-resorption-reversal-formation (ARRF) sequence and takes about 3 to 6 months to be completed in humans (60). Approximately 2% to 5% of the healthy adult skeleton is undergoing bone turnover at any given point, but most turnover is occurring in the metabolically more active trabecular elements.

Remodeling not only serves to replace dead or damaged tissue but also serves as a means for bone's capacity to adapt to changes in loading as well as to respond to nutritional and/or metabolic changes (61,62). Ultimately, the pathological processes inherent in bone diseases are reflected by inconsistencies in this remodeling sequence. For example, osteoporosis is generally viewed as an inability of osteoblasts to fully repair the resorptive defects during normal osteoclast resorption, because mean wall thickness and porosity in cortical bone are generally elevated and trabecular spacing in cancellous bone is increased (63). Perhaps as a consequence of the higher degree of remodeling observed in trabeculae, these critical structural elements are more at risk for unbalanced turnover sequences. Under conditions of aging, or changes in hormone levels, the trabeculae are at great risk of dissolving, and once connectivity is disrupted, it is very difficult to reestablish. Indeed, it is exactly this imbalance that is targeted by antiresorptive interventions for osteoporosis. It is believed that if the existing bone mineral is more difficult to resorb (or making the osteoclasts dysfunctional), the resorptive activity will no longer outpace formative activity, and bone mineral density will be maintained. There certainly is evidence of bone loss prevention or even reduced fracture rates in patients who tolerate pharmaceuticals such as hormone replacement therapy (64) and bisphosphonates (65), but some concern persists for the quality of the tissue that remains (66).

It is generally accepted that the principal responsibility of systemic peptide or steroid hormones is to regulate mineral homeostasis rather than locally control skeletal morphology. Nevertheless, PTH, for example, as the main regulator of serum calcium, has significant effects on bone remodeling. By indirectly stimulating osteoclast activity through an increase in RANKL on the osteoblast membrane and/or inhibition of OPG secretion, PTH is able to release calcium and phosphate into the blood stream while at the same time inducing net bone resorption (67).

RANKL and OPG are also implicated in vitamin D ($1,25\text{-}(OH)_2D_3$)–stimulated bone remodeling. $1,25\text{-}(OH)_2D_3$ is responsible for absorption of dietary calcium, and thus low levels lead to undermineralized bone. High levels of $1,25\text{-}(OH)_2D_3$, however, are associated with increased expression of RANKL with subsequent osteoclast activation and bone resorption and may concurrently repress circulating OPG levels.

As an example of induction of bone formation via the same effector pathway, estrogen—or, more correctly, 17β-estradiol, protects bone by increasing OPG levels in osteoblasts, thus inhibiting osteoclast differentiation and activation as well as promoting osteoclast apoptosis. Another discrete explanation for estrogen deficiency osteoporosis also points to the RANKL-RANK axis. The intracellular signaling cascade activated by the binding of RANKL to RANK is muted in the presence of estradiol (68). Therefore, using the same effector mechanism, namely the RANKL-RANK interaction, many cytokines and calciotropic hormones seem to exert their (sometimes) dual effects on bone formation and/or resorption (40).

PTH is another excellent example of a factor that, depending on levels and periodicity, can be either catabolic or anabolic to bone. Indeed, a primary function of PTH is to maintain serum ionized calcium levels within a narrow physiologic range. PTH secretion rises as calcium levels drop below 8 mg per deciliter, controlled via decreased binding of the calcium ion to the calcium receptor on the parathyroid cell (69). Thus, a serum calcium value above 10 mg per deciliter accompanied by a high level of serum PTH is diagnostic of hyperparathyroidism, with a concomitant loss of bone (70). Studies have also demonstrated, however, that PTH (1–34), when applied *intermittently*, can be strongly anabolic to bone (71). In this landmark prospective trial on 1,637 postmenopausal women with osteoporosis, it was shown that daily injections of 20 or 40 mg of PTH stimulated a 9% or 13% increase in bone mineral density, respectively. Furthermore, this enhancement of BMD was paralleled by a concomitant reduction in incidence of vertebral fractures of 65% and 69%, respectively. Although long term follow-up is not yet available and the use of this drug remains controversial, including potentiating hypercalcemia and/or gout, these data demonstrate the marked potential of a unique anabolic agent for enhancing both the quantity and quality of bone, particularly the spine. Considering that *all* interventions (e.g., bisphosphonates, calcitonin, estrogen) currently approved by the U.S. Food and Drug Administration (FDA) for treatment of osteoporosis work by inhibiting resorptive activity, this agent represents a critical new addition to the armentarium for preventing and perhaps reversing the disease. Indeed, a combinatorial therapy, which harnesses the potential of both anabolic and antiresorptive therapies, may enable physicians to effectively curb osteoporosis with much lower doses of each (72).

In addition to these hormonal regulatory mechanisms, exciting data has been gathered in support of a central control mechanism for bone mass control by the hypothalamus. In this model, leptin not only regulates body mass, but also—and at much lower serum concentrations—has an inhibitory effect on bone mass. This effect is apparently not mediated by a direct effect on bone cells and is also independent of the action of endocrine organs such as the pituitary gland, the parathyroid, and adrenal glands; instead, it suggests an additional control of bone mass solely by the central nervous system (73).

STRUCTURAL ADAPTATION IN BONE

A great deal of bone's structural success is derived not only phylogenetically (recall the deer antler and whale bullae [2]) but also through its ability to constantly redefine its mass and morphology to accommodate subtle changes in the mechanical demands of the individual. Examples for this structure-function relationship are manifold. Be it the 35% increase in cortical thickness on the humerus of the playing arm of the professional tennis player (74) or the striking bone resorption resulting from immobilization or space flight (75), it is clear that bone can quickly identify changes in its functional milieu and respond to it structurally. The "form-follows-function" concept as it pertains to the mechanical adaptation in bone was first proposed in 1892 and is widely referred to as Wolff's law (76). Even though this "law" is over a century old, it remains unclear as to what parameters in the functional environment actually control bone's adaptive response.

Certainly, one of the most attractive, and certainly inevitable, regulatory stimuli are the peak strains that bone will accommodate during functional activities. Peak strain magnitudes measured in a wide range of adult species are remarkably similar, ranging from 2,000 to -3,500 microstrain (where the yield strain of bone is approximately 7,000 microstrain and the ultimate strain is 25,000 microstrain). This generic peak strain environment has been termed *dynamic strain similarity* (77) and is one argument for the concept of bone working toward achieving a strain environment that is favorable to the cell, rather than to reduce it as far as possible, as might be ideal in the design of a concrete pillar. This is further evidence that bone is a live and viable tissue, rather than an inert material, and that—in that light—it must be considered that mechanical signals are beneficial to bone, perhaps to enhance perfusion or perifusion or to provide metabolic regulatory signals to the cell (78). Considering the biological rather structural context of these mechanical signals, it is certainly possible that the anabolic potential of a mechanical signal may derive from something other than the peak signals that arise from activity (79), as is the case with the way we recognize colors, identify tones, and distinguish textures (80).

Departing somewhat from a repair-mediated hypothesis, we have proposed that the extremely small strains that arise via muscle contraction during less vigorous but more predominant activities, such as maintaining posture, are strong determinants of bone morphology (81). We examined the regulatory potential of extremely small (0.3 G, where 1 G = earth's gravitational field), high-frequency (30 Hz) mechanical accelerations by subjecting the hind limbs of adult sheep to a ground-based vertical oscillation 20 minutes per day, 5 days per week (82). When the animals were not being treated, they joined the controls to freely roam a pasture area. This signal generated peak-to-peak strains of approximately 5 microstrain in the tibia, one thousandth of the strain magnitude necessary to cause yield failure in bone (83).

After 1 year of mechanical stimulation, the density of trabecular bone in the proximal femur was 34.2% greater in experimental sheep than in controls (probability less than 0.01), achieved by a 32% increase in trabecular bone volume, a 45% increase in trabecular number, and a 36% decrease in trabecular spacing. This anabolic response resulted in a 12% increase in stiffness, and 27% increase in strength, of the trabecular bone (84). The anabolic effect was highly selective for cancellous bone, inasmuch as there were no significant histomorphometric changes in any cortical bone parameters (85). No differences in any bone indices were detected in the radius of either control or experimental animals, which indicates that the anabolic effect was specific to that region of the skeleton subject to the mechanical signal. These low-level signals have also been shown to be effective in reversing the osteoporosis of disuse (86): 10 minutes per day of the stimulus led to retention of bone mass in suspended limbs, whereas 10 minutes per day of normal weight bearing failed to stop the resorption.

The anabolic potential of such a high-frequency strain signal indicates that it can readily influence bone mass and architecture, and thus skeletal morphology may be sculpted by omnipresent, low-level muscle activity as well as by the peak impacts inherent in load bearing. In terms of clinical relevance, the strong osteogenic capacity of these low-level signals suggests that a biomechanical intervention could provide a therapy for osteoporosis without the concomitant risks of pharmacological treatment. The attributes of such biomechanical prophylaxes are that they are native to the bone tissue, they are safe at low intensities, and mechanical signals incorporate all aspects of a complex remodeling cycle (61) and ultimately induce lamellar bone (59), which implies benefit to both bone quantity and quality. Preliminary results from measurements of bone mineral density of the spine in postmenopausal women (87) and in children with cerebral palsy (88) are encouraging in this regard.

Whatever signal transduction pathway is used for transforming physical information into something the cell population can perceive and respond to (89), it is clear that the capacity of bone tissue to adapt to its functional demands is critical to the skeleton's structural success. Indeed, as we attempt to evaluate the cellular mechanisms responsible for the positive control of bone mass, the osteogenic potential of physical stimuli cannot be ignored.

SUMMARY

In this review of the means by which bone integrates the fundamental tasks of providing skeletal structure while managing the metabolic responsibilities of an organ under endocrine, and possibly central, control, it is hoped that at the same time, the physician and scientist will have gained some insight into the challenges—and opportunities—that musculoskeletal science faces. The era after the decoding of the human genome should provide our disciplines with even more powerful tools; through transgenic approaches, the contributions of individual proteins within bone to its structural and functional integrity can and will continue to be determined. The advent of the molecular tools capable of genome-wide gene expression analyses, the search for single-nucleotide polymorphisms (SNPs), and the proteomics will certainly lead to discoveries identifying the responsible genes and proteins for many diseases affecting the bone phenotype. Advances in new biocompatible materials, both osteoconductive and osteoinductive, will also aid in the treatment of bone disorders, and new diagnostic modalities will aid in identifying persons at risk of disease perhaps before symptoms are evident.

Of course, the basic biology of bone is also of relevance to the clinician and spine surgeon. Even in a field of medicine in which hands-on experience cannot be overrated, new treatment modalities for diseases and problems of the musculoskeletal system are certain to be derived from the aforementioned studies. For example, local gene delivery systems to achieve spinal fusion between hypermobile segments in spondylolisthesis are conceivable; tissue engineering approaches to replace and augment bone, cartilage, and muscle are receiving a great deal of attention; and many of the drugs to treat arthritis, osteoporosis, and other diseases of the musculoskeletal system will be based on SNPs and complex gene interactions. Unquestionably, these are exciting times for everyone working in the musculoskeletal disciplines, and the interdisciplinary nature of the research, which has brought us tremendous insight into bone's complexity on a structural and functional level, will serve us well in the future.

REFERENCES

1. Raisz LG. Local and systemic factors in the pathogenesis of osteoporosis. *N Engl J Med* 1988;318:818–828.
2. Currey JD. Mechanical properties of bone tissues with greatly differing functions. *J Biomech* 1979;12:313–319.
3. Currey JD. The design of mineralized hard tissues for their mechanical functions. *J Exp Biol* 1999;202: 3285–3294.
4. NIH Consensus Development Conference. Osteoporosis prevention, diagnosis, and therapy. Bethesda, MD: National Institutes of Health Press, 2000:1–45.
5. Service RF. Tissue engineers build new bone. *Science* 2000;289:1498–1500.
6. Aubin JE. Bone stem cells. *J Cell Biochem Suppl* 1998;30–31:73–82.
7. Kahn AJ, Simmons DJ. Investigation of cell lineage in bone using a chimaera of chick and quail embryonic tissue. *Nature* 1975;258:325.
8. Ferrari SL, Traianedes K, Thorne M, et al. A role for N-cadherin in the development of the differentiated osteoblastic phenotype. *J Bone Miner Res* 2000;15:198–208.
9. Lecanda F, Towler DA, Ziambaras K, et al. Gap junctional communication modulates gene expression in osteoblastic cells. *Mol Biol Cell* 1998;9:2249–2258.
10. Owen TA, Aronow M, Shalhoub V, et al. Progressive development of the rat osteoblast phenotype *in vitro:* Reciprocal relationships in expression of genes associated with osteoblast proliferation and differentiation during formation of the bone extracellular matrix. *J Cell Physiol* 1990;143:420–430, 1990.
11. Martin TJ, Allan EH, Fukumoto S. The plasminogen activator and inhibitor system in bone remodeling. *Growth Reg* 1993;3:209–214, 1993.
12. Yasuda H, Shima N, Nakagawa N, et al. (1998) Osteoclast differentiation factor is a ligand for osteoprotegerin /osteoclastogenesis-inhibitory factor and is identical to TRANCE/RANKL. *Proc Natl Acad Sci USA* 1998;95: 3597–3602.
13. Reinholt FP, Hultenby K, Oldberg A, et al. Osteopontin—a possible anchor of osteoclasts to bone. *Proc Natl Acad Sci USA* 1990;87:4473–4475.
14. Ducy P, Desbois C, Boyce B, et al. Increased bone formation in osteocalcin-deficient mice. *Nature* 1996;382: 448–452.
15. Mundlos S, Otto F, Mundlos C, et al. Mutations involving the transcription factor CBFA1 cause cleidocranial dysplasia. *Cell* 1987;89:773–779.
16. Otto F, Thornell AP, Crompton AD, et al. CBFA1, a candidate gene for cleidocranial dysplasia syndrome, is essential for osteoblast differentiation and bone development. *Cell* 1997;89:765–771.
17. Gong Y, Slee RB. LDL receptor-related protein 5 (LRP5) affects bone accrual and eye development. *Cell* 2001;107(4):513–523.
18. Owen M. Cellular dynamics of bone. In: Bourne G, ed. *The biochemistry and physiology of bone,* 2nd ed. New York: Academic Press, 1973:271.
19. Jowsey J. *Metabolic diseases of bone.* Philadelphia: WB Saunders, 1977:61.
20. Mitchell RD, Edwards HM. Effects of phytase and 1,25-dihydroxycholecalciferol on phytate utilization and the quantitative requirement for calcium and phosphorus in young broiler chickens. *Poultry Sci* 1996;75: 95–110.
21. Turner C, Owan I, Brizendine EJ, et al. High fluoride intakes cause osteomalacia and diminished bone strength in rats with renal deficiency. *Bone* 1996;6:595–601.
22. Rubin C, Sun Y, Hadjiargyrou M, et al. Increased expression of matrix metalloproteinase-1 in osteocytes precedes bone resorption as stimulated by disuse: evidence for autoregulation of the cell's mechanical environment? *J Orthop Res* 1999;17:354–361.
23. Cowin SC, Weinbaum S, Zeng Y. A case for bone canaliculi as the anatomical site of strain generated potentials. *J Biomechanics* 1995;28:1281–1297.
24. Curtis TA, Ashrafi SH, Weber DF. Canalicular communication in the cortices of human long bones. *Anat Rec* 1985;212:336–344.
25. Donahue HJ, McLeod KJ, Rubin CT, et al. Cell-to-cell communication in osteoblastic networks: cell line-dependent hormonal regulation of gap junction function. *J Bone Miner Res* 1995;10:881–889.
26. Mosley JR. Osteoporosis and bone functional adaptation: mechanobiological regulation of bone architecture in growing and adult bone, a review. *J Rehabil Res Dev* 2000;37:189–199.

27. Mason DJ, Suva LJ, Genever PG, et al. Mechanically regulated expression of a neural glutamate transporter in bone: a role for excitatory amino acids as osteotropic agents? *Bone* 1997;20:199–205.
28. Burger EH, Klein-Nulend J. Mechanotransduction in bone—role of the lacuno-canalicular network. *FASEB J* 1999;13(Suppl):S101–S112.
29. Teitelbaum SL. Bone resorption by osteoclasts. *Science* 2000;289:1504–1508.
30. Walker DG. Enzymatic and electron microscopic analysis of isolated osteoclasts. *Calcif Tissue Res* 1972;9:296–309.
31. Blair HC, Teitelbaum SL, Ghiselli R, et al. Osteoclastic bone resorption by a polarized vacuolar proton pump. *Science* 1989;245:855–857.
32. Gelb BD, Shi GP. Pycnodysostosis, a lysosomal disease caused by cathepsin K deficiency. *Science* 1996;273 (5279):1236–1238.
33. Albright J, Skinner H. Bone: structural organization and remodeling dynamics. In: J Albright, R Brand, eds. *The scientific basis of orthopaedics,* 2nd ed. East Norwalk, CT: Appleton & Lange, 1987:161–198.
34. Lacey DL, Timms E, Tan HL, et al. Osteoprotegerin ligand is a cytokine that regulates osteoclast differentiation and activation. *Cell* 1998;93(2):165–176.
35. Felix R, Cecchini M, Fleisch H. MCSF restores *in vivo* bone resorption in the *opop* osteopetrotic mouse. *Endocrinology* 1990;127:2592.
36. Hume DA, Favot P Is the osteopetrotic mouse completely deficient in expression of MCSF? *J Interferon Cytokine Res* 1995;15:279–284.
37. Niida S, Kaku M, Tanne K, et al. Vascular endothelial growth factor induces osteoclast differentiation in *opop* mice. *Bone* 1998;23(5):F078.
38. Simonet WS, Lacey DL, Dunstan CR, et al. Osteoprotegerin: a novel secreted protein involved in the regulation of bone density. *Cell* 1997;89:309–319.
39. Burgess TL, Qian Y, Kaufman S, et al. The ligand for osteoprotegerin (OPGL) directly activates mature osteoclasts. *J Cell Biol* 1999;145:527–538.
40. Hofbauer LC, Khosla S, Dunstan CR, et al. The roles of osteoprotegerin and osteoprotegerin ligand in the paracrine regulation of bone resorption. *J Bone Miner Res* 2000;15:2–12.
41. Zhang J, Dai J. Osteoprotegerin inhibits prostate cancer-induced osteoclastogenesis and prevents prostate tumor growth in the bone. *J Clin Invest* 2001;107:1235–1244.
42. Pearse RN, Sordillo EM. Multiple myeloma disrupts the TRANCE/osteoprotegerin cytokine axis to trigger bone destruction and promote tumor progression. *Proc Natl Acad Sci USA* 2001;98(20):11581–11586.
43. Aubin JE, Bonnelye E. Osteoprotegerin and its ligand: a new paradigm for regulation of osteoclastogenesis and bone resorption. *Medscape Womens Health* 2000;5(2):5.
44. Hofbauer LC, Heufelder AE. The role of receptor activator of nuclear factor-kappaB ligand and osteoprotegerin in the pathogenesis and treatment of metabolic bone diseases. *J Clin Endocrinol Metab* 2000;85:2355–2363.
45. Robey PG, Fedarko NS, Hefferan TE, et al. Structure and molecular regulation of bone matrix proteins. *J Bone Miner Res* 1993;8:S483–S487.
46. Delany AM, Amling M, Priemel M, et al. Osteopenia and decreased bone formation in osteonectin-deficient mice [published erratum appears in *J Clin Invest* 2000;105:1325]. *J Clin Invest* 2000;105:915–923.
47. Aszodi A, Bateman JF, Gustafsson E, et al. Mammalian skeletogenesis and extracellular matrix: what can we learn from knockout mice? [In Process Citation]. *Cell Struct Funct* 2000;25:73–84.
48. Coetzer H, Claassen N, Van Papendorp DH, et al. Calcium transport by isolated brush border and basolateral membrane vesicles: role of essential fatty acid. *Prostaglandins* 1994;50:257–266.
49. Christoffersen J, Landis WJ. A contribution with review to the description of mineralization of bone and other calcified tissues *in vivo. Anat Rec* 1991;230:435–450.
50. Yagami K, Suh JY, Enomoto-Iwamoto M, et al. Matrix GLA protein is a developmental regulator of chondrocyte mineralization and, when constitutively expressed, blocks endochondral and intramembranous ossification in the limb. *J Cell Biol* 1999;147:1097–1108.
51. Weiner S, Traub W. Bone structure: from angstroms to microns. *FASEB J* 1992;6:879–885.
52. Rizzoli R, Slosman D, Bonjour JP. The role of dual energy X-ray absorptiometry of lumbar spine and proximal femur in the diagnosis and follow-up of osteoporosis. *Am J Med* 1995;98:33S–36S.
53. Beddington RS, Robertson EJ. Axis development and early asymmetry in mammals. *Cell* 1999;96:195–209.
54. Olsen BJ. Bone morphogenesis and embryonic development. In: Favus MJ, ed. *Primer on the metabolic bone diseases and disorders of mineral metabolism,* 4th ed. Philadelphia: Lippincott, Williams & Wilkins, 1999: 11–14.
55. Carter D, Wong M, Orr TE. Musculoskeletal ontogeny, phylogeny, and functional adaptation. *J Biomechanics* 1996;24:3–16.
56. Chiang C, Litingtung Y, Lee E, et al. Cyclopia and defective axial patterning in mice lacking *sonic hedgehog* gene function. *Nature* 1996;383:407–413.
57. Izpisua-Belmonte JC, Duboule D. Homeobox genes and pattern formation in the vertebrate limb. *Dev Biol* 1992; 152:26–36.
58. Martin R, Burr D. *Structure, function, and adaptation of compact bone.* New York: Raven Press, 1989:1–275.
59. Rubin CT, Gross TS, McLeod KJ, et al. Morphologic stages in lamellar bone formation stimulated by a potent mechanical stimulus. *J Bone Miner Res* 1995;10:488–495.
60. Frost H. *Bone remodeling dynamics.* Springfield, IL: Charles C Thomas, 1963

61. Bain SD, Rubin CT. Metabolic modulation of disuse osteopenia: endocrine-dependent site specificity of bone remodeling. *J Bone Miner Res* 1990;5:1069–1075.
62. Qin YX, Rubin CT, McLeod KJ. Nonlinear dependence of loading intensity and cycle number in the maintenance of bone mass and morphology. *J Orthop Res* 1998;16:482–489.
63. Darby AJ, Meunier PJ. Mean wall thickness and formation periods of trabecular bone packets in idiopathic osteoporosis. *Calcif Tissue Int* 1981;33:199–204.
64. Brunelli MP, Einhorn TA. Medical management of osteoporosis. Fracture prevention. *Clin Orthop* 1998;348: 15–21.
65. Watts NB. Treatment of osteoporosis with bisphosphonates. *Endocrin Metab Clin North Am* 1998;27:419–429.
66. Hirano T, Turner C, Forwood MR, et al. Does suppression of bone turnover impair mechanical properties by allowing microdamage accumulation? *Bone* 2000;27:13–20.
67. Lee SK, Lorenzo JA. Parathyroid hormone stimulates TRANCE and inhibits osteoprotegerin messenger ribonucleic acid expression in murine bone marrow cultures: correlation with osteoclast-like cell formation. *Endocrinology* 1999;140:3552–3561.
68. Shevde NK, Bendixen AC. Estrogens suppress RANK ligand-induced osteoclast differentiation via a stromal cell independent mechanism involving *c-Jun* repression. *Proc Natl Acad Sci USA* 2000;97:7829–7834.
69. Brown, EM, Gamba G, Riccardi D, et al. Cloning and characterization of an extracellular Ca^{2+} sensing receptor from bovine parathyroid. *Nature* 1993;366:575–580.
70. NIH Consensus Development Conference. Diagnosis and management of asymptomatic primary hyperparathyroidism: Consensus Development Conference Statement. *Ann Intern Med* 1991;1145:593–597.
71. Neer RM, Arnaud CD, Zanchetta JR, et al. Effect of parathyroid hormone (1-34) on fractures and bone mineral density in postmenopausal women with osteoporosis. *N Engl J Med* 2001;344:1434–1441.
72. Cosman F, Nieves J, Woelfert L, et al. Parathyroid hormone added to established hormone therapy: effects on vertebral fracture and maintenance of bone mass after parathyroid hormone withdrawal. *J Bone Min Res* 2001; 16:925–931.
73. Ducy P, Amling M, Takeda S, et al. Leptin inhibits bone formation through a hypothalamic relay: a central control of bone mass. *Cell* 2000;100:197–207.
74. Jones HH, Priest JD, Hayes WC, et al. Humeral hypertrophy in response to exercise. *J Bone Joint Surg [Am]* 1977;59:204–208.
75. Donaldson CL, Hulley SB, Vogel JM, et al. Effect of prolonged bed rest on bone mineral. *Metabolism* 1970;19: 1071–1084.
76. Wolff J. *Das gesetz der transformation des knochens.* Berlin: Hirschwald Verlag, 1892.
77. Rubin CT, Lanyon LE. Dynamic strain similarity in vertebrates, an alternative to allometric limb bone scaling. *J Theor Biol* 1984;107:321–327.
78. Lanyon LE, Skerry TM. Postmenopausal osteoporosis as a failure of bone's adaptation to functional loading: a hypothesis. *J Bone Miner Res* 2001;16:1937–1947.
79. Weinbaum S, Cowin SC, Zeng Y. A model for the excitation of osteocytes by mechanical loading-induced bone fluid shear stresses. *J Biomech* 1994;27:339–360.
80. Rubin C, Sommerfeldt D, Judex S, et al. Inhibition of osteopenia by low magnitude, high frequency mechanical stimuli. *Drug Discovery Today* 2001;6:848–858.
81. Huang RP, Rubin CT, McLeod KJ. Changes in postural muscle dynamics as a function of age. *J Gerontol A Biol Sci Med Sci* 1999;54:B352–B357.
82. Rubin C, Turner AS, Bain S, et al. Anabolism: low mechanical signals strengthen long bones. *Nature* 2001;412:603–604.
83. Carter D, Harris W, Vasu R, et al. The mechanical and biological response of cortical bone to in vivo strain histories. In: Cowin S, ed. *Mechanical properties of bone.* Am Soc Mech Eng 1981;45:81–95.
84. Rubin C, Turner AS, Müller R, et al. Quantity and quality of trabecular bone in the femur are enhanced by a strongly anabolic, non-invasive mechanical intervention. *J Bone Miner Res* 2002;17:349–357.
85. Rubin C, Turner S, Mallinckrodt C, et al. Mechanical strain, induced non-invasively in the high frequency domain, is anabolic to cancellous—but not cortical—bone. *Bone* 2002;30:445–452.
86. Rubin C, Xu G, Judex S. The anabolic activity of bone tissue, suppressed by disuse, is normalized by brief exposure to low magnitude mechanical stimuli. *FASEB J* 2001;15:2225–2229.
87. Rubin C, Recker R, Cullen D, et al. Prevention of bone loss in a post-menopausal population by low-level biomechanical intervention. *Am Soc Bone Miner Res* 1998;23:1106.
88. Ward K, Alsop C, Brown S, et al. A randomized, placebo controlled, pilot trial of low magnitude, high frequency loading treatment of children with disabling conditions who also have low bone mineral density. *Trans Am Soc Bone Miner Res* 2001;16s:1148.
89. Rubin J, Rubin C. Interdependence of genetic and epigenetic factors in determining bone strength. In: Adams J, Lukert B, eds. *Osteoporosis: genetics, prevention and treatment.* Newton, MA: Kluwer, 1999:57–72.

2

Biomechanics of Compression Fractures

Malcolm H. Pope

Liberty Safework Centre, University of Aberdeen, Foresterhill, Aberdeen, United Kingdom

BIOMECHANICS OF TRABECULAE

Trabecular bone is a porous cellular solid, made of an irregular three-dimensional array of bony rods and plates, which are themselves a composite material. Trabecular bone is a mineralized, open-cell structure that lies inside the cortical shell; a typical trabecular thickness is about 100 μm. Bone marrow fills the spaces of the pores. In addition, because all free bone surfaces are covered with bone cells, bone is a living tissue that is self-healing and has the ability to adjust its morphology in response to changes in its mechanical environment. The structure of trabecular bone meets the mechanical function very well and is arranged in such a way that it optimally bears the internal and external body loads (probably the average mechanical loads). The theory is that the trajectorial structure of bone has arisen from functional adaptation, by which unloaded bone is resorbed and highly loaded bone requires bone formation (Wolff's law). Wolff (1) thought that an implication of his trajectorial theory was that trabeculae would always intersect perpendicularly because internal stress directions must always intersect perpendicularly for any given loading case. Because trabeculae were proposed to align with these stress directions, it followed that cancellous bone architecture must form a network of perpendicular intersections. Wolff criticized the anatomical drawings of Hermann von Meyer—which were based solely on observations of cadaver specimens—for not reflecting this perpendicular architecture. Modern investigations of cancellous bone suggest that in some cases the activities of daily living lead to a dynamic mechanical environment that cannot be supported effectively by a perpendicular trabecular structure. In this regard, Wolff may have been limited by restricting his thinking to the ideal situation of a single or predominant loading environment.

In order to describe the bone architecture, several groups have developed methods with which to determine the principal bone directions in three dimensions. Three-dimensional images obtained from serial two-dimensional images are shown in Fig. 2.1 (2).

It has been established that (a) trabecular bone is linearly elastic and yields at relatively low strains; (b) failure strains in trabecular bone are largely independent of its density, are asymmetric (different in tension versus compression), and may be isotropic; (c) strength asymmetry (tension versus compression) increases with increasing modulus of the specimen; (d) loading past yield causes reductions in modulus and strength (see later discussion for more details); and (e) torsional behavior mimics tensile and compressive behaviors, but with larger failure strains and lower strengths (3).

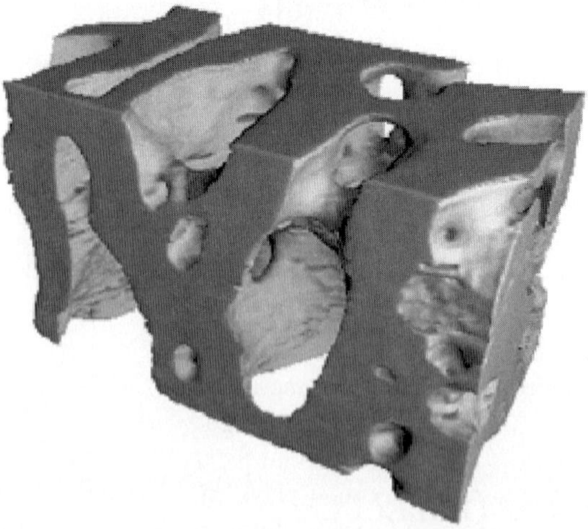

FIG. 2.1. High-resolution computer model of trabecular bone. The geometric resolution of this model is 10 μm (2).

Kopperdahl and Keaveny (4) found that for bone that is loaded along the direction of the principal orientation of the trabeculae, bending of trabeculae is negligible; trabecular deformations are dominated by axial extension or compression of the vertical trabeculae; compressive failure occurs primarily by buckling at low density and by axial yielding at high density; and tensile failure occurs by axial yielding for all densities.

There is evidence that damage occurs to individual trabeculae *in vivo* and that this damage may be a stimulus for bone remodeling. Keaveny et al. (5) studied the mechanical behavior of damaged trabecular bone. Figure 2.2 shows that after reloading that follows damage, there are marked decreases in modulus and strength. It was also found that reduction in modulus and strength depended on applied strain and not on the density.

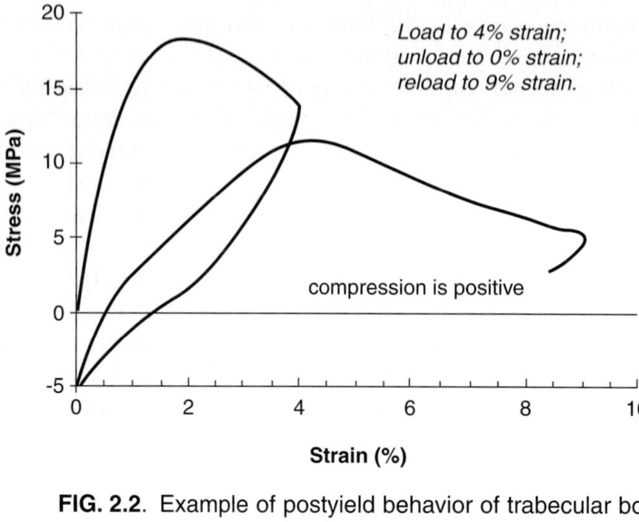

FIG. 2.2. Example of postyield behavior of trabecular bone.

BIOMECHANICS OF OSTEOPOROSIS

Although loss of bone mass is strongly correlated with increased fracture risk, only about 50% of persons with the clinical definition of osteoporosis ever suffer a fracture. Furthermore, of those who do suffer a fracture, about 50% have normal bone density. The incidence of vertebral fracture has increased threefold to fourfold for women and more than fourfold for men since the early 1970s. These data are age adjusted and therefore highlight the decrease in bone mass or bone quality from generation to generation. Mosekilde (6) studied the normal age-related changes in human bone and demonstrated that age by itself is the major determinant of vertebral bone strength, mass, and microarchitecture. At the age of 20 to 30 years, men have a higher peak bone mass and strength than do women. Men show an age-related compensatory increase in bone size (cross-sectional area of the vertebral bodies) that cannot be found in women. There is, after the age of 50 years (the menopausal stage in women), a higher tendency for disconnection of the trabecular network in women than in men. Furthermore, it was shown that loading plays an important role in the maintenance of trabecular connectivity (through the remodeling process) and in the periosteal apposition and thereby increases in cross-sectional area (through the modeling process). Loading affects bone mass, microarchitecture, and size throughout life. Loading is therefore important for the maintenance of bone strength during normal aging, and exercise plays an important role in the prevention of osteoporotic fractures.

Ladd et al. (7) combined a synchrotron x-ray imaging system with large-scale finite-element models (FEMs) to analyze the relationship between bone architecture and mechanical function. Predicting the mechanical behavior of trabecular bone requires a detailed understanding of how architecture affects the distribution of stress in the sample. With knowledge of the stress field throughout the sample and a local failure criterion, Ladd et al. determined the failure process by successive relaxation of the nodal displacements, as shown in Fig. 2.3.

Figure 2.3 shows the distribution of different load paths in one sample of trabecular bone. Three-dimensional images of the largest principal stresses are shown, for longitudinal and transverse loadings. In each image, the elements whose stress exceeds a preset value are illuminated; the variation in brightness is only to enhance the perspective. Images are shown at three different stress levels, corresponding to moderate compression, high compression, and high tension. The moderate-compression images (left) contain 50% of the occupied voxels; the high-compression images (center) and high-tension images (right) each contain 5% of the occupied voxels. At the lowest stress level (upper left and lower left images), the load paths clearly outline the trabecular structure, as can be seen by comparison with image of the structure. At higher stress levels (center images), the load paths are fewer and are distributed inhomogeneously; the orientations of the load paths are readily identifiable. There is a concentration of tension near the center of the sample, where thicker trabeculae begin to distribute the load more uniformly.

Both density and structural characteristics are of importance in structural failure. Figure 2.4 shows two specimens of human trabecular bone, taken from the L1 vertebra. Although these two specimens have almost the same bone densities, the specimen on the left was found to be twice as stiff as the one on the right. Part of this difference is architectural; the specimen on the left has a more plate-like structure, which gives it greater rigidity along the important vertical axis. However, FEMs show that architectural effects account for only about 50% of the difference; the remainder can be attributed to variations in stiffness of the bone tissue itself.

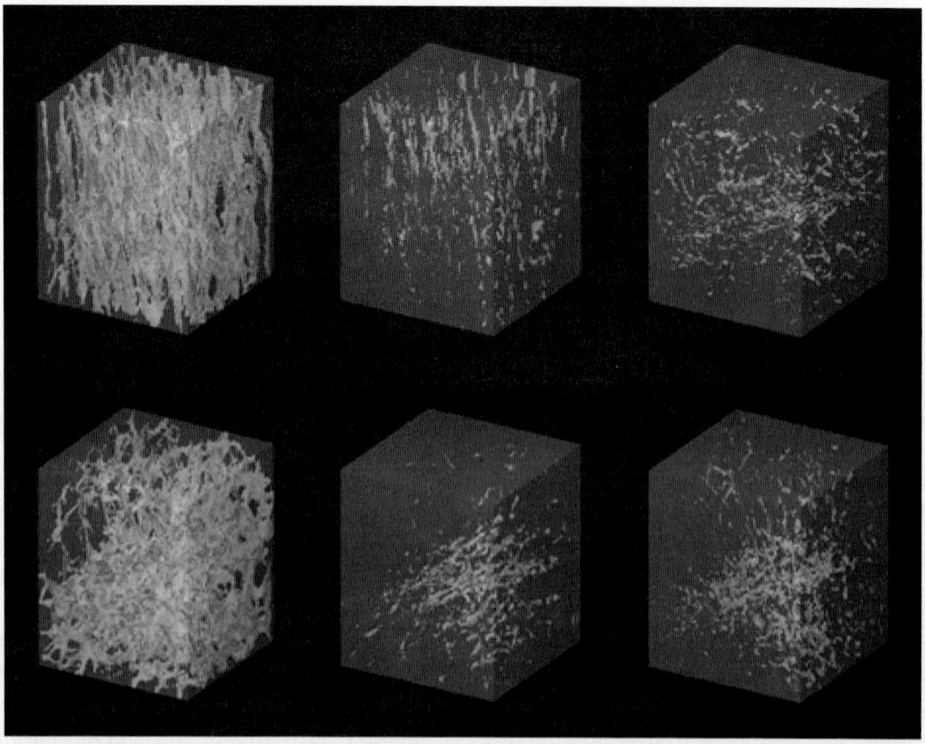

FIG. 2.3. The distribution of load paths in one sample of trabecular bone.

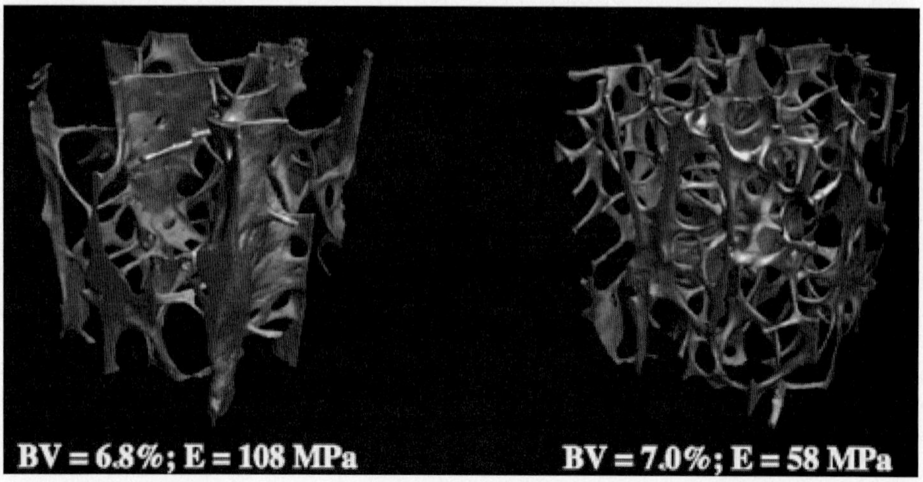

FIG. 2.4. Two specimens of human trabecular bone, taken from the L1 vertebra. (From Ladd AJC, Kinney JH, Haupt DL, et al. Finite-element modeling of trabecular bone: comparison with mechanical testing and determination of tissue modulus. *J Orthop Res* 1998;16:622-628.).

BIOMECHANICS OF COMPRESSION FAILURE

Studies of the spine in adolescents who have sustained trauma have shown injuries to the growth zone, whereas injuries to the vertebral body have been described in studies of adults. Lundin et al. (8) compressed porcine lumbar functional spine units (FSUs) to the point of failure. In the adolescents, a fracture was consistently found in the endplate through the posterior part of the growth zone, displacing the annulus fibrosus with a bone fragment at the point of insertion to the vertebra. This type of injury could not be detected in any of the adults; instead, there was a fracture of the vertebra in four cases, and in two cases, a rupture of the annulus fibrosus without a bone fragment was seen.

In the thoracic spine, the incidence of anterior wedge fractures increases with the severity of kyphosis. It has been unclear whether the role of anterior osteophytes in the thoracic spine is to restrict progressive kyphosis or to conduct axial load anteriorly. Toh et al. (9) found that there were no dramatic changes in the spatial distribution of strains after removal of anterior osteophytes; however, after removal of the osteophytes and orienting the specimen in 5 degrees of additional flexion, the strain distribution shifted anteriorly and the magnitude increased. This study demonstrated that osteophytes seem to restrict progressive kyphosis rather than conduct axial load anteriorly.

Gilsanz et al. (10) reported that neither cancellous nor cortical vertebral bone densities differed by gender in healthy adults. However, vertebral bodies in women had smaller cross-sectional areas (8.22 cm^2 versus 10.98 cm^2 in men) and volumes (22.42 cm^3 versus 30.86 cm^3 in men). Haidekker et al. (11) reported that the average compressive fracture loads were 3,533 N for nonosteoporotic cases (range, 2,602 to -5,802 N) and 1,725 N for osteoporotic cases (range, 1,311 to -2,490 N). Ching et al. (12) created thoracolumbar compression fractures, burst fractures, and flexion-distraction injuries in human thoracolumbar FSU's in order to compare residual stability as a function of type of injury. Of the three groups, bones with burst fractures retained the least residual stability. Those with compression fractures retained the most residual stability, with increases in motion of 40% in flexion-extension, 56% in lateral bending, and 3% in torsion.

Osteoporotic compression fractures are associated with minimal trauma and with loads no greater than those encountered during normal activities of daily living. With osteoporosis, there is progressive resorption of bone, resulting in reductions in bone density, thinning of trabeculae, and loss of trabecular contiguity. These changes in trabecular bone structure are associated with losses in bone strength that are disproportionate to the reductions in bone mass alone. It has been suggested that that density reductions in the vertebral centrum are accompanied by a reduction in the number of trabeculae, by preferential resorption of horizontal trabeculae, and by hypertrophy of the remaining vertical trabeculae. Snyder et al. (13) performed three-dimensional stereological analysis of trabecular bone from midsagittal sections of vertebral bodies. Both the number and thickness of trabeculae decreased linearly with density (as expressed by bone volume fraction), whereas the spacing between the trabeculae increased reciprocally. There were more vertical trabeculae with transverse trabeculae at all densities, and the number of vertical trabeculae changed with density at twice the rate of the number of transverse trabeculae. These data do not support the prevailing view that there is preferential resorption of horizontal trabeculae or hypertrophy of the remaining vertical trabeculae.

Andresen et al. (14) measured cortical and spongy bone mineral density which were matched with the vertebral body fractures. A finite element model was used to study the variation in structural and material parameters of the vertebral body. These investigations showed that, in addition to the spongiosa, the cortical shell plays an important role in the load-bearing capacity of the vertebral body. If the spongiosa is weakened as a result of a loss of bone mineral density, the residual load-bearing capacity of the vertebral bodies is increasingly assumed by the cortical bone. The lower susceptibility to fracture in men in comparison with women when spongy bone mineral density is reduced can thus be attributed to the lack of a reduction in cortical bone mineral density.

BIOMECHANICS OF PREVENTION

Myers and Wilson (15) pointed out that the ability of the spine to carry load depends on the structural capacity of the vertebrae and on the loading conditions that arise from activities of daily living or from trauma. The ratio of the load on the spine to the failure load of the bone is called the *factor of risk,* a value that indicates whether fracture is likely to occur during a given activity. A high factor of risk can result from weak bone that has a low failure load or from a risk activity that generates a large force. The failure load of the vertebral body depends on the density and architecture of the trabecular bone and on the shape, size, and organization of the vertebral body. The magnitude of a load applied to the spine depends on the specific activity. Bending and lifting activities generate loads on the spine that exceed the failure load of vertebrae with very low bone mineral density. Biomechanical indications for prevention of age-related fractures point to the need to strengthen bone by maintaining or increasing density and the need to lower the magnitude of forces applied to the spine in elderly persons by avoiding such risk activities as lifting.

Not only are the vertebrae weak in these patients but there is also muscle weakness and poor endurance.

Chronic back tiredness or fatigue is a common complaint of people who have a history of osteoporotic vertebral fracture. Trunk muscle endurance was studied in people with vertebral osteoporosis by Shipp et al. (16). Combined trunk and arm endurance is a measure of the time a person can stand while holding a two-pound dumbbell in each hand with the arms at 90 degrees of shoulder flexion and the elbows extended. Moderately strong and statistically significant correlations were found between this test and 16 measures of physical impairment and function.

It is important that osteoporotic patients receive instructions on the biomechanics of safe lifting and on dangerous postures. Many postures can produce a change in the geometry of the spine, but moving from standing up to bending down and then from bending down to standing up (during which the lumbar spine changes from lordotic to kyphotic to lordotic), in combination with lifting or lowering a load, creates a particular risk for a compression fracture. The patient should be given the safe lifting guidelines listed in Table 2.1.

Medical professionals should also be aware of the recommendations embedded in the 1991 National Institute of Occupational Safety and Health (NIOSH) Lifting Equation. In 1991 the NIOSH equation was revised to account for the effects of other variables, such as asymmetrical lifting, good or poor handles, and the total time spent lifting during the workday. Another lifting equation yields a recommended weight limit (RWL) as follows:

$$RWL = LC \times HM \times VM \times DM \times AM \times FM \times CM,$$

where LC is a load constant (51 lbs.); HM is a horizontal multiplier, 10/H; VM is a vertical multiplier, $[1 - (0.0075\ [V - 30])]$; DM is a distance multiplier, $[0.82 + (1.8/D)]$; AM is an asymmetric multiplier, $[1 - (0.0032A)]$, in which A is the angle of asymmetry, which is angular displacement of the load from the sagittal plane, measured at the origin

TABLE 2.1. *Safe lifting guidelines*

Lifting safely will protect your back while you lift. Before you lift an object, ask yourself the following questions:

Do you think you can lift it alone?
Is the load too big or too awkward?
Does the load have good handles or grips?
Is there anything to obstruct proper lifting?
Could the contents of the load shift while being lifted?

For safe lifting, remember to:

Stand as close to the load as possible.
Bend at your knees, not your waist.
Hug the load close to your body; don't hold it away from you.
Raise yourself up with the strong thigh muscles.

and destination of the lift; FM is a frequency multiplier (from NIOSH guidelines) and CM is a coupling multiplier (from NIOSH guidelines).

Further work is necessary to determine how these recommendations should be modified for patients with osteoporosis. In the meantime, physicians must be wary about the factors listed earlier (asymmetry and so forth).

CONCLUSIONS

As mentioned earlier, trabecular bone is a porous cellular solid that comprises bony rods and plates, which are themselves a composite material. A typical trabecular thickness is about 100 μm. The trajectorial structure of cancellous bone has arisen from functional adaptation, by which unloaded bone is resorbed and highly loaded bone forms more bone.

It has been established that (a) trabecular bone is linearly elastic and yields at relatively low strains; (b) failure strains in trabecular bone are largely independent of its density, are asymmetrical (different in tension versus compression), and may be isotropic; (c) strength asymmetry (tension versus compression) increases with increasing modulus of the specimen; (d) loading past yield causes reductions in modulus and strength; and (e) torsional behavior mimics tensile and compressive behaviors but with larger failure strains and lower strengths. For bone that is loaded along the direction of the principal orientation of the trabeculae, bending of trabeculae is negligible; trabecular deformations are dominated by axial extension or compression of the vertical trabeculae; compressive failure occurs primarily by buckling at low density and by axial yielding at high density; and tensile failure occurs by axial yielding for all densities.

Loss of bone mass is strongly correlated with increased fracture risk. The incidence of vertebral fracture has increased threefold to fourfold for women and more than fourfold for men since the early 1970s. After menopause, women demonstrate a higher tendency for disconnection of the trabecular network than do men at the same age. Loading affects bone mass, microarchitecture, and size throughout life. Loading is therefore important for the maintenance of bone strength during normal ageing, and exercise plays an important role in the prevention of osteoporotic fractures. In the thoracic spine, the incidence of anterior wedge fractures increases with the severity of kyphosis. Osteophytes seem to restrict progressive kyphosis rather than conduct axial load anteriorly. Vertebral bodies in women have lower cross-sectional areas and volumes than do those in men. Osteoporotic compression fractures are associated with minimal trauma and with loads no greater than those encountered during normal activities of daily living. With osteoporosis, there is progressive resorption of bone, resulting in reductions in bone density, thinning of trabeculae, and loss of trabecular contiguity. These changes in trabecular bone structure are associated with losses in bone strength that are disproportionate to the reductions in bone mass alone. It has been suggested that density reductions in the vertebral centrum are accompanied by a reduction in the number of trabeculae, by preferential resorption of horizontal trabeculae, and by hypertrophy of the remaining vertical trabeculae.

Biomechanical indications for prevention of age-related fractures point to the need to strengthen bone by maintaining or increasing density and the need to lower the magnitude of forces applied to the spine in the elderly. Chronic back tiredness or fatigue is a common complaint of people who have a history of osteoporotic vertebral fracture. Therefore, exercise can help to maintain both bone mass and muscle tone. It is important that osteoporotic patients receive instructions on the biomechanics of safe lifting and on dangerous postures. Recommendations can be based on the 1991 NIOSH Lifting Equation.

REFERENCES

1. Wolff J. *Das gesetz der transformation der knochem.* Berlin: Hirschwald, 1892.
2. Beck JD, Keaveny TM: A serial-grinding technique for high-resolution imaging of trabecular bone. *Trans ORS* 1996; p. 709.
3. Keaveny TM, Borchers RE, Gibson LJ, et al. Theoretical analysis of the experimental artifact in trabecular bone compressive modulus. *J Biomech* 1993;26:599–607.
4. Kopperdahl DL, Keaveny TM. Compressive and tensile elastic and failure properties of human vertebral trabecular bone. ASME Summer Bioengineering Conference 1995:357–358.
5. Keaveny TM, Wachtel EF, Guo XE, et al. Mechanical behavior of damaged trabecular bone. *J Biomech* 1994;27:1309–1318.
6. Mosekilde L. Age-related changes in bone mass, structure, and strength— effects of loading. *Z Rheumatol* 2000;59(Suppl 1):1–9.
7. Ladd AJC, Kinney JH, Haupt DL, et al. Finite-element modeling of trabecular bone: comparison with mechanical testing and determination of tissue modulus. *J Orthop Res* 1998;16:622–628.
8. Lundin O, Ekstrom L, Hellstrom M, et al. Exposure of the porcine spine to mechanical compression: differences in injury pattern between adolescents and adults. *Eur Spine J* 2000;9(6):466–471.
9. Toh E, Yerby SA, Bay BK, et al. The effect of anterior osteophytes and flexural position on thoracic trabecular strain. *Spine* 2001;26(1):22–26.
10. Gilsanz V, Boechat MI, Gilsanz R, et al. Gender differences in vertebral sizes in adults: biomechanical implications. *Radiology* 1994;190(3):678–682.
11. Haidekker MA, Andresen R, Werner HJ. Relationship between structural parameters, bone mineral density and fracture load in lumbar vertebrae, based on high-resolution computed tomography, quantitative computed tomography and compression tests. *Osteoporos Int* 1999;9(5):433–440.
12. Ching RP, Tencer AF, Anderson PA, et al. Comparison of residual stability in thoracolumbar spine fractures using neutral zone measurements. *J Orthop Res* 1995;13(4):533–541.
13. Snyder BD, Piazza S, Edwards WT, et al. Role of trabecular morphology in the etiology of age-related vertebral fractures. *Calcif Tissue Int* 1993;53(Suppl 1):S14–S22.
14. Andresen R, Werner HJ, Schober HC. Contribution of the cortical shell of vertebrae to mechanical behaviour of the lumbar vertebrae with implications for predicting fracture risk. *Br J Radiol* 1998;71(847):759–765.
15. Myers ER, Wilson SE. Biomechanics of osteoporosis and vertebral fracture. *Spine* 1997;22(24 Suppl):25S–31S.
16. Shipp KM, Purse JL, Gold DT, et al. Timed loaded standing: a measure of combined trunk and arm endurance suitable for people with vertebral osteoporosis. *Osteoporos Int* 2000;11:914–922.

3

Biomechanics and Physiology of Fragile Vertebrae

Tommy Hansson

Department of Orthopaedics and School of Medicine, Sahlgren Academy at Göteborg University, Göteborg, Sweden

The amount of bone mineral in the vertebral body is by far the most important factor determining its strength (1). The importance of the bone mineral for the strength of the human vertebrae has been shown in biomechanical studies in which the variations in the amount of bone mineral have been found to explain almost 80% of the variation in strength of the tested vertebrae (1). Currently, bone mineral values two or two and half standard deviations lower than a population average are used to define pathologically low bone mineral levels. Such a definition of osteoporosis or bone fragility rather arbitrarily includes both false-positive and false-negative values. It is not surprising that such a definition is imprecise especially for a condition such as bone fragility, in which not only does the amount of bone mineral matter but also a trauma is needed for a fracture to occur. For a physician on duty at an emergency department with no available bone scanners, a practical and useful "screening" method could be to use Frost¥s definition for bone fragility (2). He suggested several decades ago that fragility is present when a *minor everyday trauma* is enough to cause a fracture. By combining both strength (bone mineral) of the bone and the fracture causing load (minor everyday trauma), the well-known intimate interrelation between those two factors is applied to form a reliable predictor of bone fragility (2).

At a certain point, many people, usually elderly and most frequently women, experience a sudden stabbing, excruciating pain caused by compression of a vertebral body. It is obvious that a better understanding of all the different factors will one day prevent this from happening. This chapter discusses some aspects of the intricate interactions between important properties of vertebral fragility fractures, such as

- The technique for determination of bone mineral density
- The strength of human vertebrae
- Fatigue properties of vertebrae
- Microscopic failures and healing trabecular microfractures

DETERMINATION OF THE BONE MINERAL DENSITY IN THE HUMAN SKELETON

For a long time, regular radiography was the only noninvasive technique for estimating the density of the skeleton *in vivo.* This method is inaccurate, allowing only rough

TABLE 3.1. *The relative proportions of cancellous and cortical bone in different parts of the human skeleton*

Bone	Cancellous bone/Ratio of cortical bone
Calcaneus	90/10
Distal radius	60/40
Femoral neck	45/55
Lumbar spine	50/50
Lumbar vertebral body	90/10

quantitative estimates of the amount of calcified tissue. New techniques developed during the 1960s and 1970s, such as x-ray spectrophotometry, single-photon and dual-photon absorptiometry (DPA), and dual x-ray absorptiometry (DEXA), made both precise and accurate measurements of the bone mineral density in the human skeleton possible for the first time (3,4). DPA and DEXA could be used for measurements even in the central axial skeleton, such as the spine (3,5–7).

The lifelong and continuous remodeling process of the skeleton in which old bone mineral is replaced occurs predominantly as a surface phenomenon of the actual skeletal part. Simplified cortical bone can be regarded as having two surfaces: one inner (endosteal) and one outer, (periosteal). Cancellous bone, in contrast, is made up of an intricate construction consisting primarily of tiny bony trabecular columns and crossties that have many surfaces and is therefore said to have a high ratio of surface to volume. For this reason, remodeling and the effects of remodeling are most likely to be detected in skeletal parts with a high inclusion of spongy or cancellous bone. As can be seen in Table 3.1, the lumbar vertebral body with its 90/10 ratio of cancellous to cortical bone has far more cancellous bone than do other skeletal parts. Changes in the amount of bone mineral are, for that reason, most likely to be detectable first in the spine.

Computed tomography and ultrasonography are other techniques developed more recently and used for bone mineral determination (Table 3.2). The photon absorptiometric technique in particular has been developed further, and its use in both research and clinical practice has become widespread.

The development has increased the precision in bone mineral determinations. The precision of a measurement is associated with the random error in measuring; also, when in repeat measurements the variation is low, the precision or reproducibility is regarded as high. Accuracy, however, reflects the agreement between the true value and the measured value. The continuous development of new ways for determining the bone mineral density of the skeleton has not led to an improvement of the accuracy as it has for the preci-

TABLE 3.2. *Precision and accuracy in bone mineral determinations at different locations with the most commonly used measuring technique (percentage:)*

Technique	Bone	Precision	Accuracy
Single photon absorptiometry	Forearm	2.5	9.4
Dual photon absorptiometry	Vertebra	3.0	10.3
Dual photon absorptiometry	Calcaneus	1.8	6.3
Dual x-ray absorptiometry	Vertebra	1.0	9.0
Triple x-ray absorptiometry	Vertebra	3.4	1.2
Quantitative CT	Vertebra	4.0	19.0
Ultrasound attenuation	Calcaneus	2.9	21.6

sion (see Table 3.2). One explanation for the relatively poor accuracy is that fat tissue and fat-like tissues influence the transmitted photons in a similar way as does bone. This is particularly important if the fat or fat-like tissues are unevenly distributed outside or inside the measured bone (7,8).

THE STRENGTH OF HUMAN THORACIC AND LUMBAR VERTEBRAE

There are several ways in which the bone mineral density has an effect on the strength of the bone. In experiments with the compressive strength in human cadaver vertebrae, a linear relationship repeatedly has been found between the compressive strength and the amount of bone mineral (Fig. 3.1) (1). A more recent and advanced analysis of the relations between compressive strength and the amount of bone mineral has shown that the best calculation is obtained through a power function (Fig. 3.2). In an early study performed before the advent of noninvasive techniques for bone mineral determinations, it was suggested that in vertebrae with extremely low densities, this relation could be a nonlinear one (9). More recent studies with DPA technique on world-class power lifters—who represent the other extreme of bone mineral values—have also revealed a nonlinear relation between compressive vertebral strength and the amount of bone mineral (10). These results, if correct, suggest that in vertebrae with extremely low or high bone mineral values, even a minor change of the bone mineral density causes a considerable change in strength. In people with average densities, it is possible that the bone mineral values constitute the "transition range" between a linear and a nonlinear relation, the lowest values being the border below which a fracture readily can or will occur. It would not be surprising if the architecture and especially variations in the architecture of the cancellous bone could explain those changing relations. It is well established that a reduction in bone mineral density parallels not only a thinning of the trabecular columns but

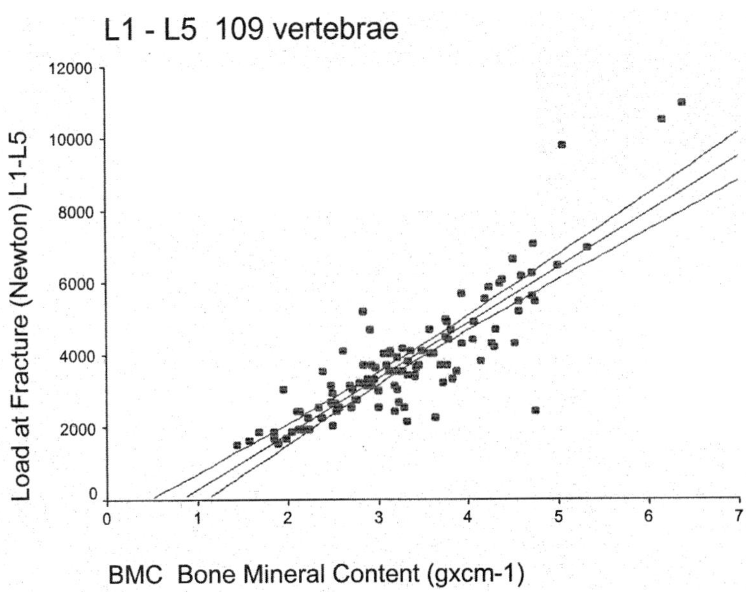

FIG. 3.1. The relation between bone mineral content and ultimate compressive strength in 109 lumbar vertebrae.

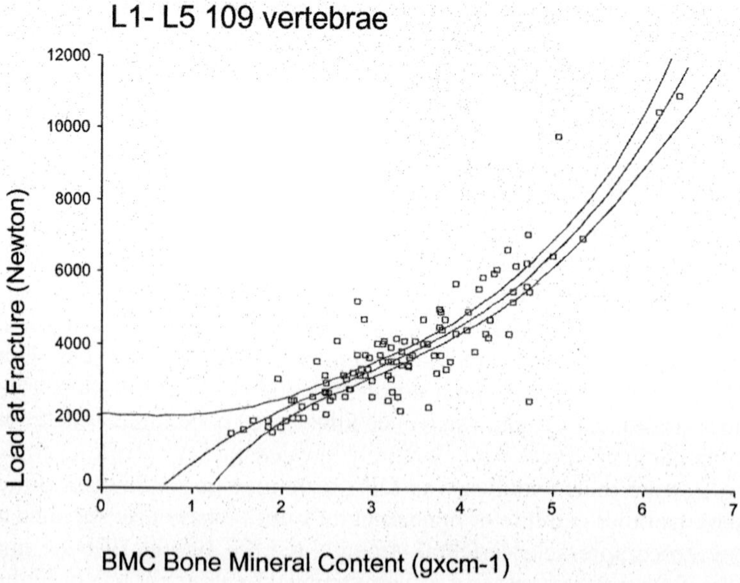

FIG. 3.2. When the relation between the bone mineral content and ultimate compressive strength is fitted to a power equation (cubic), the knee in the lower end of the curve could indicate that minor bone mineral changes induce structural changes within the cancellous bone, profoundly affecting ultimate strength.

also an additional reduction of trabecular crossties between the vertical columns. Because a reduction of the number of crossties or horizontal trabeculae, as well as a reduction of the circumference of the vertical columns, lowers the mechanical strength according to power functions, bone mineral losses inducing those architectural changes will have a detrimental effect on the bones strength properties.

FATIGUE PROPERTIES OF THE LUMBAR MOTION SEGMENT

The introduction of nondestructive techniques for determination of the amount of bone mineral in the human vertebrae allowed not only strength testing in intact vertebrae but also repetitive loading at loads below an estimated ultimate strength level (11,12). As for a single load, the ability of the vertebral body to resist repeat loading in compression was found to be closely related to its bone mineral density. Because several vertebral compression fractures seem to occur without any obvious external trauma or excessive load, it is possible that they develop as a result of fatigue. In these cases, the loading history causing such a fatigue failure should consist only of the loads of the trunk above the actual vertebra.

THE FIRST VISIBLE COMPRESSION FRACTURE

When intact vertebral bodies and adjacent intact intervertebral discs have been tested for ultimate strength in compression, three different failure modes have been detected. All three involve the disc, the endplate, and the spongy bone adjacent to the endplate (1). The most common failure type typically involves the nucleus pulposus, the neighboring endplate, and the underlying spongy bone. These fractures are apparent and distinct when analyzed histologically; however, it has been a common experience in several studies that these fractures caused at ultimate strength testing have been very difficult to reveal with advanced radiographic or other imaging techniques *in vitro.* For that reason, the clinical significance of this or similar types of fractures still must be clarified. It is obvious that these endplate and spongy bone fractures are even harder to discover *in vivo,* located as they are in the center of the vertebral body, which, being in the lumbar spine, is situated almost at the level of the middle of the bowel.

TRABECULAR MICROFRACTURES

The finding that healing trabecular microfractures in many vertebrae are abundant in exactly the same regions of the vertebral bodies as are the experimental fractures seems to prove that similar failures do occur *in vivo* as experimentally *in vitro* (Fig. 3.3). The healing trabecular fractures, visible as microcalluses (Fig. 3.4), are related to the amount of bone mineral in the vertebral bodies (13). The finding that these healing microfractures were far from uncommon, even in vertebrae with at least average or normal bone mineral values, was somewhat confusing (13). This latter finding indicated that their significance at least hypothetically could be manifold.

They may, for example, be indicative of a first but clinically indeterminable endplate and trabecular bone fracture complex of the same type as those caused during ultimate strength testing. In persons with low bone mineral values, those endplate fractures might be the predecessors of the gross osteoporotic crush or compression fracture. In such fragile vertebrae, the presence of "soft" healing calluses may undermine part of the endplate, concentrating more load (stress) to other regions of the endplate. In doing so, they may be a part of a continuous yielding process of fragile vertebral bodies, resulting, for example, in centrally compressed "cod fish" type of vertebral defect.

For spines with normal amounts of bone mineral, it has been suggested that the effect of endplate fractures and fractures of the adjacent trabeculae could be a factor in disc degeneration: for example, changing the stiffness of the bone (14).

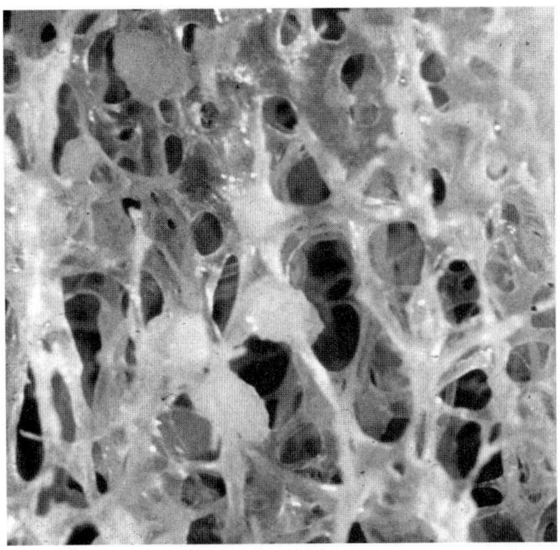

FIG. 3.3. Healing trabecular fractures (microcalluses) in close vicinity to the vertebral endplate.

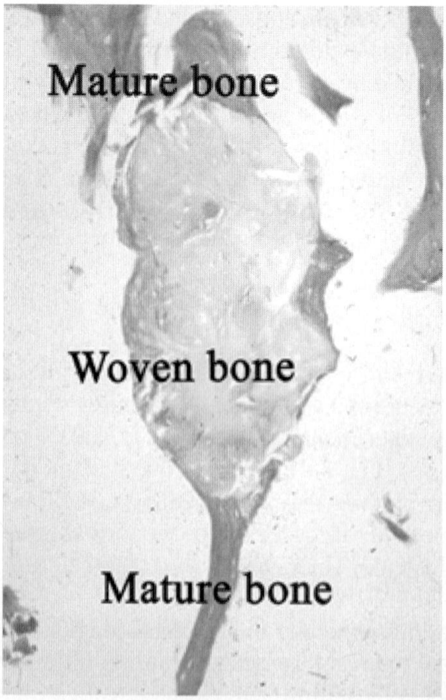

FIG. 3.4. Histological view of one single trabecular microcallus from a lumbar vertebral body, showing mature well-organized bone in the normal trabecula, whereas the callus consists of woven, less well-organized bone.

Because gross vertebral body compression fractures are much more unlikely to occur in spines with normal or above-normal bone mineral values, their presence may suggest a different significance. In normally mineralized vertebrae, those healing trabecular fractures may indicate that the actual vertebral body has been subjected to an overload, resulting in a "typical" endplate fracture complex similar or identical to the fractures caused during an ultimate strength testing.

Whether the endplate fracture generates acute back pain, for example, is not proven. The presence of free nerve endings within the involved spongy bone, among other areas, makes such a scenario far from unrealistic (15).

One last hypothesis is that the endplate and trabecular fractures are the micro-cracks suggested by Frost as being a way in which the remodeling process of the skeleton—in this case, the vertebral body—is propagated (2).

THE FIRST VERTEBRAL FRACTURE *IN VIVO*

By relating the actual fracture-causing forces in recently fractured spines to the amount of bone mineral, it should be possible to define a relatively narrow fracture risk range. This range would mark the bone mineral level below which a compression fracture is more or less likely to occur. The validity in analyzing the magnitude of the fracture-causing trauma together with the patient and relating that to her or his spine mineral content to obtain a relevant and narrow fracture risk threshold has been confirmed clinically.

The predilection site for the occurrence of the first vertebral compression fracture, a fragility fracture, is at the T12 or L1 level. Because neither the amount of bone mineral nor the shapes of these two vertebral bodies differ significantly from those of neighboring vertebrae, their readiness to fail most probably reflects their anatomical position as a fulcrum between the relatively stiff thoracic spine and the more moveable lumbar spine.

Interrelated to the bone mineral and the fracture-causing load is the velocity of the trauma (the strain rate). Results of experiments at different strain rates have suggested that the vertebrae are stronger at higher rates, which indicates a hydraulic effect in the rapidly loaded vertebral body.

Other influences on the susceptibility of the vertebral bodies may include differences in strength determined by size, location in relation to the spine, and normal kyphosis or lordosis (4).

SUMMARY

Several biomechanical properties determine the occurrence of a vertebral compression or crush fracture. Except for the fracture-causing trauma or load, the amount of bone mineral seem to be of decisive importance. The amount of bone mineral in the vertebral body determines its capacity not only for resisting a peak load but also for resisting repeat loading (fatigue). The presence of healing trabecular microfractures, especially in the cancellous bone adjacent to the endplate, indicates that the gross, radiographically detectable crush fracture probably has a predecessor involving the same regions of the vertebral body.

REFERENCES

1. Hansson T, Roos B, Nachemson A. The bone mineral content and ultimate compressive strength of lumbar vertebrae. *Spine* 1980;5(1):46–55.
2. Frost HM. The pathomechanics of osteoporoses. *Clin Orthop* 1985;(200):198–225.
3. Roos BO, Skoldborn H. Dual photon absorptiometry in lumbar vertebrae: I. Theory and method. *Acta Radiol Ther Phys Biol* 1974;13(3):266–280.
4. Swanpalmer J, Kullenberg R, Hansson T. Determination of bone mineral density in the third lumbar vertebral body using photon absorptiometry techniques. *Appl Radiat Isot* 1998;49(12):1511–1518.
5. Roos BO, Hansson TH, Skoldborn H. Dual photon absorptiometry in lumbar vertebrae. Evaluation of the baseline error. *Acta Radiol Oncol* 1980;19(2):111–114.
6. Swanpalmer J, Kullenberg R, Hansson T. Measurement of bone mineral using multiple-energy x-ray absorptiometry. *Phys Med Biol* 1998;43(2):379–387.
7. Szucs J, Jonson R, Granhed H, et al. Accuracy, precision, and homogeneity effects in the determination of the bone mineral content with dual photon absorptiometry in the heel bone. *Bone* 1992;13(2):179–183.
8. Mazess RB, Vetter J. The influence of marrow on measurement of trabecular bone using computed tomography. *Bone* 1985;6(5):349–351.
9. Bell GH, Dunbar O, Beck JS, et al. Variations in strength of vertebrae with age and their relation to osteoporosis. *Calcif Tissue Res* 1967;1(1):75–86.
10. Granhed H, Jonson R, Hansson T. The loads on the lumbar spine during extreme weight lifting. *Spine* 1987;12(2):146–149.
11. Hansson TH, Keller TS, Spengler DM. Mechanical behavior of the human lumbar spine: II. Fatigue strength during dynamic compressive loading. *J Orthop Res* 1987;5(4):479–487.
12. Brinckmann P, Biggemann M, Hilweg D. Fatigue fracture of human lumbar vertebrae. *Clin Biomech* 1988; pp. 1–23.
13. Hansson T, Roos B. Microcalluses of the trabeculae in lumbar vertebrae and their relation to the bone mineral content. *Spine* 1981;6(4):375–380.
14. Adams MA, Freeman BJ, Morrison HP, et al. Mechanical initiation of intervertebral disc degeneration. *Spine* 2000;25(13):1625–1636.
15. Brown MF, Hukkanen MV, McCarthy ID, et al. Sensory and sympathetic innervation of the vertebral endplate in patients with degenerative disc disease. *J Bone Joint Surg Br* 1997;79(1):147–153.

4

Modeling of Bone Damage and Fracture in Osteoporosis

*Tony S. Keller, *Victor Kosmopoulos, and †Michael A.K. Liebschner

**Department of Mechanical Engineering, University of Vermont, Burlington, Vermont, and †Department of Bioengineering, Rice University, Houston, Texas*

This chapter provides a general overview of the biomechanics of osteoporotic compression fractures. Experimental, analytical, and numerical studies of vertebral bone loss and spinal deformity are discussed. A structural, anatomically accurate, finite-element model of vertebral damage and repair is also presented.

OSTEOPOROSIS

Osteoporosis is a skeletal disorder characterized by weakened skeletal architecture caused by suboptimal bone development or a reduction in bone mass. It is a disease that weakens the structural properties of bone in both men and women and results in fracture when loads applied to bone exceed its ability to support those loads. Thus, osteoporosis is a significant risk factor for fracture. Fracture, especially in load-bearing structures such as the vertebral bodies in the spinal column, causes pain and deformity and can lead to immobilization and death (1). In the United States, ten million persons have been diagnosed with osteoporosis, and another 18 million have low bone mass, which renders them at increased risk for osteoporosis and fracture. Treatment of osteoporotic fracture is estimated to be as high as $15 billion annually (2). To date, a considerable amount of research has focused on the diagnosis and prevention of vertebral osteoporosis, but less attention has been directed toward improving treatment for patients with vertebral compression fractures and spinal deformity.

STRUCTURAL AND MECHANICAL BEHAVIOR OF VERTEBRAL BONE

The design or structure of bone in human vertebrae and elsewhere in the body varies, ranging from a very porous solid (trabecular bone) to a very dense solid (compact bone). The anterior column, or centrum, of human vertebrae comprises only a very thin cortical shell (<2 mm), which is virtually indistinguishable from the trabeculae that constitute the bulk of the vertebral centrum (Fig. 4.1). In view of the porous nature of bone, the relative amount of bone tissue is described histologically in terms of the apparent density (ρ_a). Apparent density is defined as the mass of bone tissue present within a given volume. Clinically, bone mass is estimated from dual energy x-ray absorptiometry (DEXA). This low-radiation method provides measures of the distributions of bone mineral con-

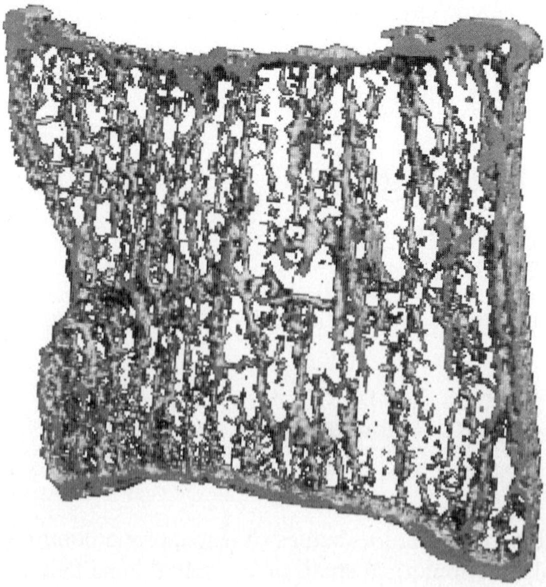

FIG. 4.1. Volume rendering of micro–computed tomography scan image of T10 osteopenic vertebral body (1.8-mm–thick section).

tent (BMC), in grams per centimeter, and bone mineral density (BMD), in grams per square centimeter, within the body (3).

Although BMC and BMD are not true volumetric measures of tissue mass or apparent density, both have been shown to be useful predictors of bone fragility (4–7). Hansson (5) performed *in vitro* mechanical compression tests on 109 intact L1–L4 vertebral centra from subjects aged 31 to 79 years). In this test series, the BMC ranged from 1.44 to 6.39 g/cm (mean, 3.33 g/cm), and the compressive force at failure ranged from 1,520 to 10,987 N (mean, 3,850 N). From these data, the following linear correlation between vertebral strength (ultimate force, F_{ult}, in newtons) and BMC (in grams per centimeter) is obtained:

$$F_{ult} = 1{,}535\text{BMC} - 1{,}258.$$

This linear relationship indicates that the ultimate compressive force of the human lumbar vertebral centrum can be as low as 952 N (BMC = 1.44 g per centimeter). As described later, when the vertebral strength decreases to this level or lower, the vertebral structures can fail under loads imposed by the weight of the body above the vertebrae.

From a mechanical point of view, ultimate force is a structural property that is dependent on both the size (geometry) and composition (material) of the tissue. Thus, the ultimate forces of vertebrae from different regions in the spine cannot be compared because the sizes of the cervical, thoracic, and lumbar vertebrae vary appreciably from one another and from one level to another. For this reason, material property measurements, such as stress or the ratio of force to area, are often preferred, because they account for geometric variations of different size structures. An estimate of the apparent stress at failure (σ_{ult}, MPa or 10^6 N/m^2) can be obtained for Hansson's data by dividing the ultimate force (in newtons) by the cross-sectional area (in square millimeters) reported for the vertebral endplate. The apparent stress at failure of the lumbar vertebrae is found to range from 0.95 to 4.95 MPa (mean, 2.29 MPa). In this case, apparent stress refers to the fact that the porosity of the vertebral centrum is still unaccounted for: Two vertebrae with the same endplate area can have very different structural properties if their porosities or apparent densities differ appreciably.

Mechanical properties not only vary from vertebrae to vertebrae and from level to level but can also vary dramatically within a given vertebral body (see Fig. 4.1). Trabeculae tend to be more dense, rod-like structures in the inferior and superior sections, in contrast to the less dense, plate-like trabeculae that are associated with the central region of the lumbar vertebral centrum (8). Studies of the physical and mechanical properties of lumbar vertebral trabecular bone have also shown that trabecular bone underlying the normal intervertebral disc nucleus is significantly stronger, stiffer, and denser than trabecular bone underlying the disc annulus (7,9,10). Such intravertebral variations in trabecular bone properties have been attributed, in part, to adaptation to the heterogeneous pressure distribution within the normal intervertebral disc (10): The pressurized disc nucleus exerts higher stresses on the underlying endplate and trabecular bone in comparison with pressure transmitted by the disc annulus. Keller et al. (10) also noted that disc degeneration reduces intravertebral variations in the apparent strength and apparent density of trabecular bone in regions adjacent to the endplate, which presumably reflects a more uniform or homogeneous distribution of pressure and stress within the degenerated disc.

Keller (11) published empirical relationships from *in vitro* mechanical tests that can be used to calculate the compressive apparent strength (σ_a, MPa) of trabecular and cortical bone:

$$\sigma_a = 46.1\rho_a^{1.93}$$

where ρ_a is the apparent density ($0.05 < \rho_a < 1.9$ g/cm^3). The approximately square exponent means that a relative reduction in apparent density of one half will produce a corresponding relative reduction in compressive apparent strength of one fourth. In elderly subjects (aged >70 years), the apparent density of human vertebral trabecular bone can be as low as 0.05 g/cm^3, which corresponds to an ultimate compressive strength of only 0.05 MPa. In the numerical simulations that follow, stresses much greater than 0.05 MPa are produced in vertebrae when subjected to forces associated with weight bearing in upright postures.

BIOMECHANICS OF VERTEBRAL COMPRESSION FRACTURES

Vertebral compression fractures occur when the loads applied to the vertebral structures exceed their ability to support that load. Although apparent density and its clinical counterparts (BMC, BMD) provide good estimates of bone mechanical properties, they are not absolutely definitive. From a mechanical point of view, the load-bearing or structural capacity (force at failure) of the vertebrae depends on both material properties (mineral content, tissue density, and apparent density) and geometric properties (size, orientation, and connectivity of bone elements). The load-bearing capacity of the vertebrae, coupled with the applied loads (magnitude, duration, rate), determines the fracture risk (Fig. 4.2).

Four characteristic types of fractures are formed during overloading of the vertebral body: central endplate fracture, Schmorl's node, wedge fracture, and burst fracture. Central endplate fractures are often the first sign of failure as observed during *in vitro* compression fatigue loading experiments conducted on normal and osteopenic human lumbar vertebral motion segments, such as that of Hansson et al. (8). This study also

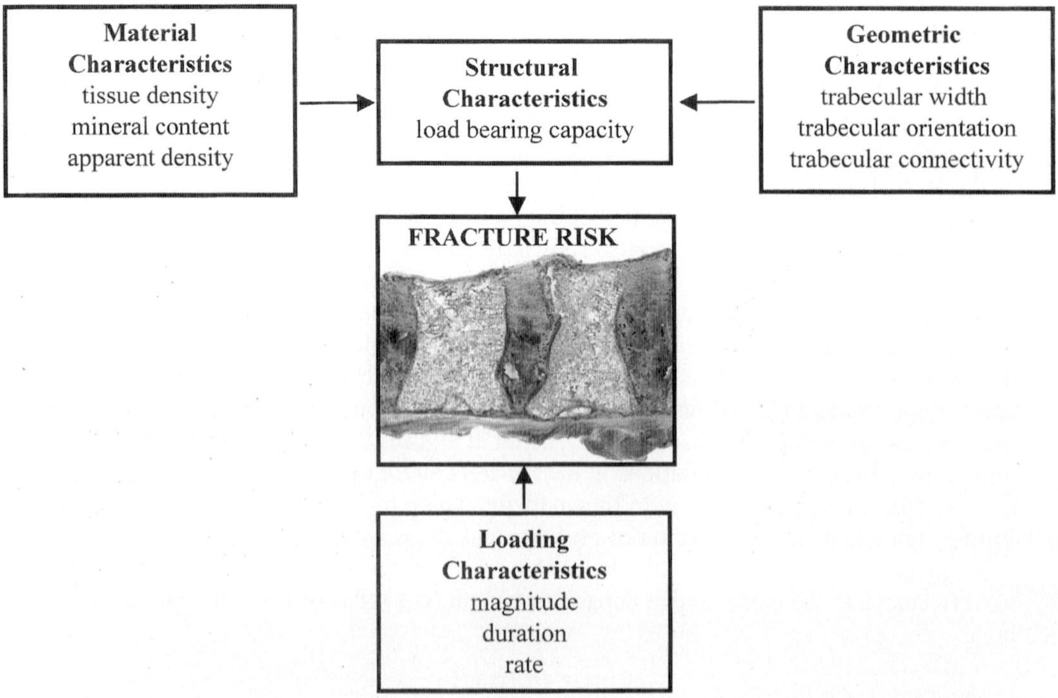

FIG. 4.2. Biomechanical determinants of fracture risk.

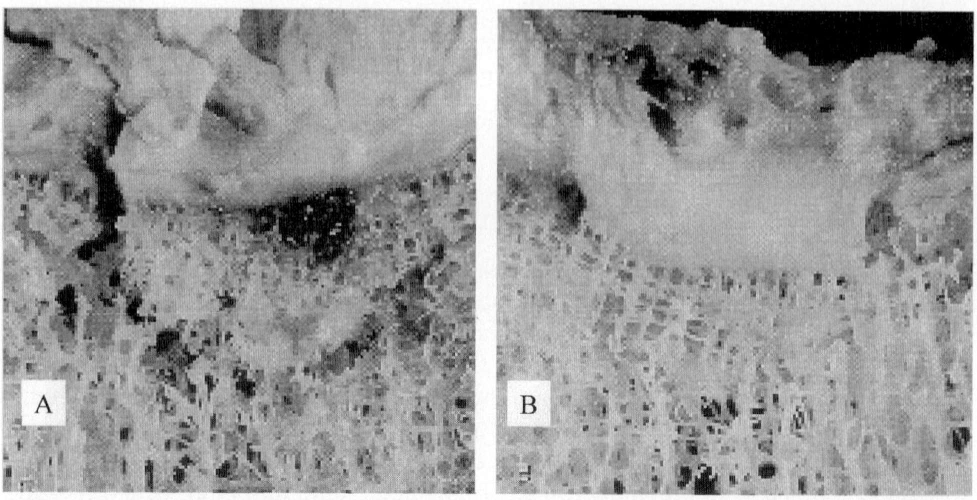

FIG. 4.3. Vertebral endplate fractures produced during *in vitro* dynamic axial compressive fatigue loading experiments. **A:** Central end-plate fracture. **B:** Schmorl node fracture. (Adapted from Hansson T, Keller T, Jonson R. Fatigue fracture morphology in human lumbar motion segments. *J Spinal Disord* 1988;1:33–38.)

demonstrated how remarkably close to failure the human spine is when it comes to repetitive loading: Compressive forces as low as 50% of the failure strength of the vertebrae produce fatigue fractures after fewer than 1,000 cycles. Hansson et al. (12) also noted that Schmorl's nodes were associated predominantly with segments from younger patients with less degenerated discs, whereas central endplate fractures were associated predominantly with older, more degenerated discs (Fig. 4.3). A combination of central endplate fracture and anterior wedge fracture is formed during compression-flexion loading of lumbar vertebrae (13).

In normal and osteopenic vertebrae, compression fractures that result from fatigue damage or low-force trauma are generally undetectable on conventional radiographs (1). As the severity of endplate fractures and Schmorl's nodes increases, however, the characteristic biconcave curvature of the endplates and vertebral body height reduction become evident on radiographs (14) (Fig. 4.4). Other radiographically detectable fractures include burst fractures, which typically result from direct trauma such as a fall from a height. Burst fractures involve compressive failure of the anterior and middle columns of the vertebral body and may result in a large anterior-superior fragment and significant loss of vertebral body height. For most clinicians, radiographically detectable compression fractures represent the first verified presence of osteoporosis or bone fragility (see Fig. 4.4).

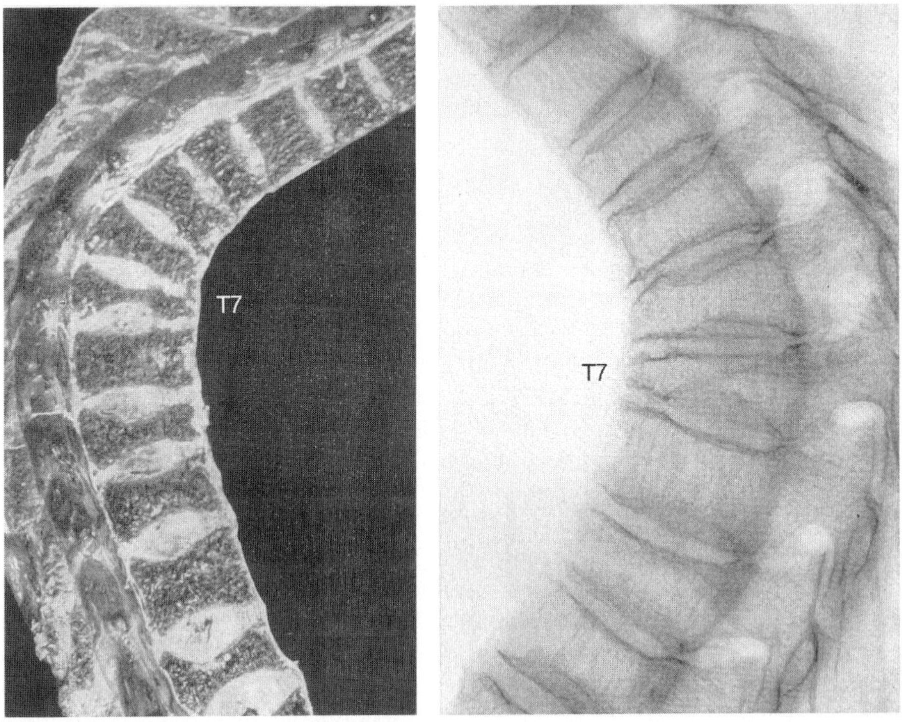

FIG. 4.4. Left: Photomicrograph of the thoracic spine of a 63-year-old woman with a thoracic kyphosis (≈80 degrees) produced by vertebral wedge fractures (T6, T7). Right: Radiograph of same specimen. (From Schmorl G, Junghanns H. *The human spine in health and disease.* New York: Grune & Stratton, 1957.)

VERTEBRAL DEFORMITY

Vertebral compression and compression-flexion fractures, particularly anterior wedge fractures in the middle and lower thoracic regions, produce spinal deformities characterized by increased thoracic kyphosis. The normal spine is characterized by a thoracic curvature of approximately 40 degrees. A single anterior wedge fracture can increase thoracic curvature by 10 degrees or more, and thoracic curvatures greater than 70 degrees are common in elderly subjects with multilevel compression fractures (see Fig. 4.4). In a study of 98 elderly, postmenopausal women, Cortet et al. (15) reported a mean increase in thoracic curvature of 11 degrees in osteoporotic women with radiographic evidence of fracture in comparison with women without radiographic evidence of fracture (mean curvature, 52 degrees). Moreover, the severity of thoracic kyphosis has been shown to increase with decreasing BMD (16). In advanced osteoporosis, compression fractures result in a loss of vertebral height and formation of a kyphotic deformity, or "dowager's hump." This deformity is often associated with severe pain and loss of mobility.

In spite of the fact that noninvasive technology can be used to determine precisely the amount of bone mineral in different parts of the human skeleton, practical techniques for measuring the fracture-generating forces and stresses are still not available. However, it is possible to estimate the magnitude of forces acting on the spine by using biomechanical models. Keller and Nathan (17) developed an upright posture, sagittal plane model of the region of C2 to S1, which they used to estimate disc forces and stresses and concomitant diurnal changes in disc height and stature. Vertebral body (VB) and intervertebral disc (IVD) geometries were modeled as quadrilaterals. Static equilibrium forces and moments were computed about each IVD centroid for forces associated with the body weight (line of gravity) and activity of the antigravity muscles (such as the musculus erector spinae). This model predicted that IVD compressive forces and stresses associated with upright posture weight bearing were greatest in the middle and lower thoracic regions of the spine.

VERTEBRAL DEFORMITY MODEL

Figure 4.5 illustrates the quadrilateral element biomechanical model of Keller and Nathan (17), which has been adapted to predict anterior and posterior VB deformations and to account for age-related bone loss and stiffness reduction (18). In this analysis, the neutral, upright spine geometry is based on digitized lateral radiographs of a person with a height of 176.8 cm and a weight of 76.6 kg. Anterior VB deformation (d_A) and posterior VB deformation (d_P) were computed by using the following equations obtained from static equilibrium of forces and moments about the quadrilateral element centroid:

$$d_P = 9.81W(l_W/l_E + \cos\alpha)/\{k(h_A/h_p)(1 + l_A/l_E)\text{-}l_p/l_E + 1]\};\ d_A = d_P(h_A/h_P)p$$

where W is body weight, l_W is body weight moment arm, l_E is posterior muscle moment arm, α is quadrilateral anterior-posterior bisector angle in relation to horizontal, h_A is anterior VB height, h_P is posterior VB height, l_A is anterior VB force moment arm, l_P is posterior VB force moment arm, k is VB stiffness, and p=2 is an empirical constant. The deformed vertebral body geometry (h_A and h_P) of each segment was computed as $h_P - d_P$ and $h_A - d_A$, and a coordinate transformation (rotation, translation) was applied to each vertebral quadrilateral in order to restore the original disc geometry. Aging (age in years) was simulated by varying the L3 vertebral compressive force at failure (F_{ult}, in Newtons) according to empirical data published by Hansson (5):

$$F_{ult} = -75\text{age} + 8{,}199.$$

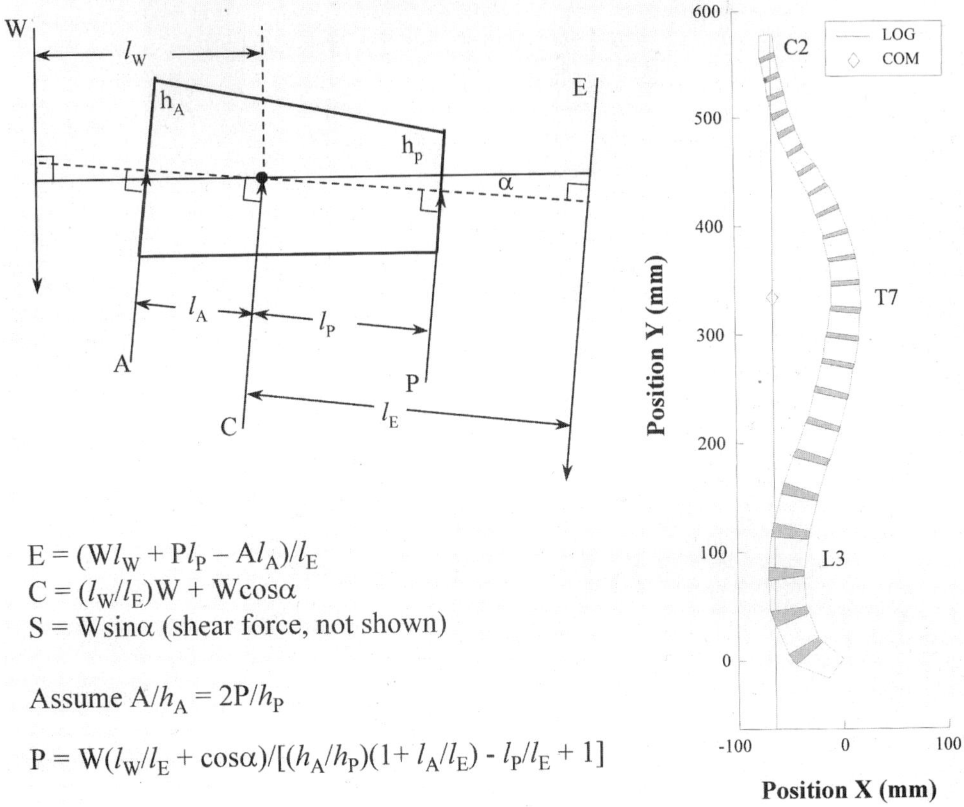

FIG. 4.5. Quadrilateral element intervertebral disc (IVD) and vertebral body (VB) deformity model of the region C2 to S1. W, body force vector; E, extensor muscle force; C, compressive force at centroid; S, shear force at centroid; A, anterior element force; P, posterior element force; LOG, line of gravity; COM, trunk center of mass.

This linear relationship indicates that by age 80, the force required to produce failure of the L3 lumbar vertebrae is only 2,200 N, or about one third of the compressive failure force at age 30 (F_{ult} = 5,949 N). In the following analyses, forces representative of elderly subjects (aged >80 years, F_{ult} < 2,250 N) were simulated and compared to a baseline model approximating a 30-year-old subject (F_{ult} > 6,000 N).

IVD and VB material and structural properties were derived from the model of Keller and Nathan (17). VB midheight cross-sectional area was modeled as 90% of the adjacent IVD area. The ultimate compressive force of each of the other VB segments was adjusted to the L3 value multiplied by the IVD area ratio (segment disc area/L3 disc area) squared. Likewise, the VB structural stiffness values were obtained by multiplying the VB modulus (L3 = 25 N/m^2) by the VB cross-sectional area/VB height. The VB modulus was then decreased through a stiffness reduction algorithm based on perfect plasticity theory (19), and the ensuing new vertebral body geometries and orientations were computed.

The analytical model reproduces the salient features of spinal deformities caused by osteoporotic wedge fractures: namely, an increased thoracic curvature (Fig. 4.6).

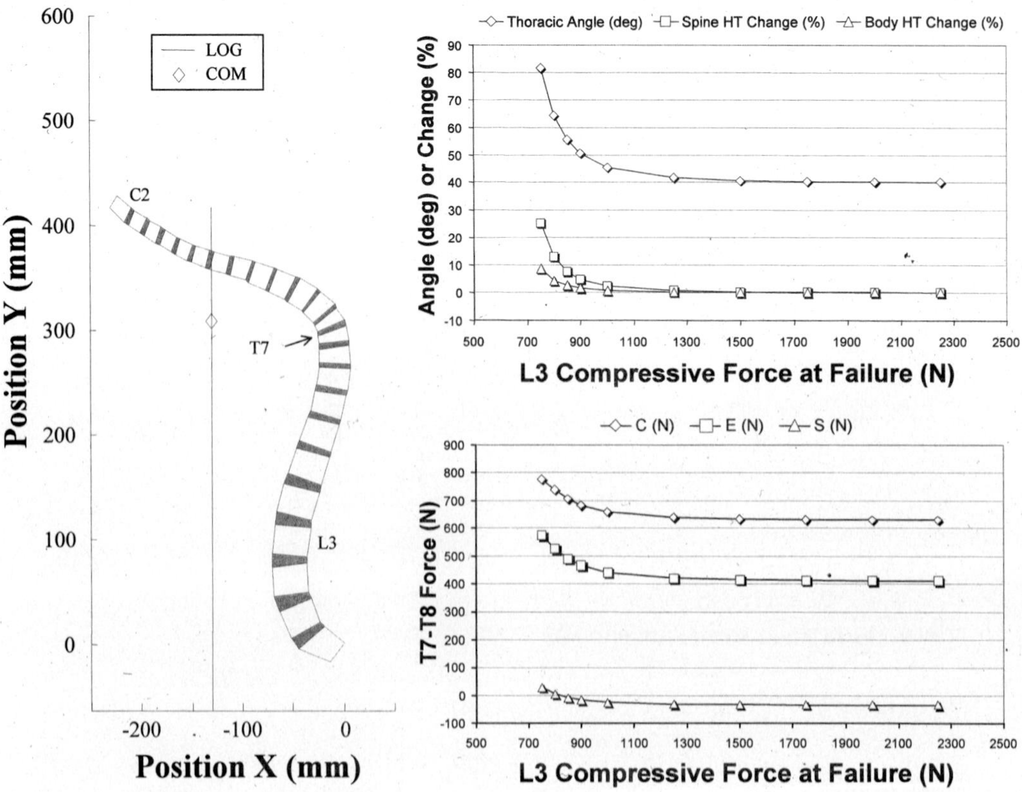

FIG. 4.6. Summary of vertebral deformity simulation results. Left: Graphical depiction of 750 N ultimate compressive force model. Vertebral body (VB) compression fractures, including T7 and T8 crush-like deformities, resulted in a 15.1-cm decrease in stature. Upper right: Changes in thoracic angle (degrees), spine height (percentage) and body height (percentage) associated with age-simulated variations in VB ultimate compressive force. Lower right: Changes in T7-T8 intervertebral disc (IVD) forces (C, S) and extensor muscle force (E) associated with age-simulated variations in VB ultimate compressive force.

Changes in thoracic angle and the concomitant spinal height changes were most apparent when the ultimate compressive force was less than 1,250 N. The most osteopenic model (F_{ult} = 750 N) produced gross deformities of the spine, including anterior wedge fracture deformities at T7 and T8 (>10 degree kyphotic deformity at T7). In this model, increases in thoracic curvature (41.7-degree increase) and decreases in VB height (7.7% total height reduction) resulted in a 25.2% decrease in spinal height (region of C2 to S1) and an 8.6% decrease in total body height. The resulting deformity produced a 15.1-cm anterior translation of the cervical-thoracic spine, which in turn was associated with a 19% increase in compressive force, a 24% increase in compressive stresses, and a 40% increase in paraspinal extensor muscle force at the T7–T8 level. In Table 4.1, the baseline model geometry predictions are compared with deformity predictions representative of the osteopenic (F_{ult} = 750 N) patient (apparent age of 99 years). Note that the thoracic deformity (81.6-degree° kyphotic angle) associated with the 750 N ultimate compressive force model corresponds very closely with clinical osteoporotic kyphosis deformities (see Fig. 4.4).

TABLE 4.1. *Geometry characteristics of the baseline (Fult = 6000 N) and osteopenic (Fult = 750 N) vertebral deformity models*

Model F_{ult} (N)	Total Spine height (mm)	Anterior VB height (mm)	Posterior VB height (mm)	C2s Shift (mm)	L4 Shift (mm)	Cervical Angle C2–C7 (degrees)	Thoracic Angle T2–T10 (degrees)	Lumbar Angle T12–L5 (degrees)
6,000	596.3	497.6	507.1	0	0	-11.2	39.9	-52.6
750	445.8	447.3	479.8	-151	-4.49	-10.3	81.6	-52.3
Change	150.5	50.3	27.3	-151	-4.49	-0.9	-41.7	-0.3

VB, vertebral body.

The vertebral deformity model presented here suggests that initiation of spinal deformity is primarily the result of vertebral deformity and exacerbated by anterior translation of the spinal column. Fractures and marked deformities are predicted to occur when the ultimate compressive strength of the vertebral column (L3) falls below 1,250 N. According to the *in vitro* mechanical test and densitometry data of Hansson (5), the latter corresponds to an L3 vertebral BMC of 1.63 g per centimeter and an apparent age of 93 years. Additional work is needed to study the combined effects of VB height reduction (osteoporotic kyphosis) and IVD height reduction (senile kyphosis), as well as mechanical overload caused by activities such as lifting and exercise.

VERTEBRAL DAMAGE

Analytical models such as the vertebral deformity model presented here provide a basic understanding of the apparent forces and stresses acting on the vertebral structures, but they do not tell us anything about the magnitude of tissue stresses and strains. Characterization of trabecular bone tissue stresses and strains is important for understanding basic skeletal mechanics, fracture risk, damage, and fracture repair. Measures of more explicit mechanical stress-strain behavior are obtained through the use of numerical techniques such as the finite-element analysis (FEA) method.

FEA is a computer-based procedure that provides approximate answers to the deformations, stresses, and strains in physical structures with complex geometry that are acted upon by external forces. In contrast to classical methods in which structures are considered along a continuum, the structure is considered in FEA to be an assembly of finite-sized particles or "elements." Points where the elements are interconnected are termed *nodes,* and the procedure in selecting the nodes is termed *discretization* or *modeling.* Measures of the mechanical behavior of the elements and overall structure are obtained by solving a system of algebraic equations for the node displacements. Solution accuracy depends on the degree to which the structure is discretized. In typical FEA models, mathematical descriptions of geometry and material properties based on a few thousand elements are used. FEA is well suited for computer-based analysis of complex geometry structures and yields important information about internal stresses and strains that cannot be determined easily by other means.

Currently, there are two basic approaches to FEA of trabecular bone structures:

apparent density models, which can be used to obtain information regarding apparent stresses and strains in vertebral structures [for a review, see Gilbertson et al. (20)], and

structural models, which give information about vertebral trabecular tissue stresses and strains [for a review, see Saxena and Keller (21)].

FEA studies of the human spine have demonstrated that the most sensitive parameter influencing solution accuracy is the selection of the trabecular bone modulus (22). Because of the inherent computational demands required for precise discretization of vertebral trabecular bone structures, most FEA studies have idealized the highly porous trabecular structure component of the vertebral centrum as a solid characterized in terms of its bulk or apparent density and modulus (22–25). This strategy reduces the complexity (number of elements) and computational costs of the analysis, but it does not capture the structural intricacies of trabecular bone.

Advances in digital imaging techniques, such as quantitative serial sectioning (QSS) and micro–computed tomography (μCT), together with dramatic improvements in computer computational power, have enabled researchers to analyze anatomically precise structural two-dimensional and three-dimensional models of vertebral trabecular bone (21,23,26,27). In addition to improved accuracy, structural FEA models provide precise estimates of tissue level stresses and strains. Using a QSS imaging approach to obtain digital images of trabecular bone, Saxena et al. (27) created precise (up to 42 thousand 20-μm resolution elements), three-dimensional, structural finite-element models of small subvolumes (1.5 × 1.5 × 2.0 mm) of normal and osteopenic vertebral trabecular bone. They found that the stress intensity (σ/σ_a = tissue stress/apparent stress) or stress concentrations in trabecular bone were up to 100 times greater than the applied apparent stress (force/surface area). In addition, they noted that the stress concentrations in trabecular bone tissue increased an additional threefold to fivefold when the volume fraction of trabecular bone was reduced by 50% (corresponding to a reduction in apparent modulus E_a from 61 to 5.2 MPa). A reduction in volume fraction of this magnitude is typical of age-related bone loss and osteoporosis. These findings indicate that vertebral trabecular bone is a highly loaded structure and, in the case of osteopenic bone, may be damaged by relatively low loads such as load magnitudes associated with upright-posture weight bearing.

VERTEBRAL DAMAGE MODEL

A structural finite-element model of vertebral damage illustrates numerical simulation of vertebral damage and repair (28). The osteopenic T10 vertebral model, shown in Fig. 4.7, couples a two-dimensional (plane stress) FEA with a modulus reduction algorithm derived from perfect plasticity theory (19). In perfect plasticity theory, a hyperbolic tangent function is used to characterize the nonlinear, stress-strain behavior of vertebral trabecular bone tissue as follows:

$$\sigma = \sigma_0[\tanh(E_0\varepsilon/\sigma_0)^4]^{1/4},$$

where σ is the tissue stress, ε is the tissue strain, σ_0 is the tissue strength, and E_0 is the tissue modulus. Taking the derivative of this equation with regard to strain yields an expression that can be used to characterize trabecular bone tissue damage in terms of the decrease in tissue modulus with increasing tissue strain (28).

On the basis of the aforementioned power function relationship (11), the strength (σ_0) of dense trabecular bone tissue (ρ = 1.9 g/cm^3) is estimated as 159 MPa. In the FEA simulation that follows, the trabecular bone, intervertebral disc, and bone marrow tissues of the T10 vertebral body are modeled as isotropic, linear elastic materials with elastic modulus values of 10 GPa, 2.16 MPa, and 10 kPa, respectively. Previous FEA stress-strain studies have shown that model results are relatively insensitive to Poisson ratio variations

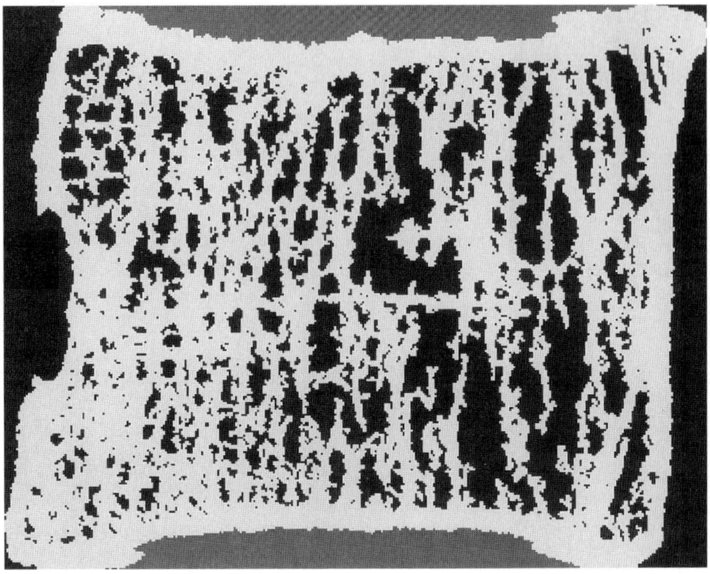

FIG. 4.7. Structural, two-dimensional, sagittal plane, finite-element model of an osteopenic T10 vertebral body derived from micro-computed tomographic scan images (83 μm/element resolution). Bone elements (37,828) are shown in white, marrow elements (27,176) are black, and intervertebral disc elements (5,261) are shaded light gray. Dimensions are 24.82 (anterior-posterior) × 19.51 × 1.8 mm thick.

(22,27); therefore, a value of 0.3 is assumed for all 299 × 235 (70,265), four-node isoparametric elements. The model is loaded with a compressive load ranging from −50 N to −500 N (in 10 increments) applied uniformly to a rigid, laterally constrained top plate. The vertebral body is simply supported at its base. The peak load was chosen to represent the compressive force at T10 for a 76.6 kg person in an upright posture (17). The FEA was performed with the use of custom MATLAB® programs (The MathWorks, Boston, Massachusetts).

Figure 4.8A illustrates the nonlinear compressive stress-strain behavior and modulus reduction of the T10 vertebral body predicted by the structural finite-element model. The apparent compressive stress increased in a relatively linear manner with increasing compressive strain up to about 6.7 MPa (0.66% apparent strain). At this stress level, the reduction in the apparent compressive modulus was 10%, which indicates that very little bone tissue damage occurred. At the maximum apparent compressive stress level (11.2 MPa, corresponding to a peak compressive load of 500 N and a peak compressive strain of 10.9%), however, the apparent modulus reduction was 90%, which indicates that substantial damage to the vertebral body occurred. At this stress level, 21.1% of the trabecular bone elements showed a modulus reduction of 10% or more. The corresponding height reduction of the damaged T10 vertebral body was 2 mm. Stress concentrations in the trabecular bone tissue increased with increasing apparent stress and concomitant modulus reduction (see Fig. 4.8). Stresses in the trabecular bone elements ranged from five times (tension) to 25 times (compression) the apparent compressive stress in the undamaged vertebra (Fig. 4.8B), increasing to 30 times (tension) to 50 times (compression) the apparent stress at the 11.2 MPa apparent stress level (Fig. 4.8C).

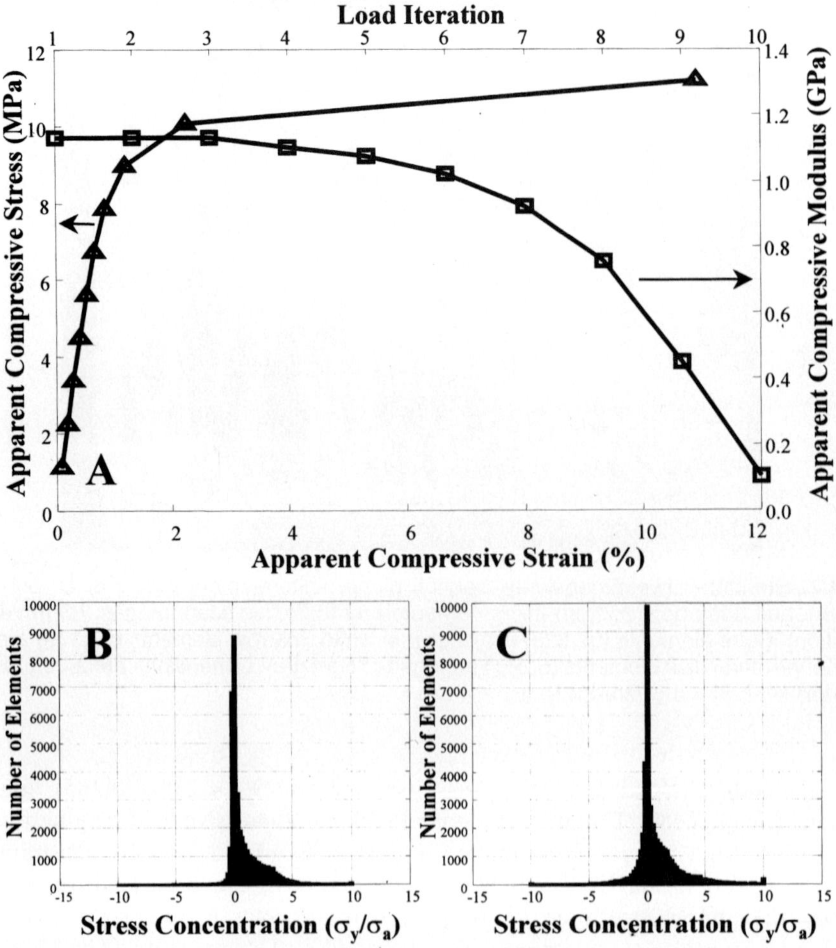

FIG. 4.8. Stress-strain behavior obtained from the structural finite-element analysis damage simulation of the T10 osteopenic vertebra: ten iterations from 50 to 500 N. **A:** Apparent compressive stress and modulus versus compressive strain. Trabecular bone stress concentrations are shown for undamaged vertebra **(B)** (first iteration = 50 N) and damaged vertebra **(C)** (last iteration = 500 N).

The normal human spinal column is a highly loaded structure. Compressive forces as high as 7,000 N are predicted for lumbar vertebrae during the performance of maximum-exertion isometric trunk-extension tasks (29). In a young, healthy person, such forces are readily tolerated by the VB and IVD. The finite-element simulations of osteopenic vertebrae presented here and elsewhere (21,26,27) indicate that a substantial amount of trabecular tissue damage occurs at compressive forces less than 600 N. This load level is equivalent to forces acting on the spine during quiet, upright standing (see Fig. 4.4). Thus, structural damage to osteopenic vertebrae during everyday activities is most likely a common occurrence. Additional study is needed to characterize trabecular bone mechanical behavior and damage initiation in response to nonuniform loading conditions such as combined compression and bending.

VERTEBROPLASTY AND KYPHOPLASTY

Vertebroplasty and kyphoplasty are two newly developed minimally invasive techniques for the treatment of vertebral compressive fractures that, unlike traditional treatments, help restore spinal alignment and decrease chronic pain (30). Vertebroplasty involves the forced injection of polymethylmethacrylate (PMMA) through one or two bone biopsy needles into the closed space of a collapsed vertebral body (30,31). This technique provides pain relief and stabilization but typically does not restore the height of the collapsed vertebral body. Kyphoplasty involves the insertion of a bone balloon into the vertebral body under biplanar fluoroscopic image guidance. The balloon is then inflated, causing the trabecular bone to compact, resulting in a suitable cavity in which to reexpand the vertebral body. PMMA is then injected with more control and less pressure than during a vertebroplasty. Two advantages of kyphoplasty are the restoration of vertebral body height and reduction of thoracic kyphosis (30,31). Biomechanical studies have demonstrated that treatment of experimentally created compression fractures with vertebroplasty is an effective means by which to restore the strength and, to a lesser extent, the stiffness of the damaged vertebrae (32). These authors noted that 2 to 4 mL of PMMA cement restored the strength of thoracolumbar vertebrae, but 4 to 8 mL of cement was necessary to restore the stiffness of the vertebrae to predamage levels. The biomechanical aspects of kyphoplasty are not as well understood.

Use of computer models and numerical tools to simulate and guide surgical repair is becoming increasingly routine and is rapidly advancing the state -of -the art in treatment of musculoskeletal disorders (33,34). Liebschner et al. (23) used an anatomically precise, three-dimensional apparent density finite-element model to simulate the effects of vertebroplasy on the apparent stiffness of a damaged L1 vertebral body. They found that only a small amount of bone cement (15% of the vertebral bone volume fraction) was necessary to restore the apparent modulus of the vertebral body to predamage levels. Use of smaller cement values will in theory, restore the mechanical integrity of the vertebral body while minimizing surgical complications such as cement leakage.

VERTEBROPLASTY MODEL

With an anatomically precise fracture damage model of osteoporotic bone, it is possible to investigate clinical treatment of vertebral fractures. The structural, two-dimensional finite-element model of the osteopenic T10 vertebral body described previously is used to illustrate how to study apparent modulus and trabecular tissue stress changes in the vertebral body after vertebroplasty (28). For this analysis, six different distributions of PMMA cement were simulated with the vertebral body model overloaded to 10.9% compressive apparent strain (apparent compressive modulus reduction of 90%). Variations in PMMA location (anterior, posterior, superior, and inferior) and amount (area fraction = cement area/vertebral area) were examined. Asymmetrical (anterior) placement of the PMMA was modeled with six cement area fractions ranging from 4.2% to 34.7% of the total vertebral body area. Because this was a two-dimensional simulation, the PMMA distribution was assumed to produce a cylindrical cement volume configuration within the vertebral body cavity, from which the cement volume could be estimated (Table 4.2). The PMMA was assumed to have a modulus of 2.16 GPa (35,36) and a Poisson ratio of 0.3. Changes in apparent modulus and trabecular

TABLE 4.2. *Characteristics of the damaged (model A) and polymethylmethacylate vertebroplasty models (B to G)*

Model	Marrow Area Fraction (%)	Cement Area Fraction (%)	Effective Cement Volume (cm³)	Mean Apparent Modulus (MPa)	Stress Concentration ( )	Stress Concentration >3 (% elements)
A	34.7	0.0	0.0	102.4	1.33	12.2
B	30.4	4.23	0.66	107.6	1.31	12.0
C	26.9	7.81	1.21	117.9	1.26	11.3
D	21.3	13.4	2.07	132.0	1.21	10.5
E	15.7	19.0	2.95	169.9	1.12	9.3
F	10.2	24.5	3.80	442.5	0.91	7.7
G	0.0	34.7	5.38	1470	0.79	2.7

bone tissue stress concentrations were determined for a single iteration of a uniform compressive force of 500 N.

Figure 4.9 summarizes the results of the vertebroplasty simulation. Anterior and inferior placement of cement (4.2% of total vertebral body area) within the vertebral body centrum resulted in the greatest increase (up to 12.2%) in the damaged vertebral body apparent modulus (see Fig. 4.9A). A cement area fraction between 25% (model F) and 35% (model G) of the total vertebral body area was required to restore the vertebral body stiffness (apparent modulus) to the intact or predamage stiffness level (see Fig. 4.9B). Models F and G correspond to an effective cylindrical cement volume of 3.8 cm^3 (3.8 mL) and 5.4 cm^3 (5.4 mL), respectively (see Table 4.2). Addition of PMMA cement was

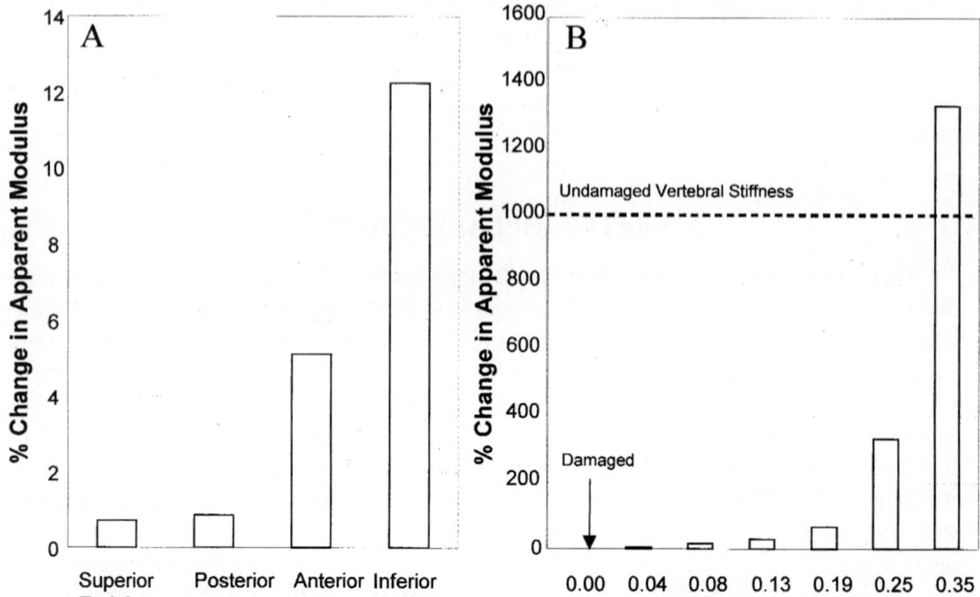

FIG. 4.9. Results of the vertebroplasty simulation in terms of cement location **(A)** and cement fraction **(B).** Values reflect the percentage of change with regard to the damaged vertebral body's apparent compressive modulus.

also found to significantly reduce the stress concentrations within the trabecular bone (see Table 4.2).

In terms of restoration of apparent stiffness and reduction of trabecular bone tissue stress concentration, the structural FEA results support the idea that an optimal vertebroplasty surgical solution can be achieved with appropriate cement placement and the use of 3 to 5 mL of cement (23,32). In this study, replacement of the entire marrow volume with PMMA cement (model G) resulted in restoration of the vertebral body stiffness to above predamage levels. In addition to simulation of vertebral damage and repair, current FEA modeling efforts are focusing on stress-adaptation of trabecular bone (37) and simulation of trabecular adaptation after vertebroplasty and kyphoplasty.

CONCLUSION

Mechanical testing, analytical modeling, and numerical analysis are useful tools with which to study vertebral mechanical properties, deformity, tissue damage, and repair. The ability to create anatomically precise structural models of vertebral trabecular bone should provide researchers and clinicians with valid computational tools with which to study osteoporotic vertebral compression fractures and repair.

ACKNOWLEDGMENTS

This work was supported by the Whitaker Foundation, the National Aeronautic and Space Administration Experimental Program to Simulate Competitive Research (EPSCoR), the Department of Energy EPSCoR, Chiropractic Biophysics Non Profit, and the University of Vermont Stimulate Undergraduate and Graduate Research/Faculty Mentoring (SUGR/FaMe) program.

REFERENCES

1. Hansson T, Keller TS. Osteoporosis of the spine. In: Wiesel S, Weinstein J, Herkowitz H, et al., eds. *The lumbar spine,* 2nd ed. Philadelphia: WB Saunders, 1996:969–988.
2. National Institutes of Health Consensus Development Conference on Osteoporosis, Prevention, Diagnosis, and Therapy. Bethesda, MD, March 27–29, 2000.
3. Dunn WL, Wahner HW, Riggs BL. Measurement of bone mineral content in human vertebrae and hip by dual photon absorptiometry. *Radiology* 1980;136:485–487.
4. Eriksson SA, Isberg BO, Lindgren JU. Prediction of vertebral strength by dual photon absorptiometry and quantitative computed tomography. *Calc Tissue Int* 1989;44:243–250.
5. Hansson T. The bone mineral content and biomechanical properties of lumbar vertebrae. PhD Thesis, University of Göteborg, Göteborg, Sweden, 1977.
6. Hansson T, Roos B, Nachemson A. The bone mineral content and ultimate compressive strength in lumbar vertebrae. *Spine* 1980;1:46–55.
7. Keller TS, Hansson TH, Abram AC, et al. Regional variations in the compressive properties of lumbar vertebral trabeculae. *Spine* 1989;14:1012–1019.
8. Hansson TH, Keller TS, Panjabi MM. A study of the compressive properties of lumbar vertebral trabeculae: effects of tissue characteristics. *Spine* 1987;11:56–62.
9. Keller TS, Moeljanto E, Main JA, et al. Distribution and orientation of bone in the human vertebral centrum. *J Spinal Disord* 1992;5:60–74.
10. Keller TS, Ziv I, Moeljanto E, et al. Interdependence of lumbar disc and subdiscal bone properties: a report of the normal and degenerated spine. *J Spinal Disord* 1993;6:106–113.
11. Keller TS. Predicting the compressive mechanical behavior of bone. *J Biomech* 1994;27:1159–1168.
12. Hansson T, Keller T, Jonson R. Fatigue fracture morphology in human lumbar motion segments. *J Spinal Disord* 1988;1:33–38.
13. Granhed H, Hansson T, Jonson R. Mineral content and ultimate compressive strength of lumbar vertebrae. A cadaver study. *Acta Orthop Scand* 1989;60:105–109.
14. Schmorl G, Junghanns H. *The human spine in health and disease.* New York: Grune & Stratton, 1957.

15. Cortet B, Houvenagel E, Puisieux F, et al. Spinal curvatures and quality of life in women with vertebral fractures secondary to osteoporosis. *Spine* 1999;24:1921–1925.
16. Goh S, Price RI, Leedman PJ, et al. Age-independent correlation of optically determined thoracic kyphosis with lumbar spine bone mineral density. *J Musculoskeletal Res* 1999;3:267–274.
17. Keller TS, Nathan M. Height change due to creep in intervertebral discs: a sagittal plane model. *J Spinal Disord* 1999;12:313–324.
18. Keller TS, Harrison DE, Colloca CJ, et al. Prediction of spinal deformity following disc degeneration and osteoporosis. Proceedings of the International Society for the Study of the Lumbar Spine, Cleveland, OH, May 14–18, 2002.
19. Betten J. Generalization of nonlinear material laws found in experiments to multi-axial states of stress. *Eur J Mech ASolids* 1989;8:325–339.
20. Gilbertson LG, Goel VK, Kong WZ, et al. Finite element methods in spine biomechanics research. *Crit Rev Biomed Eng* 1995;23:411–473.
21. Saxena R, Keller TS. Computer modeling for evaluating trabecular bone mechanics. In: An YH, Draughn RA, eds. *Mechanical testing of bone and the bone-implant interface.* Boca Raton, FL: CRC Press, 1999:407–436.
22. Suwito W, Keller TS, Basu PK, et al. Geometric and material property study of the human lumbar spine using the finite element method. *J Spinal Disord* 1992;5:50–59.
23. Liebschner MAK, Rosenberg WS, Keaveny TM. Effects of bone cement volume and distribution on the vertebral stiffness after vertebroplasty. *Spine* 2001;26:1547–1554.
24. Mizrahi J, Silva MJ, Keaveny TM, et al. Finite-element stress analysis of the normal and osteoporotic lumbar vertebral body. *Spine* 1993;18:2088–2096.
25. Whyne CM, Hu SS, Lotz JC. Parametric finite element analysis of vertebral bodies affected by tumors. J Biomech 2001;34:1317–1324.
26. Saxena R, Keller TS. A volumetric finite element scheme to investigate the mechanical properties of normal and osteoporotic trabecular bone. In: Pedersen P, Bensøe MP, eds. *IUTAM symposium on synthesis in bio solid mechanics.* Dordrecht: Kluwer Academic Publishers, 1999:373–86.
27. Saxena R, Keller TS, Sullivan JM. A three-dimensional finite element scheme to investigate the apparent mechanical properties of trabecular bone. *Comput Methods Biomech Biomed Eng* 1999;2:285–294.
28. Kosmopoulos V, Keller TS, Liebschner MAK: Finite element modeling of vertebral damage and repair. Proceedings of the 10th Annual Symposium on Computational Methods in Orthopaedic Biomechanics, University of Texas Southwestern Medical Center, Dallas, TX, February 9, 2002.
29. Guzik DC, Keller TS, Szpalski M, et al. A biomechanical model of the lumbar spine during upright isometric flexion, extension, and lateral bending. *Spine* 1996;21:427–433.
30. Garfin SR, Yuan HA, Reiley MA. New technologies in spine: kyphoplasty and vertebroplasty for the treatment of painful osteoporotic compression fractures. *Spine* 2001;26:1511–1515.
31. Lieberman IH, Dudeney S, Reinhardt M-K, et al. Initial outcome and efficacy of "kyphoplasty" in the treatment of painful osteoporotic vertebral compression fractures. *Spine* 2001;26:1631–1638.
32. Belkoff SM, Mathis JM, Jasper LE, et al. The biomechanics of vertebroplasty. The effect of cement volume on mechanical behavior. *Spine* 2001;26:1537–1541.
33. Nolte LP, Visarius H, Arm E, et al. Computer-aided fixation of spinal implants. *J Image Guid Surg* 1995;1:88–93.
34. Poulin F, Aubin CE, Stokes IA, et al. Biomechanical modeling of instrumentation for the scoliotic spine using flexible elements: a feasibility study. *Ann Chir* 1998;52:761–767.
35. Davies JP, O'Connor DO, Greer JA, et al. Comparison of the mechanical properties of Simplex P, Zimmer Regular, and LVC bone cements. *J Biomed Mater Res* 1987;21:719–730.
36. Saha S, Pal S. Mechanical properties of bone cement: a review. *J Biomed Mater Res* 1984;14:435–462.
37. Keller TS. Finite element modeling of bone tissue stress-adaptation. In: Spillman WB, ed. *Complex adaptive structures.* Bellingham, WA: Society of Photo-Optical Instrumentation Engineers, 2001;4512:232–245.

5

Analysis of the Epidemiology and Risk Factors of Vertebral Compression Fractures

Angelo A. Licata

Department of Endocrinology, Metabolic Bone Center, The Cleveland Clinic Foundation, Cleveland, Ohio

The 1990s witnessed astonishing advancements in the scientific understanding of bone metabolism and its clinical impact on osteoporosis. Because of this progress, the development of new pharmacological therapies has been unusually rapid. Despite these advances, the incidence of osteoporotic fractures is increasing worldwide. This rising tendency is generally ascribable to hip fractures, the most obvious and worrisome of all fractures. The greatest number of fractures, however, occur in the vertebrae. Unlike hip fractures, vertebral fractures are not easily monitored. They still account for most clinical problems of acute and chronic pain that plague patients and confound practitioners. Their seemingly benign nature belies the fact that they also increase morbidity and cause premature death. In this chapter, the epidemiology and risk factors of fractures are discussed from a pathophysiological viewpoint.

EPIDEMIOLOGY

The true incidence of vertebral fractures is not known. Depending on the study cited, 50% to 80% of these fractures are clinically silent or asymptomatic. Even when present, they can be a radiological challenge to identify because in many cases, distortions of vertebral size and/or shape are not obvious.

Diagnosing a "silent" fracture is typically accomplished with the documentation of a change in radiological anatomy. Herein lies the problem: What is a fracture on the radiograph? The degree of deformity from a normal appearance is the hallmark of the fracture. The extent to which the ratio of anterior height to posterior height or the midvertebral height decreases or vertebral anatomy deviates from adjacent vertebrae determines whether the radiological fractures are diagnosed in clinical practice. These vertebral changes may or may not be associated with pain. Because there is a "normal" degree of spinal deformity in the absence of osteoporosis, it is very difficult to know whether an anatomical change is a fracture. Without prior images for comparison, any deformity may over-represent a fracture. On the other hand, if a fracture is silent, it is unlikely that imaging would be done anyway, and hence it would not be found. Underrepresentation is the other extreme. Wedge deformities may not be obvious as a clear-cut compression. Subtle changes in the ratio of anterior and posterior vertebral height are a challenge to diagnosis. Changes of more than 15% to -20% are criteria of fracture in many pharmacological studies. Smaller changes may not receive a diagnosis of fracture because normal variation in anatomy may obscure them. A small distortion or change in measurements may not be evident or may be interpreted differently from one time to the next. Such a difficulty leads to the cases in which fractures disappear or vertebral height increases. Radiological fractures are found in about 26% of women aged 50 and older (1). The incidence of these fractures increases from 5 per 1000 person-years in women aged 50 to 54 years to almost 30 per 1000 person-years in women 85 years and older. These fractures are not clinically diagnosed.

In medical practice today, the hospitalization rate for these fractures is low. Thus, accurate tracking of vertebral fractures is difficult, in contrast to data obtained from the rate of hospitalization for hip fractures. Despite these confounding issues, some facts have emerged. According to the annual hospital discharge data of the Health Care Financing Administration in the United States (1986 to 1989), regardless of age, the average hospital discharge rates for vertebral fractures were 17.7 per 10,000 white women and 3.7 per 10,000 African-American women. Among white women, the discharge rate rose from 5.3 per 10,000 at age 65 to 47.8 per 10,000 at age 90. On average, the rate for women was 1.6 times greater than that for men (2). Coupling these data with incidence figures of 170 per 10,000 at age 65 and 384 per 10,000 at ages 85 and older and diagnostic rates of 54.6 per 10,000 and 132.7 per 10,000 at ages 65 and 85 and older, respectively, it is clear how few patients are actually hospitalized for these fractures (2).

FRACTURE RISK

Osteoporosis is defined as a disease of low bone mass or density, in which destruction of microarchitecture of the bone renders it susceptible to fracture from a traumatic event, however minor. From the clinical perspective, a variety of historical factors in a patient's life increase the risk of osteoporosis and its fractures, both vertebral and nonvertebral. The most noteworthy risk factors are family history of osteoporosis, small stature, abnormal growth, poor lifestyle habits, premature menopause, tobacco use, low body weight, previous fractures, age, poor calcium intake, and lack of exercise (Table 5.1).

From the pedagogical viewpoint, all risk factors can be categorized into four major areas: genetic, hormonal, nutritional, and physical. Adolescents and adults are influenced by these factors in quite opposite directions. In youth, these four areas involve anabolic processes of the skeleton. In the adult, they give rise to the catabolic nature of aging.

TABLE 5.1. *Clinical and pathophysiological risk factors of vertebral compression fractures*

Clinical factors	Pathophysiological factors
Family history of osteoporosis	Genetics
Small stature	Nutrition
Delayed growth	Hormones
Inadequate nutrition	Activity
Low level of activity	
Age	
Early menopause	
Previous fracture	
Poor gait and balance	
Tobacco use	

YOUTH AND THE SKELETON

A low bone mass or density is a necessary component of osteoporotic fracture, but it is not sufficient in and of itself. Fractures are less likely in the adult if the skeleton has achieved a high peak bone mass during youth (3). Achieving this peak mass is contingent on optimal interplay of the four factors noted earlier.

In women, the pubertal spurt in bone development occurs earlier and ends sooner than in men. Menarche initiates skeletal growth in women at, on average, about ages 11 to 12 years if body weight and estrogen levels are appropriate (4). By the midteens, peak bone development has occurred. Very little is added thereafter (5). In men, however, skeletal development starts in the midteen years and continues into the early second decade. Attainment of peak mass is slower. Delayed puberty and growth lower the maximal peak bone mass attained (6).

The genetic endowment from the parents gives each individual the potential for a maximal achievable bone mass. Children with parents of small stature have a lower bone mass than do children with parents of large stature (7). This is often seen in the adult years when small-statured healthy premenopausal women are evaluated because of a family history of osteoporosis. "Abnormal" density is often found if the mother or both parents of such a woman are small in stature. For want of a better term, this can be classified as constitutional osteopenia—genetically endowed low peak mass—rather than osteoporosis.

Activity does have a positive effect on bone growth. Women who engage in competitive sports before puberty have greater bone mass than those who become physically active afterwards (8). This increment in bone mass can influence the adult skeleton. Women who were athletic in their youth have higher bone density than those who were not physically active (9,10).

Proper nutrition is essential for growth. Without it, skeletal problems arise, typified by disorders such as anorexia nervosa, inflammatory bowel disease, exacerbation of cystic fibrosis, and diabetes mellitus. Calcium is spoken about extensively as if it were the only important nutrient. But it is only one of the many essential nutrients, vitamins, and minerals that must be considered. Attainment of peak mass is linked to sufficient nutrition (10).

ADULTHOOD AND THE SKELETON

By the middle of the second decade or beginning of the third decade, most people have attained all the bone of the adult skeleton. After that point, the skeleton begins an inexorable decline in structure as the aging process begins. Genetic predisposition becomes a marker of risk for osteoporosis and its fractures. Deficiencies in hormones, nutrition, and exercise negatively impact the skeleton; sufficient amounts positively protect the skeleton.

Postmenopausal estrogen deficiency has been recognized as a causal agent of primary osteoporosis for over 50 years. It accelerates bone loss tenfold or more above the background rate that is caused by aging. Only in the early 1990s has the basic physiology been understood. Estrogen stops bone resorption (12). It controls osteoclast recruitment and activity, decreases activation frequency of the basic multicellular unit of remodeling, and decreases bone loss. In its absence, skeletal microarchitecture is destroyed. Herein lies the explanation for why age, prevalent fractures, and minor trauma are significant risk factors for fractures and why bone density alone can account for only 60% to -70% of the total risk for fracture. The most striking example of this concept is the difference in fracture rates of young and old persons with the same mineral density measured on dual energy x-ray absorptiometry.

Aging causes a small, slow loss of bone yearly. It impairs the normal physiological absorption of calcium that triggers a compensatory rise in parathyroid hormone and increased bone turnover. Likewise, a lack of adequate dietary calcium causes the same phenomenon even with normal absorptive physiology. Calcium supplementation protects the skeleton from this loss (11). Some clinical studies show that calcium supplementation produces a striking reduction in bone fractures in populations deficient in calcium but little effect in populations already sufficiently supplied with the mineral. Vitamin D deficiency abets this process, whether it arises from natural causes, intestinal disease, or drug-related problems.

Activity and physical loading of bone protects the skeleton and attenuates loss from aging. Contrary to the general wisdom, exercise does not build bone in the sense used for the adolescent skeleton. Its effects are small. The quality, duration, intensity, and frequency of exercise required to aid skeletal health are poorly known, despite claims to the contrary. The conundrum facing patients and clinicians is that the best exercise for the skeleton may be beyond the capability of the frail skeleton for which it is intended. There is no exercise for adults that will substitute for the pharmacological therapy used to treat osteoporosis. What exercise can accomplish is muscle strengthening and restoration of some coordination, normal gait, and balance (13). These all help control the acute fractures from falls. What is not well understood is the type of trauma needed for silent vertebral fractures and to what extent activity or exercise protects or causes such fractures. It is clear that recurring fractures follow closely behind every fracture (14).

SUMMARY

All risk factors used clinically are ascribable to the four major areas discussed earlier. Their impact on bone health is modified by age (i.e., anabolism of youth versus catabolism of aging). With the exception of genetics, all factors have been a focus of some form of therapy for prevention and treatment. In the future, therapies will be used to restore postmenopausal bone to a more structurally sound pristine form. Parathyroid hormone will be the first of these anabolic drugs. Drug therapy, however, takes months or years to be effective. In contrast, surgical treatment such as vertebroplasty and kyphoplasty seems best for the acute event. They offer hope for quick control of pain, stabilization of fractures, restoration of anatomical height, control of kyphosis, and reduction in morbidity. However, it is unlikely that they can promote long-term skeletal reconstruction. For the foreseeable future, a combination of both approaches seems the optimal solution.

REFERENCES

1. Melton LJ, Kan SH, Frye MA, et al. Epidemiology of vertebral fractures in women. *Am J Epidemiol* 1989;129:1000–1011.
2. Jacobsen SJ, Cooper C, Gottlieb MS, et al. Hospitalization with vertebral fractures among the aged: a national population-based study, 1986–1989. *Epidemiology* 1992;3:515–518.
3. Gordon CL, Halton JM, Atkinson SA, et al. The contributions of growth and puberty to peak bone mass. *Growth Dev Aging* 1991;55:257–262.
4. Lloyd T, Rollings N, Andon MB, et al. Determinants of bone density in young women: I. Relationships among pubertal development, total body bone mass, and total body bone density in premenarchal females. *J Clin Endocrinol Metab* 1992;75:383–387.
5. Bonjour JP, Theintz G, Buchs B, et al. Critical years and stages of puberty for spinal and femoral bone mass accumulation during adolescence. *J Clin Endocrinol Metab* 1991;73:555–563.

6. De Boer H, Blok GJ, van Lingen A, et al. Consequences of childhood—onset growth hormone deficiency for adult bone mass. *J Bone Miner Res* 1994;9:1319–1326.
7. Lonzer MD, Imrie R, Rogers D, et al. Effects of heredity, age, weight, puberty, activity, and calcium intake on bone mineral density in children. *Clin Pediatr* 1996;35:185–189.
8. Kannus P, Heidi-Haapasalo MB, Sievanen H, et al. Effect of starting age of physical activity on bone mass in the dominant arm of tennis and squash players. *Ann Intern Med* 1995;123:27–31.
9. Welten DC, Kemper HCG, Post GB, et al. Weight-bearing activity during youth is a more important factor for peak bone mass than calcium intake. *J Bone Miner Res* 1994;9:1089–1096.
10. Valimaki MJ, Karkkainen M, Lamberg-Allardt C, et al. Exercise, smoking, and calcium intake during adolescence and early adulthood as determinants of peak bone mass. *BMJ* 1994;309:230–235.
11. McKane WR, Khosla S, Egan KS, et al. Role of calcium intake in modulating age-related increases in parathyroid function and bone resorption. *J Clin Endocrinol Metab* 1996;81:1699–1703.
12. Riggs BL, Khosla J, Melton LJ III. A unitary model for involutional osteoporosis: estrogen deficiency causes both type I and type II osteoporosis in postmenopausal women and contributes to bone loss in aging men. *J Bone Miner Res* 1998;13:763–773.
13. Sinaki M, Wollan PC, Scott RW, et al. Can strong back extensors prevent vertebral fractures in women with osteoporosis? *Mayo Clin Proc* 1996;71:951–956.
14. Lindsay R, Silverman SL, Cooper C, et al. Risk of new vertebral fracture in the year following a fracture. *JAMA* 2001;285:320–323.

6
Natural History

*Federico Balagué, *Sieglinde Major Schumacher, and †Jean Dudler

*Service de Rhumatologie, Médecine Physique et Rééducation, Hôpital Cantonal, Fribourg, Switzerland, and †Service de Rhumatologie, Médecine Physique et Rééducation, Centre Hospitalier Universitaire Vaudois, Lausanne, Switzerland

DEFINING THE PROBLEM

In determining the natural history of a nondirectly lethal disease, it is good to keep in mind some shortcomings and problems with such an attempt.

The natural history of disease has been defined as "the evolution of disease without medical intervention; that is, how patients will fare if nothing is done for their disease" (1). Ideally, this means that physicians should be aware of all the clinically relevant events occurring from the precise moment when the fracture occurs to the patient's death. In other words, it means that physicians should first be able to diagnose confidently any occurrence of osteoporotic compression fractures from their onset, even if asymptomatic. They then should be able to follow up those cases. Such follow-up would require longitudinal studies that include enough large numbers of subjects and use standardized outcome measures (gathered by means of questionnaires as well as by tests of performance) and repeated examinations to detect incident fractures and any other relevant outcomes. This would have to be done without any intervention, while accepting, apart from the ethical point of view, that such a strict follow-up is not an intervention that modifies the outcomes by itself. It is not surprising that we have not found any study fulfilling all the methodological requirements necessary to reach general valid conclusions. Therefore, the term *natural history* should be understood more as a spontaneous clinical course without major interventions rather than true natural history.

Diagnosis is another pitfall. A generally accepted way to identify fractures with good sensitivity and specificity should be available in order to evaluate the results of such longitudinal studies. Unfortunately, there is still no internationally agreed definition for vertebral fracture (2). Three morphological types of vertebral fractures are usually recognized: wedge, concave (also called "biconcave"), and crush fractures (3,4). This variable, associated with the different definitions used to label a vertebral deformity as "fracture," the differences concerning the number of vertebrae included in radiological examinations, the different ages of patients, the frequencies of radiological evaluations, and other conditions make comparisons between studies very difficult. In their literature review, Ziegler et al. identified 20 different morphometric algorithms (5), and a gold standard for vertebral fracture simply does not exist (2,6). Grados et al. (2) compared four morphometric definitions and a semiquantitative consensus reading. They concluded that these morphometric approaches should not be employed alone but instead should be combined with a visual assessment to detect prevalent fractures. However, the semiquantitative approach can be employed alone by experienced and well-trained readers (2). It is also important to be aware that with some techniques, such as morphometric x-ray absorptiometry, the number of false-positive findings for either newly deformed vertebrae or vertebrae with reversal of deformity outnumbers the true-positive cases of fractures as diagnosed with the use of the semiquantitative radiologic assessment as the gold standard (7).

Identifying the precise time when a vertebral fracture occurs is another difficulty. From a clinical standpoint, 50% of patients have no history of pain (8), and a significant number of patients fail to report any injury or trauma. In a longitudinal study that included 15 patients with acute low back pain attributed to insufficiency fractures of the spine, 21 vertebral fractures were diagnosed by bone scan, whereas 30 vertebrae were identified on lateral radiographs (4). Overall, 35 vertebral fractures were diagnosed by either scintigraphy or radiography, but only 16 (45.7%) were consistently identified by both techniques (4).

Although radiographs can also demonstrate old deformities or images of comorbid conditions (8), bone scan is sometimes recommended for detecting fractures when standard radiographs remain questionable (9). However, the time needed for the bone scan to yield positive findings after a fracture is correlated with the age of the patient and can take a few days for an elderly patient (10). Moreover, new vertebral fractures also show increased scintigraphic uptake for approximately 6 months (9).

Maybe for all these reasons, vertebral fractures have been reported to be the most common but least understood of all osteoporotic fractures (9). Ziegler et al., in their article entitled "What Is a Vertebral Fracture?", stated that the answer is somewhat different according to what is being viewed (5). We chose to look at the natural history, or, rather, the "spontaneous clinical evolution without major interventions," of vertebral osteoporotic compression fractures with regard to two related aspects: what happened to the vertebra and the spine itself and what happened to the patient as an individual. Keeping in mind that all the aforementioned shortcomings and problems related to diagnosis, timing of diagnosis, bias of selection, and bias of recollection ultimately influences the gathering of data and the final conclusions about the natural history of osteoporotic vertebral fractures.

EFFECTS OF TIME ON THE FRACTURED VERTEBRA AND THE SPINE ITSELF

An osteoporotic fracture is not a single definite event in time but an ongoing process both at the level of the fracture but also in the rest of the spine. Among 210 women with symptomatic nontraumatic vertebral fractures, Lyritis et al. (11) distinguished two types of initial presentation. In 121 of these patients, the first radiographic examination revealed a fully collapsed vertebra, whereas among the other 89 women, they only found mild signs of vertebral fracture or even no signs at all (11). Nevertheless, definitive radiological signs of collapse appeared during subsequent (second to fifth) painful attacks in the latter subgroup, which underlined this ongoing osteoporotic process (11). Other authors have also hypothesized that large vertebral collapses may be the results of insufficiency fractures on already fractured vertebrae or the results of sequential collapses of a vertebra that initially had only a small deformity (4).

In a longitudinal study, nonspine fractures were predictive of incidental vertebral fractures. Moreover, there was a cumulative effect with prevalent vertebral fractures and decreases in bone density (12). Together with decreased bone mass, existing fractures are a strong risk factor for new vertebral fractures (13–15). Each existing fracture approximately triples the risk for subsequent fractures, and this risk is particularly high among persons with low bone mineral density (8). Two studies analyzed the iliac crest bone biopsies of both men and women with and without vertebral fractures. Two-dimensional histological findings were reported to be similar in fracture and nonfracture groups in either gender (16). However, a three-dimensional analysis of the same material showed that the fracture group had a "mass-independent trabecular discontinuity," which contributes to skeletal failure (17).

New fractures can be located at any level of the spine, above or below the previously injured one, and not only at the adjacent levels (18). In a prospective study of 721 Japanese-American women (mean age, 69.5 ± 5.3 years) with a median of 3.1 years between radiographs, it appeared that among women with prevalent fractures, the increased fracture risk extends beyond nearby vertebrae (18). Interestingly, a temporal clustering effect has been identified in rare cases, underlining again the global aspect of the osteoporotic process in the spine. Kaplan et al. (19) reported on eight patients identified during an 8-year period among the 150 to 200 new patients per year attending their facility. These patients experienced at least five vertebral compression fractures within an 8-month span instead of the one to four fractures over a period of 4 to 5 years reported in the literature. These successions of fractures occurred both below and above the initial fracture (19).

In a cross-sectional study, wedge fractures were the most frequent, and the prevalence of multiple fractures was 31% (3). Nevertheless, all the possible combinations of fracture types (wedge, crush, and concave) were observed, and it appears that the type of the first fracture is not predictive of the type of subsequent lesions. Ross et al. (20) confirmed these findings in a longitudinal study. Among the 35 women (of 203) with incident fractures, 30 had wedge fractures and 10 had crush fractures; some women had both incident fracture types (20).

Fractures can ultimately induce spinal deformities. In a prospective study of 87 women (mean age, 62.4 years; range, 35 to 95 years), there was a significant correlation between thoracic kyphosis, measured by Cobb angle, and number of prevalent vertebral fractures. However, 19% of women with no thoracic fractures nonetheless had hyperkyphosis, which suggests the presences of contributing nonskeletal factors (21).

Even if the majority of osteoporotic vertebral fractures are of the wedge type (3), cases of unstable burst fractures without any traumatic event do exist (22). Previous studies have demonstrated a favorable natural remodeling of the spinal canal after lumbar burst fractures in adults treated conservatively (23,24), and a case of lumbar vertebral "reformation" after surgical treatment of a traumatic compression fracture has been reported (25). We did not find such information for osteoporotic fractures, but there is no pathophysiological reason why such remodeling could not also take place in osteoporotic burst fractures.

CASE REPORT

A 74-year-old white woman was hospitalized for severe acute lumbosacral pain. She had a history of idiopathic osteoporosis and was known to have sustained previous fractures of several vertebrae (T3, T5, T7, and L3), the pelvis, and the femoral neck. Nevertheless, she had been able to remain independent, lived alone, and was taking care of her own household.

Pain started suddenly 48 hours before admission without any triggering event, was unresponsive to nonsteroidal antiinflammatory drugs, and required opiates. Standard

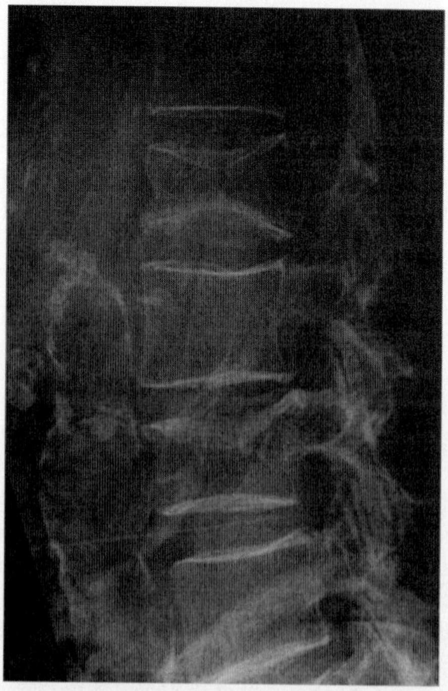

FIG. 6.1. Standard radiographs demonstrating an old known compression fracture of L3 and a new compression of L1 that was not demonstrated by a bone scan performed 2 days later.

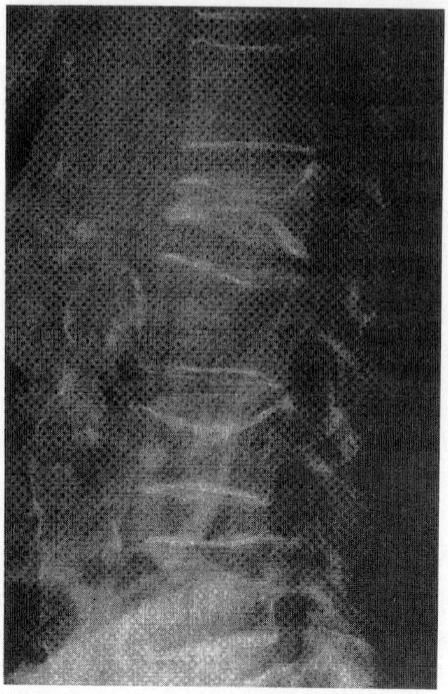

FIG. 6.2. Radiographs repeated 3 weeks later, clearly demonstrating a crush fracture

radiographs demonstrated a compression fracture of L1 not apparent on previous radiographs (Fig. 6.1), but a bone scan performed 4 days after the pain started yielded normal findings. A second bone scintigram obtained on day 16 finally demonstrated the expected increased uptake of the L1 vertebra.

Despite nasal calcitonin and high doses of opiates, severe pain persisted, and new radiographs were ordered 3 weeks after the pain had begun. At that time, a crush fracture of L1 was obvious (Fig. 6.2). It appeared that this unfavorable evolution was the result of subsequent fractures within the same vertebra occurring over a short period of time.

Despite transpedicular vertebroplasty of several vertebral bodies, the final outcome was poor. The patient ultimately required long-term transdermal fentanyl for pain control and had to be admitted definitively to a nursing home.

EFFECTS ON THE PATIENT OUTCOMES

In an editorial, Truumees (26) stated that although most patients experience improvement with conservative management of vertebral compression fractures, inactivity contributes to a spiral of further bone loss, subsequent fractures, and functional decline, often accompanied by depression, sleep disturbance, and decreased pulmonary function after multiple vertebral compression fractures (26).

Ross (8) distinguished three categories of consequences from vertebral fractures: pain, physical changes and impairment, and psychosocial decline. Some studies published during the late 1990s gave a better idea of the evolution of vertebral fractures over time (13,14), especially as quality of life and specifically health-related quality of life have gained importance in terms of outcomes (27).

Pain

Up to 50% of vertebral fractures could be asymptomatic, and the consequences of vertebral fractures are traditionally believed to resolve in a few weeks to months as the fractures heal (8,13). From their study, Lyritis et al. (11) concluded that in a majority of cases and particularly in aged patients, the natural history of the vertebral fracture is "exhausted" after the first episode of pain. Typically, this clinical episode develops with pain that is severe (mean VAS score among the 121 patients with this type of fracture: 9 ± 0.2; range, 0 to 10) but has a short duration (4 to 8 weeks). This type of fracture was labeled type I by the authors. Another type of fracture, type II, occurs in younger patients with better bone mineral density. These fractures appear progressively; a radiological vertebral collapse is visible only after two to five episodes of pain, and in these cases the whole course can then be extended for up to 20 months (11).

Nevertheless, it is more likely that chronic pain persist for years, and physical impairment increases progressively with the number and severity of vertebral fractures (8). A longitudinal study showed that women with incidental fractures reported mean levels of back pain frequency three times higher during the first 600 days after fracture. The level of pain then dropped but stayed to approximately twice the baseline level for the rest of the follow-up period (maximum duration of follow-up, 1,439 days) (20). In a study of 645 postmenopausal Japanese-American women, the prevalence of back pain during the previous 12 months was 32.9%; the prevalences in all age groups up to 79 years of age were similar to this percentage but increased to almost 42% among women aged 80 years and older (28). An incidental fracture during the previous 4 years was associated with a 2.8-fold increase in the risk for back pain; the risk increased to 7.8-fold for women with two recent fractures and to 21.7-fold for women with three recent fractures (28). Finally, another prospective study of more than 7,000 white women underlines again the ongoing and relentless process of osteoporotic disease and its natural history. It is reported that 3 to 4 years after a vertebral fracture, new symptoms probably result from the occurrence of new fractures (14), slightly more than two thirds of which are not diagnosed clinically despite being identified on new radiographs. However, these fractures were not coming to medical attention, despite the fact that they were associated with a twofold to threefold increase in back pain and functional limitation (14). This study looked at the confounding effect of aging on increased back pain and disability during follow-up. Back pain and disability increased from 23% and 15% respectively in women with neither prevalent nor incidental fractures. These numbers were much lower than in any groups with incidental fractures, which emphasizes the role of new fractures for those outcomes (14).

This grim evolution is not limited to women; a study of 63 men with symptomatic vertebral fractures concluded that vertebral fractures in men were associated with considerable morbidity (29).

Physical Changes

One of the obvious physical changes resulting from fractures is stature loss. In a prospective study of 504 postmenopausal Japanese-American women monitored for an average of 7.7 years, the average stature loss was 2.1 cm among women with at least one incidental fracture, in contrast to 0.4 cm among those without fractures. Each wedge and crush fracture resulted in an estimated height reduction of 0.86 cm and 1.08 cm, respectively, whereas endplate fractures did not significantly contribute to stature loss. Interestingly, among women after age 80 without incidental fractures, the mean rate of physiological stature loss was less than 1 mm per year (30).

Function and Quality of Life

Another important aspect of the natural history of vertebral fractures is the impact of such lesions on functional capacity and quality of life. Gold (31) called attention to the psychological and social impact of vertebral fractures, particularly in women with multiple fractures. Excellent reviews on these consequences of vertebral fractures, including a large bibliography, have been published (8,32).

Numerous studies on various aspects of the subject have been published. Recent fractures certainly have an impact on both function and quality of life. A prospective study of 569 postmenopausal Japanese-American women showed that recent fractures (defined as having occurred sometime during, on average, the previous 4.3 years) were significantly correlated with poor physical functioning (13). In a cross-sectional study of 50 patients, subjects were divided into two groups according to time after fracture (less than 24 months versus more than 24 months), and their qualities of life were compared. The differences were significant; subjects with "recent" fractures had lower scores for perception of average pain, social extroversion, and well-being (33). However, another case-control study of 145 female patients with vertebral osteoporotic fractures (average number of vertebral fractures, 2.9 ± 1.6; estimated time since last fracture, 5.1 ± 4.8 years) showed that quality of life and functionality were significantly reduced among these subjects in comparison with matched controls (34).

It also appears that fractures per se, not just pain, are correlated with this decline in function and quality of life. In a case-control study of ten women with vertebral fractures (range, two to ten) and ten matched controls without fractures, the physical, functional, and psychosocial performances of both groups were compared by means of different tests. Compression fractures were associated with impaired function in the three domains tested (35), but, interestingly, both groups were similar in terms of the amount of pain medication taken, number of current illnesses, participation in physical activities, and the number of lumbar degenerative disorders. In another interesting cross-sectional study, a group of 63 osteoporotic patients (mean age, 65 ± 7.9 years) was compared with a group of patients with chronic low back pain (approximately 9 years younger). Back pain intensity and frequency were not different between these two groups of women; however, disability scores were significantly higher in osteoporotic patients, independently of age (36). Moreover, this study showed that there was a significant linear relationship between quality of life and clinical measures of spinal deformation; osteoporotic patients with two or more fractures had more functional limitations than did women with one fracture. This was confirmed by a cluster analysis (36). A cross-sectional study also demonstrated that women with vertebral fractures were significantly more dependent on help in different daily activities than were women of the same mean age without vertebral fractures but suffering from low back pain. However, it was not possible to distinguish between the effect of pain from that of other confounders in this study (37). In a longitudinal (follow-up ranging from 6 months to 5 years), nonrandomized study to develop a new questionnaire to evaluate disability in osteoporotic patients with vertebral fractures, Helmes et al. (38) demonstrated persistent long-term disability despite significant improvement in back pain.

It is also important to note that patients with a single fracture already have a significant decrease quality of life (27). Some authors found a correlation between decreased health-related quality of life and increasing number of prevalent vertebral fractures, particularly lumbar fractures (27); others, however, did not found such statistical relationship between the number and severity of fractures and the severity of symptoms (39).

Finally, it is usually stated that among all the fractures identified on radiographs, 50% have been reported to be symptomatic (back pain), 33% are clinically diagnosed, and 8% necessitate hospitalization (8). Two percent of affected patients also need long-term nursing care (8), which is another way to look at the potential dramatic functional impact of fractures. Any length of hospitalization is also increased by a direct contribution of a vertebral fracture, independently of any comorbid conditions such as age, gender, or any major disorders (40).

All the previous data are drawn from clinical and epidemiological research. Another way of collecting information is the descriptive phenomenological approach. One article reporting on the interviews of five women who had experienced vertebral fractures (8 weeks to 6 years earlier) shows the tremendous impact of such a fracture, lasting sometimes many years. This is one sentence from the author's abstract summarizing these experiences: "Constant pain, loss of independent function, changes in physical appearance, feelings of isolation, a sense of vulnerability, and an uncertain future were the hallmarks of the experience" (41).

Mortality

An excess rate of mortality after vertebral fractures has been reported (42). In one study, women with one or more prevalent compression fractures (defined as a reduction of at least 20% in the posterior height in comparison to that of adjacent vertebrae) showed an age-adjusted risk of total mortality of 1.6 per compression fracture. A nonsignificant association was found for wedge fractures (defined as at least 20% reduction in the anterior height). When only deaths from cardiovascular disease were considered, the relative risk was 3.9 for compression fractures and 2.0 for wedge fractures for people with two or more fractures versus none (43). It appears, according to the published survival curves, that the death rates among patients with no, one, and two fractures start diverging about 8 years after menopause (43). One prospective study of more than 6,000 women demonstrated that after adjustment for incidental fractures (and several other potential confounders), bone loss—evaluated by means of bone mineral density at the hip and the calcaneum—was an independent predictor of mortality (44). Thus, it appears that fractures are rather an indicator of comorbidity (42).

CONCLUSIONS

In conclusion, even if a significant number of osteoporotic fractures (even collapsed vertebrae) are not diagnosed and induce no significant complaint, each new vertebral fracture has a well-defined negative effect. In terms of pain, acute onset and high-intensity pain lasting for several weeks are common with acute fractures. The long-term outcome is characterized on average by moderate levels of pain persisting for several years after the fracture. The decreased frequency of pain with time after fracture has been attributed to fracture healing, gradual adaptation to pain, or a combination of both (20).

In terms of functional capacity, there is a significant negative effect (comparable to being 10 years older) that lasts for several years. According to Helmes et al. (38), the natural history of disability in osteoporotic patients is not favorable, despite specialized advice, education, and treatment directed at restoring bone mass.

Each fracture is also associated with a significantly increased risk of subsequent fractures, which leads to a poor long-term prognosis with regard to pain, function, quality of life, and psychosocial factors.

Moreover, vertebral fractures are associated with a significant excess rate of mortality mainly from cardiovascular disorders.

REFERENCES

1. Fletcher RH, Fletcher SW, Wagner EH, eds. *Clinical epidemiology. The essentials,* 2nd ed. Baltimore: Williams & Wilkins; 1988.
2. Grados F, Roux C, de Vernejoul M, et al. Comparison of four morphometric definitions and a semiquantitative consensus reading for assessing prevalent vertebral fractures. *Osteoporos Int* 2001;12:716–722.
3. Ismail A, Cooper C, Felsenberg D, et al. Number and type of vertebral deformities: epidemiological characteristics and relation to back pain and height loss. *Osteoporos Int* 1999;9:206–213.
4. Kawaguchi S, Yamashita T, Koshio H, et al. Insufficiency fracture of the spine: a prospective analysis based on radiographic and scintigraphic diagnosis. *J Bone Miner Metab* 2001;19:312–316.
5. Ziegler R, Scheidt-Nave C, Leidig-Bruckner G. What is a vertebral fracture? *Bone* 1996;18:169S–177S.
6. Cranney A, Tugwell P, Cummings S, et al. Osteoporosis clinical trial endpoints: candidate variables and clinimetric properties. *J Rheumatol* 1997;24:1222–1229.
7. Ferrar L, Jiang G, Eastell R. Longitudinal evaluation of morphometric x-ray absorptiometry for the identification of vertebral deformities. *Osteoporos Int* 2001;12:661–671.
8. Ross P. Clinical consequences of vertebral fractures. *Am J Med* 1997;103:30S–43S.
9. Wasnich RD. Vertebral fracture epidemiology. *Bone* 1996;18:179S–183S.
10. Palmer EL. Nuclear medicine. In: Weissleder R, Rieumont M, Wittenberg J, eds. *Primer of diagnostic imaging,* 2nd ed. St. Louis: Mosby; 1997:817–863.
11. Lyritis GP, Mayasis B, Tsakalakos N, et al. The natural history of the osteoporotic vertebral fracture. *Clin Rheumatol* 1989;2:66–69.
12. Wasnich RD, Davis JW, Ross PD. Spine fracture risk is predicted by non-spine fractures. *Osteoporos Int* 1994;4:1–5.
13. Huang C, Ross PD, Wasnich RD. Vertebral fracture and other predictors of physical impairment and health care utilization. *Arch Intern Med* 1996;156:2469–2475.

14. Nevitt M, Ettinger B, Black D, et al. The association of radiographically detected vertebral fractures with back pain and function: a prospective study. *Ann Intern Med* 1998;128:793–800.
15. Ross P, Davis J, Epstein R, et al. Pre-existing fractures and bone mass predict vertebral fracture incidence in women. *Ann Intern Med* 1991;114:919–923.
16. Hordon LD, Raisi M, Aaron JE, et al. Trabecular architecture in women and men of similar bone mass with and without vertebral fracture: I. Two-dimensional histology. *Bone* 2000;27:271–276.
17. Aaron J, Shore P, Shøre R, et al. Trabecular architecture in women and men of similar bone mass with and without vertebral fracture: II. Three-dimensional histology. *Bone* 2000;27:277–282.
18. Davis JW, Grove JS, Wasnich RD, et al. Spatial relationships between prevalent and incident spine fractures. *Bone* 1999;24:261–264.
19. Kaplan F, Scherl J, Wisneki R, et al. The cluster phenomenon in patients who have multiple vertebral compression fractures. *Clin Orthop* 1993;297:161–167.
20. Ross PD, Davis JW, Epstein RS, et al. Pain and disability associated with new vertebral fractures and other spinal conditions. *J Clin Epidemiol* 1994;47:231–239.
21. De Smet A, Robinson R, Johnson B, et al. Spinal compression fractures in osteoporotic women: patterns and relationship to hyperkyphosis. *Radiology* 1988;166:497–500.
22. Arciero R, Leung K, Pierce J. Spontaneous unstable burst fracture of the thoracolumbar spine in osteoporosis. *Spine* 1989;14:114–117.
23. Fidler M. Remodelling of the spinal canal after burst fracture. *J Bone Joint Surg Br* 1988;70:730–732.
24. Ha K, Han S, Chung M, et al. A clinical study of the natural remodeling of burst fractures of the lumbar spine. *Clin Orthop* 1996;323:210–214.
25. Beerman R, Batt HD, Green BA. Lumbar vertebral reformation after traumatic compression fracture. *AJNR Am J Neuroradiol* 1985;6:455–456.
26. Truumees E. Osteoporosis [Editorial]. *Spine* 2001;26:930–932.
27. Oleksik A, Lips P, Dawson A, et al. Health-related quality of life in postmenopausal women with low BMD with or without prevalent vertebral fractures. *J Bone Miner Res* 2000;15:1384–1392.
28. Huang C, Ross PD, Wasnich RD. Vertebral fractures and other predictors of back pain among older women. *J Bone Miner Res* 1996;11:1026–1032.
29. Scane A, Sutcliffe A, Francis R. The sequelae of vertebral crush fractures in men. *Osteoporos Int* 1994;4:89–92.
30. Huang C, Ross PD, Lydick E, et al. Contributions of vertebral fractures to stature loss among elderly Japanese-American women in Hawaii. *J Bone Miner Res* 1996;11:408–411.
31. Gold DT. The clinical impact of vertebral fractures: quality of life in women with osteoporosis. *Bone* 1996;18:185S–189S.
32. Cooper C. The crippling consequences of fractures and their impact on quality of life. *Am J Med* 1997;103:12S–17S; discussion, 17S–19S.
33. Begerow B, Pfeifer M, Pospeschill M, et al. Time since vertebral fracture: an important variable concerning quality of life in patients with postmenopausal osteoporosis. *Osteoporos Int* 1999;10:26–33.
34. Hall SE, Criddle RA, Comito TL, et al. A case-control study of quality of life and functional impairment in women with long-standing vertebral osteoporotic fracture. *Osteoporos Int* 1999;9:508–515.
35. Lyles KW, Gold DT, Shipp KM, et al. Association of osteoporotic vertebral compression fractures with impaired functional status. *Am J Med* 1993;94:595–601.
36. Leidig-Bruckner G, Minne HW, Schlaich C, et al. Clinical grading of spinal osteoporosis: quality of life components and spinal deformity in women with chronic low back pain and women with vertebral osteoporosis. *J Bone Miner Res* 1997;12:663–675.
37. Galindo-Ciocon D, Ciocon JO, Galindo D. Functional impairment among elderly women with osteoporotic vertebral fractures. *Rehabil Nurs* 1995;20:79–83.
38. Helmes E, Hodsman A, Lazowski D, et al. A questionnaire to evaluate disability in osteoporotic patients with vertebral compression fractures. *J Gerontol A Biol Sci Med Sci* 1995;50:M91-M98.
39. Cook DJ, Guyatt GH, Adachi JD, et al. Quality of life issues in women with vertebral fractures due to osteoporosis. *Arthritis Rheum* 1993;36:750–756.
40. Papaioannou A, Adachi JD, Parkinson W, et al. Lengthy hospitalization associated with vertebral fractures despite control for comorbid conditions. *Osteoporos Int* 2001;12:870–874.
41. Paier G. Specter of the crone: the experience of vertebral fracture (living with chronic illness). Adv Nurs Sci 1996;18:27–36.
42. Walker-Bone K, Dennison E, Cooper C. Epidemiology of osteoporosis. *Rheum Dis Clin N A* 2001;27:1–18.
43. von der Recke P, Hansen M, Hassager C. The association between low bone mass at the menopause and cardiovascular mortality. *Am J Med* 1999;106:273–278.
44. Kado DM, Browner WS, Blackwell T, et al. Rate of bone loss is associated with mortality in older women: a prospective study. *J Bone Miner Res* 2000;15:1974–1980.

7

Clinical Presentation and Differential Diagnosis

Björn Rydevik and Helena Brisby

Department of Orthopaedics, Sahlgrenska University Hospital, Göteborg University, Göteborg, Sweden

Osteoporosis is mostly a silently progressive disease, which at its end stage can culminate in fracture. In spinal osteoporosis, this is usually seen as a vertebral body compression fracture.

CLINICAL PRESENTATION

The patient may present with an acutely painful fracture in not only the spine but also the rib, wrist, or hip. In the spine, normal physical activity may exceed the stress tolerance of the osteoporotic bone tissue, leading to vertebral fracture. Such fracture may be painless, but usually there is severe regional pain, which may last 3 to 4 weeks (1). In the thoracic spine, this may result in accentuation of the thoracic kyphosis, which in turn can be later compensated for by an increased lumbar lordosis. Such changes may result in altered spinal biomechanics, which may contribute to the production of low back pain. Typically, patients with osteoporotic compression fractures may have symptoms for 6 to 9 months, and thereafter the pain may gradually disappear if no further fracture occurs. Also, not all patients report an episode of acute pain. An asymptomatic thoracic or lumbar compression fracture is frequently noted on radiographic examinations performed for unrelated purposes. Such macroscopic fractures can represent development over time of a series of small and, individually, clinically insignificant microfractures. Osteoporosis in itself does not seem to predispose affected patients to back pain at ages of less than 80 years (2). However, the prevalence of back pain has been described to be greater (about 50%) among women who lost over 2 cm of height than among those (about 20%) who lost less than 2 cm of height (2). Stooping of the spine, usually reflecting one or more compression fractures, can also predispose the patient to back pain, in comparison with a normally configured back. However, a previous history of hip fracture or Colles' fracture has no correlation with osteoporotic back pain (2).

The clinical symptomatology of osteoporotic spine problems has been analyzed by Patel et al. (3). They noted that after an acute vertebral compression fracture, pain frequently radiated into the flank or anteriorly (66%). However, radiation of pain into the lower extremities was very rare (6%). Patel et al. also pointed out that other associated symptoms such as nausea (26%), abdominal pain (20%), chest pain (30%), and strain-exacerbated pain (60%) were common. In addition, they found that pain was reported to

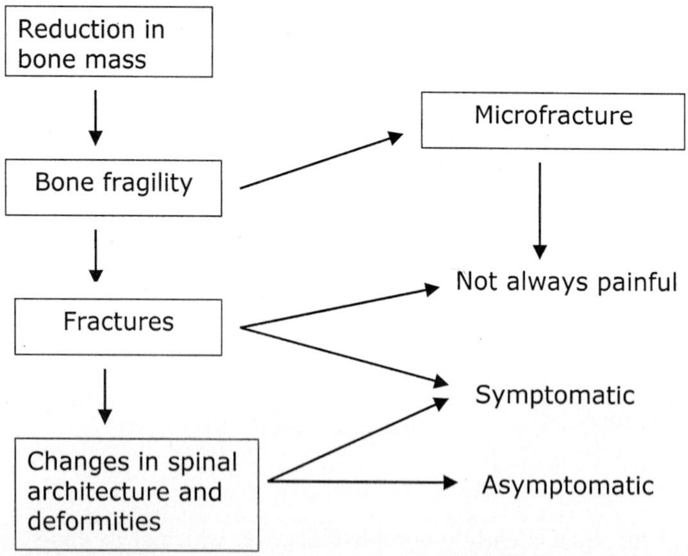

FIG. 7.1. Model of spinal pain in osteoporosis. (From Hadjipavlou AG, Lander PH. Osteoporosis of the spine and its management. In: White AH, Schofferman JA, eds. *Spine care.* St. Louis: Mosby, 1995:847–869.)

improve with positions such as recumbency (43%), sitting (36%), and standing and walking (16%).

As pointed out earlier, gradual osteoporotic compression fractures may be clinically asymptomatic, which suggests that microfractures, when they occur, may not necessarily be a source of spinal pain (4). However, the knowledge regarding the pathophysiology of pain production in these conditions is incomplete. Some data indicate that microfractures could be the origin of back pain in severe osteopenia and after the age of 80 (5). In the thoracic spine, both asymptomatic and painful fractures usually occur in the ventral aspect of the vertebrae. Progressive fractures thus lead to shortening of the anterior height of the vertebral bodies in relation to the posterior height. This results in a gradual increase of the thoracic kyphosis. In the lumbar region, the fractures are distributed equally throughout the vertebral body without wedge formation, and the combined effects of compression and wedge fractures lead to a spinal deformity with excessive thoracic kyphosis and loss of spinal height.

A reduction in bone mass is not always painful, but such a reduction may lead to bone fragility, in turn predisposing affected patients to painful or asymptomatic vertebral fractures (Fig. 7.1) (6). Vertebral fragility and fractures can result in structural changes in the spine that may become pronounced with deformities such as scoliosis and kyphosis (7). Low back pain in a patient with such structural changes is likely to have a mechanical component that will not respond to osteoporotic pharmacological treatment.

DIFFERENTIAL DIAGNOSIS

When these patients are evaluated clinically, it should be noted that the symptoms are often complex and varying. The patients are usually elderly and can be sick with other conditions. Other causes such as visceral pain from abdominal organs and cardiopulmonary conditions should be regarded as possible differential diagnostic entities. Such conditions are especially important to consider because the pain picture in patients with osteoporotic compression fractures often involves abdominal pain and chest pain (3).

SUMMARY

When patients with suspected osteoporotic compression fractures are evaluated, the following main points should be taken into account:

- Local pain, often (>60%) radiating to the flank or anteriorly, is the most common symptom.
- Associated symptoms such as nausea, abdominal pain, and chest pain are common (20% to 30% of patients).
- It is important to consider the possible coexistence of visceral pain from abdominal organs and/or cardiopulmonary conditions.

REFERENCES

1. Frost HM. The spinal osteoporosis: mechanism of pathogenesis and pathophysiology. *J Clin Endocrinol Metab* 1973;2:257–275.
2. Finsen V. Osteoporosis and back pain among the elderly. *Acta Med Scand* 1988;223:443–449.
3. Patel U, Skingle S, Campbell GA, et al. Clinical profile of acute vertebral compression fractures in osteoporosis. *Br J Rheumatol* 1991;30:418–421.
4. Vernon-Robert B, Pirie CJ. Healing trabecular micro fractures in the bodies of lumbar vertebrae. *Ann Rheum Dis* 1973;32:406–412.
5. Frost HM. *Bone remodeling and skeletal modeling errors.* Springfield, IL: Charles C Thomas, 1973.
6. Hadjipavlou AG, Lander PH. Osteoporosis of the spine and its management. In: White AH, Schofferman JA, eds. *Spine care.* St. Louis: Mosby, 1995:847–869.
7. Healey JH, Lane JM. Structural scoliosis in osteoporotic women. *Clin Orthop* 1985;195:216–223.

8

Consequences of Kyphotic Deformity

Stephen Eisenstein

Centre for Spinal Studies, Robert Jones and Agnes Hunt Orthopaedic Hospital, Oswestry, Shropshire, United Kingdom

"I grow old...I grow old... I shall wear the bottoms of my trousers rolled."
T.S. Eliot, *The Love Song of J. Alfred Prufrock* (1915)

DEFORMITY AND QUALITY OF LIFE

Vertebral osteoporotic fracture has a devastating effect on the quality of life and functional capacity of its victims, not yet adequately recognized and measured only as recently as the late 1990s (1). The kyphosis itself has a number of consequences common to all kyphosing conditions. In English, and as applied to women, the kyphosis is often referred to disparagingly as a "dowager's hump"—that is, the hump expected to be seen on an aged widow. The associated loss of stature is not only physical but also perceived as a loss of social standing. Consequences include diminished ability to reach up for items stored at a height; loss of horizontal gaze and associated loss of walking mobility; reduced respiratory capacity and function; increased compression on the abdominal cavity, which is more likely to produce various perineal prolapses in this relatively aged population; and an increased tendency to fall as a result of the need to induce hyperextension of the cervical spine, which in turn is associated with vertebral artery constriction (M. Davie, *personal communication,* 2001).

PAIN

Pain in kyphotic deformity has four origins:

Musculoligamentous, resulting from the loss of segmental support of the vertebral body and putting disproportionate load on the posterior and lateral "guy ropes" of the spine.
Intercostal neuralgia, usually bilateral, intractable, and severe, probably the result of a relative descent of the pedicles of the compressed vertebra or the vertebra above, putting traction on the segmental nerve roots passing under those pedicles.
Continuing microfractures within the collapsing vertebral body.
Direct pressure on the kyphotic gibbus from sitting against the back of a chair or from lying supine on a mattress.

NEUROLOGICAL DEFICIT

This complication is, fortunately, extremely rare, for reasons that are difficult to explain in view of the high prevalence of osteoporotic fractures in the increasing aged population. Most experienced spine surgeons and physicians have encountered at least one such case in which the posterior wall of the vertebra has ballooned onto the dura sufficiently to produce an upper or lower motor neuron syndrome.

FURTHER FRACTURE AND KYPHOSIS

There is evidence that fracture kyphosis by itself predisposes affected patients to further fracture and kyphosis deformity (2,3). This is easily explained from the fact that some kyphosis imposes pressure greater than previous compressive forces on vertebral bodies not yet compressed but all equally weakened by osteoporosis. Osteoporotic vertebral deformity in women is also a strong predictor for fracture of the femoral neck (3). It is possible that compensatory hyperlordosis in the cervical spine could result in odontoid fractures and fractures of the posterior arch of the atlas (4).

REFERENCES

1. Hall SE, Criddle RA, Comito TL, et al. A case-control study of quality of life and functional impairment in women with long-standing vertebral osteoporotic fracture. *Osteoporos Int* 1999;9:508–515.
2. Klotzbuecher CM, Ross PD, Landsman PD, et al. Patients with prior fractures have an increased risk of future fractures: a summary of the literature and statistical synthesis. *J Bone Miner Res* 2000;15:721–739.
3. Ismail AA, Cockerill W, Cooper C, et al. Prevalent vertebral deformity predicts incident hip though not distal forearm fracture: results from the European Prospective Osteoporosis Study. *Osteoporos Int* 2001;12:85–90.
4. Nagashima H, Morio Y, Hasegawa K, et al. Odontoid fractures of the posterior arch of the atlas in the elderly over 85 years with severe thoracic kyphosis secondary to osteoporosis. *Injury* 2001;32:501–504.

9

Mechanisms of Pain in Osteoporotic Vertebral Compression Fracture

Charles E. Pither

Pain Management Department and Pain Input Unit, St. Thomas's Hospital, London, United Kingdom

Osteoporosis is similar to various other painful medical illnesses such as endometriosis and low back pain in that the pain is not clearly related to the degree of tissue damage. Radiographs, magnetic resonance imaging (MRI) scans, and measures of bone density give no indication of the amount of pain (1).

To understand this better, it is important to appreciate the complexity of the pain experience. Pain is never simply a sensation; it is always a perception, which is the end point of a complex process of cortical appraisal (2). Pain in osteoporosis is unlikely to occur in the absence of nociception, but troublesome pain does not imply high levels of nociception or worse tissue damage. Low levels of nociception can produce troublesome distress and disability in unfavorable circumstances.

Osteoporosis is usually painless until a fracture occurs, but only one third of fractures is diagnosed clinically. Fracture rate increases steadily with age, and further fractures are more likely once one has occurred (3).

PATTERNS OF PAIN

The disease of osteoporosis, however, is seldom a problem for the orthopedic surgeon in the absence of pain; complaints of pain are almost always the presenting symptom. The pattern of pain can vary considerably, however, and different mechanisms are responsible for the pain in different clinical situations.

Three major patterns of pain can be distinguished:

1. Relatively sudden onset of pain in a previously pain-free but at-risk person, in whom subsequent investigations reveal a compression fracture. This is essentially the acute pain of a bone injury and is probably no different in genesis from any other fracture. The pain is *acute* and includes an inflammatory component. Treatment is the same as for an acutely painful fracture (4).
2. Persistent pain that may have started with a single, clearly defined episode but does not settle with therapy and continues to trouble the patient, developing into a pattern of "chronic pain." This pain is variously related to pathological processes in the spine but is best treated as a *chronic pain* problem through a multimodal approach.
3. Complaints of poorly localized pain in the presence of osteoporosis that does not clearly correlate with a compression fracture. This pattern of pain poses problems

diagnostically, centering on whether the pain is caused by osteoporotic collapse or other mechanisms. The exact source of pain often cannot be identified, but multiple mechanisms of pain generation and sources of pain are probably involved.

It must also be remembered that osteoporotic collapse frequently occurs in the absence of significant pain, as exemplified by the so-called dowager's hump.

SOURCES OF PAIN

Discussion of the pain processes in osteoporosis must include the various potential sources of pain within the spine and surrounding tissues. Pain can arise only from innervated tissue. Various potential sources of pain can be identified in the perispinal tissues (5).

Pain Caused by Nociceptors in Bone Itself

People definitely feel pain when bone is fractured. A fracture disrupts the periosteum, which is densely innervated and can be a source of nociception through either injury or mechanical deformation. A fracture that disrupts the periosteum provokes pain.

Similarly, the endplate is well innervated and probably has some pressure transduction properties. Alteration of loading across the endplate produces pain (6); therefore, disruption of the endplate by a fracture produces pain. However, it is uncertain whether this is always the case. Schmorl's nodes represent a herniation of the disc through the endplate, and these are generally thought to be asymptomatic. The acute inflammation and hemorrhage that accompany the injury increase pain by mechanisms described as follows.

Although it is generally agreed that the periosteum is sensitive to pain, and all health care providers familiar with performing perivertebral injections in conscious patients will testify to this, it is less clear whether medullary bone is sensitive to pain. Although nerves have been viewed as traversing through the medullary bone of the vertebral body (7), these nerves are probably not nociceptive (8). Clinical experience suggests that injection or progression of an instrument through the body itself does not provoke pain. In particular, vertebroplasty involving the injection of bone cement into the cavity can be performed painlessly with local anesthesia alone (see Chapter 26). The question about the sensitivity of medullary bone has not been completely resolved but has important bearings on the management of osteoporosis (see later discussion).

The Disc Complex

Much back pain arises from the disc and closely related structures (5). The disc margin is innervated, and pressure on this area and surrounding tissue has been suggested as a source of pain in discal injury (9). Not only can a fractured vertebra directly impinge on the disc margin and maybe disrupt the integrity of the disc, but changes in angulation alter loading across the disc, which has been shown to be a source of pain (6).

Ligamentous and Soft Tissue Pain Arising from the Perivertebral Structures Close to the Fracture Site

In the acute phase, structures local to the fracture site are irritated and may be injured. These include longitudinal ligaments anteriorly and posteriorly and the radiate and costotransverse ligaments. Other muscular and soft tissue structures such as pleura are close enough to the vertebra to be irritated by local hemorrhage. This will similarly trigger pain by initiation of the algesic cascade, to be described.

Nerve Compression Pain Caused by Local Collapse

Pain of a radicular nature is frequently encountered in both the acute and chronic phases of vertebral collapse. This is usually identifiable because it has the characteristic quality of neuropathic pain and radiates in the distribution of a somatic sensory nerve, usually an intercostal nerve.

It is reasonable to assume that such pain arises from the compression or irritation of the nerve root as it emerges through the vertebral foramen. Compression can arise from the fracture extending posteriorly towards the foramen, with perhaps a fragment pressing on the nerve, and also, in severe collapse, from compromise of the foramen caused by severely abnormal angulation. Such processes are more prominent when preexisting degenerative changes are present, with osteophytosis and facet hypertrophy causing a degree of foramenal stenosis. It must be realized that radicular pain does not arise from only nerve compression: various other mechanisms have been postulated, including inflammation resulting from the release of kinins and peptides from discs and other structures. Tumor necrosis factor has been proposed as a potent source of inflammation in disc herniation (10). Similar mechanisms are likely to be involved in vertebral collapse.

Joint Pain

Both the facet and costovertebral joints are well innervated and are agreed to be a source of pain in many spinal conditions. Any significant abnormal angulation of the spine caused by collapse causes alteration to the neutral position and stresses the joint capsule and the articular cartilage. This alters the local biomechanics, causing pain. It is also likely to provoke spinal reflexes in the affected segment, causing paraspinal muscle spasm.

Muscle Pain

Any significant abnormal angulation of the spine causes an alteration in the neutral posture with a consequent change in the muscle balance required to maintain a normal upright stance. Adverse or sustained muscle contracture is a potent source of pain in many conditions, including spinal disorders. Furthermore, if the abnormal angulation is significant enough in the thoracic region to cause kyphosis, secondary changes are necessary in the cervical spine to restore neutral bias to the cranium. This can provoke additional excess contraction in the cervical musculature, leading to neck pain and headache.

Muscle pain can also arise from fatigue caused by activity after excessive rest. Patients with pain and the knowledge that they have weak bones are prone to rest excessively, and this may make matters worse, not better. In such cases, deconditioned fatigues muscles may be a more likely source of pain than are weak bones (11).

In addition to this anatomical analysis of sources of pain, some general pain mechanisms are also important.

Acute Pain Mechanisms

The processes of this phase of pain development are well understood and are summarized in Fig. 9.1. Rapid changes occur not only in the peripheral environment but also

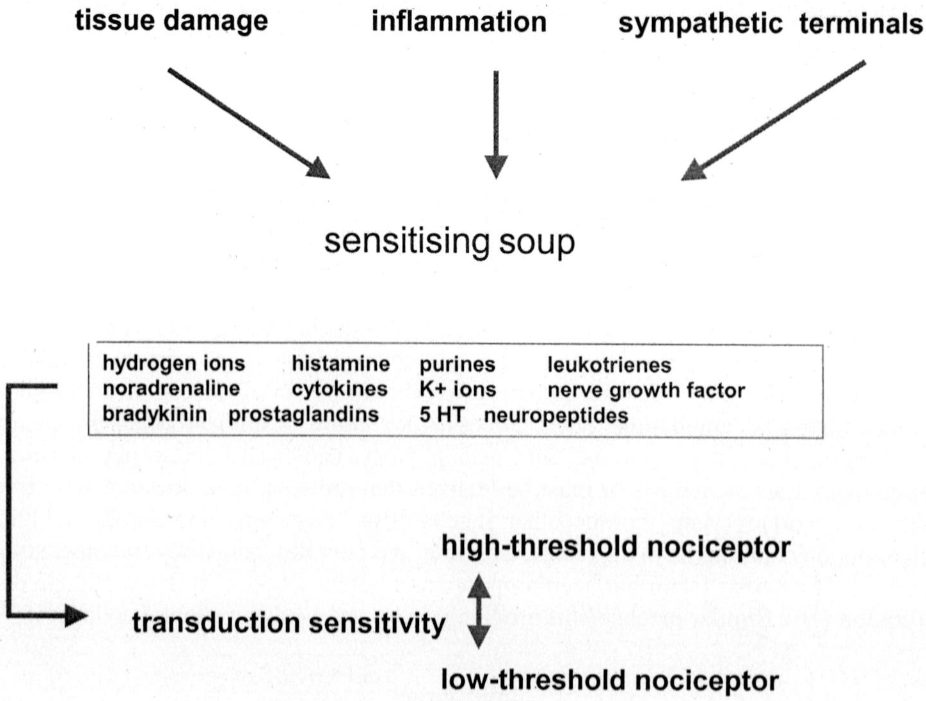

FIG. 9.1. Peripheral sensitization.

within the central nervous system. An acute fracture is a tissue injury that causes hemorrhage and an inflammatory exudate. Various ions and chemical mediators such as peptides and hormones contribute to the peripheral sensitization of nociceptors, with a resultant up-rating of their sensitivity. This produces a higher neuronal firing rate for any given stimulus.

Nerves not only are electrical conduits but also transmit chemical signals. Tissue trauma in the periphery causes a discharge that provokes changes in the chemical environment in the dorsal horn within hours of its occurrence. These processes diminish, with a return to the pre-accident situation, as the acute inflammation resolves and healing takes place.

Chronic Pain Mechanisms

With persistent stimuli arising from tissues, central sensitization develops, as depicted in Fig. 9.2. Important changes occur in the dorsal horn of the spinal cord, which have the effect of producing a greater central effect for any given stimulus (12). In particular, activation of the *N*-methyl-D-aspartate (NMDA) and neurokinin 1 (NK1) receptors by glutamate increases the responsiveness of the interneurons, causing "wind-up" (13). This results in magnification of the effects of the original stimulation.

The extent to which these mechanisms extend centrally into those areas of the brain responsible for pain processing, such as the periaqueductal gray area and the limbic system remains uncertain. In neurological pain syndromes, such as phantom limb pain, major changes in the brain's processing of pain can be demonstrated. The effect is the

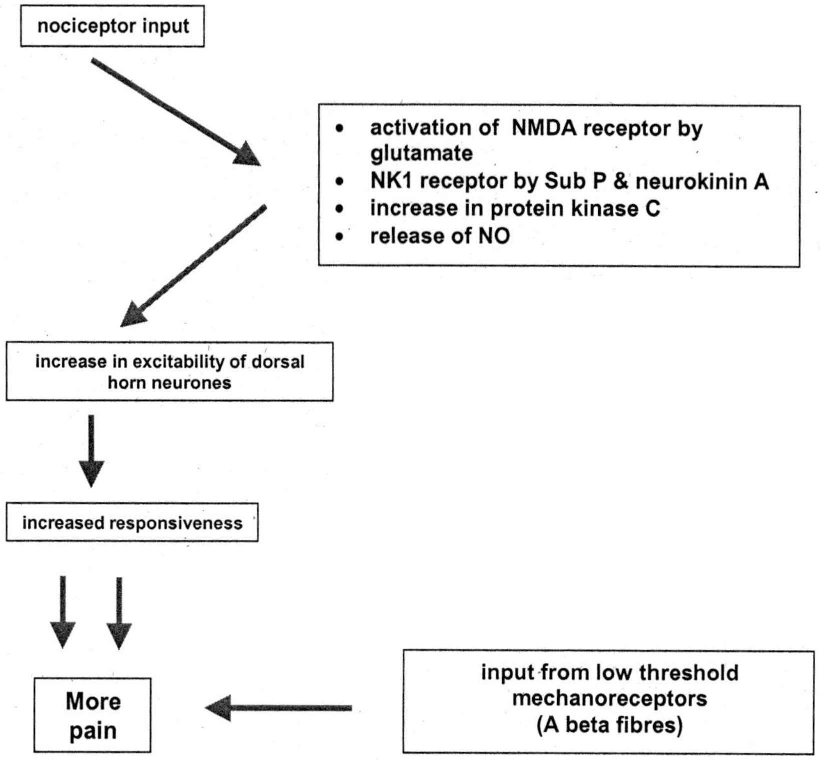

FIG. 9.2. Central sensitization.

activation of a pain matrix by stimuli not normally noxious. This is sometimes termed "pain memory." In effect, the stereotypic pain can be triggered by a variety of stimuli or situations. It is agreed that these processes can develop in chronic pain syndromes of non-neurological origin.

Secondary Deconditioning

Although it is difficult to ascertain to what extent the prolonged effects of changes in posture, fitness, and range of movement contribute to the development of chronic pain, it is certain that such effects are not beneficial and probable that they act in an adverse manner. Frost described the crucial interaction of bone density and muscle strength, in which deterioration in the latter causes further demineralization of bone (11). Even if these mechanisms do not necessarily produce pain, they certainly contribute to the disability that follows. For example, fear-avoidance mechanisms, in which fear of causing further damage leads to avoidance of activity, leading in turn to a further diminution of fitness and perpetuation of deformity, worsens the overall suffering and increases complaints of pain.

Psychological Effects

It must also be realized that all the pain mechanisms just described are modified by the general status and mood of the patient and are subject to behavioral contingencies (14).

Depression and chronic pain are closely related. Pain frequently causes depression in vulnerable patients, and once this occurs, the processing and perception of pain is adversely affected. This is not simply a question of coping poorly with a stressor, which chronic pain is, once depression has intruded; instead, it is a more fundamental issue concerning the threat and unpleasantness of the pain experience.

The complexity of these mechanism necessitates a holistic interdisciplinary assessment of the pain in all cases in which the pain has become chronic.

IS OSTEOPOROSIS PAINFUL IN THE ABSENCE OF CLEAR-CUT VERTEBRAL COLLAPSE?

Osteoporosis is frequently blamed for pain in the spine in patients with diagnosed osteoporosis but without clear-cut fracture. The question arises as to whether osteoporosis is painful even in the absence of a visible fracture. Undoubtedly, the processes involved within osteopenic bone are complex and involve metabolic, neural, hormonal, and structural changes (15).

Many osteoporosis sufferers are old, and the elderly frequently complain of pain in the spine and elsewhere. It seems clear that minor demineralization per se does not produce pain. Among the population without spinal pain, there is a range of bone mineralization; it is therefore clear that at normal levels of bone density, there is no link between generalized pain and mineralization.

In spite of this, bone pain is an undoubted reality in a number of metabolic bone conditions, such as renal failure (16) and liver disease (17). However, it has been suggested that the bone pain seen in hemodialysis is related more to osteomalacia than to osteoporosis (18). Microtrauma has been postulated as a mechanism for the genesis of pain in osteoporosis, with the suggestion that with loss of strength, bone can become pain sensitive to normal loads that stress the weakened architecture. Experimental explanations to support this postulate have not been forthcoming.

Bone pain that follows renal disease has been correlated with bone edema on MRI scanning. Although peptide neuromodulators have been implicated, the mechanism remains unclear (19).

It is possible that at more severe degrees of osteoporosis, pain could be generated from microfractures within the vertebral body (20), which are not visible on radiographs. Evidence of this must be evaluated with considerable scrutiny because of the multiplicity of factors at play. Some general treatments for osteoporosis, such as the biphosphonates, have been shown to reduce general pain (21,22); they may do this through mechanisms other than that of increasing bone mineral content. Similarly, calcitonin (23), can also be of value as a treatment for bone pain (24), through uncertain mechanisms of action.

Musgrave (25), in a study of postmenopausal women, found that back pain levels were higher in women who were currently taking or had previously taken estrogen supplements than in those who had never taken hormone replacement therapy. Increased levels of pain corresponded with higher bone density. These data, too, suggest that lower bone density per se is not associated with pain.

There are few data available to inform the scientific debate on this subject. It is this author's view that, except in very serious osteoporosis in which bony integrity in the spine is likely to be compromised even if frank collapse has not occurred, osteoporosis alone does not cause pain and that most patients with pain and osteoporosis have commoner mechanical mechanisms to account for their symptoms.

REFERENCES

1. Boos N, Rieder R, Schade V, et al. 1995 Volvo Award in clinical sciences. The diagnostic accuracy of magnetic resonance imaging, work perception, and psychosocial factors in identifying symptomatic disc herniations. *Spine* 1995;20:2613–2625.
2. Price DD. Psychological and neural mechanisms of the affective dimension of pain. *Science* 2000;288:1769–1772.
3. Haczynski J, Jakimiuk A. Vertebral fractures: a hidden problem of osteoporosis. *Med Sci Monit* 2001;7:1108–1117.
4. Frost HM. Personal experience in managing acute compression fractures, their aftermath, and the bone pain syndrome, in osteoporosis. *Osteoporos Int* 1998;8:13–15.
5. Kuslich SD, Ulstrom CL, Michael CJ. The tissue origin of low back pain and sciatica: a report of pain response to tissue stimulation during operations on the lumbar spine using local anesthesia. *Orthop Clin North Am* 1991;22:181–187.
6. McNally DS, Shackleford IM, Goodship AE, et al. *In vivo* stress measurement can predict pain on discography. *Spine* 1996;21:2580–2587.
7. Antonacci MD, Mody DR, Heggeness MH. Innervation of the human vertebral body: a histologic study. *J Spinal Disord* 1998;11:526–531.
8. Gronblad M, Korkala O, Konttinen YT, et al. Silver impregnation and immunohistochemical study of nerves in lumbar facet joint plical tissue. *Spine* 1991;16:34–38.
9. Brown MF, Hukkanen MV, McCarthy ID, et al. Sensory and sympathetic innervation of the vertebral endplate in patients with degenerative disc disease. *J Bone Joint Surg Br* 1997;79:147–153.
10. Olmarker K. Radicular pain—recent patholophysiologic concepts and therapeutic implications. *Schmerz* 2001;15:425–429.
11. Frost HM. Changing views about "Osteoporoses" (a 1998 overview). *Osteoporos Int* 1999;10:345–352.
12. Zimmermann M. Pathobiology of neuropathic pain. *Eur J Pharmacol* 2001;429:23–37.
13. Parsons CG. NMDA receptors as targets for drug action in neuropathic pain. *Eur J Pharmacol* 2001;429:71–78.
14. Eccleston C. Role of psychology in pain management. *Br J Anaesth* 2001;87:144–152.
15. Kiebzak GM. Age-related bone changes. *Exp Gerontol* 1991;26:171–187.
16. Monier-Faugere MC, Mawad H, Qi Q, et al. High prevalence of low bone turnover and occurrence of osteomalacia after kidney transplantation. *J Am Soc Nephrol* 2000;11:1093–1099.
17. Hay JE, Lindor KD, Wiesner RH, et al. The metabolic bone disease of primary sclerosing cholangitis. *Hepatology* 1991;14:257–261.
18. Alvarez-Ude F, Feest TG, Ward MK, et al. Hemodialysis bone disease: correlation between clinical, histologic, and other findings. *Kidney Int* 1978;14:68–73.
19. Grotz WH, Breitenfeld MK, Braune SW, et al. Calcineurin-inhibitor induced pain syndrome (CIPS): a severe disabling complication after organ transplantation. *Transplant Int* 2001;14:16–23.
20. Frost HM. The pathomechanics of osteoporoses. *Clin Orthop* 1985;(200):198–225.
21. Crandall C. Risedronate: a clinical review. *Arch Intern Med* 2001;161:353–360.
22. Fitton A, McTavish D. Pamidronate. A review of its pharmacological properties and therapeutic efficacy in resorptive bone disease. *Drugs* 1991;41:289–318.
23. Rifat SF, Kiningham RB, Peggs JF. Calcitonin in the treatment of osteoporotic bone pain. *J Fam Pract* 1992;35:93–96.
24. Gennari C, Agnusdei D, Camporeale A. Use of calcitonin in the treatment of bone pain associated with osteoporosis. *Calcif Tissue Int* 1991;49(Suppl 2):S9–S13.
25. Musgrave DS, Vogt MT, Nevitt MC, et al. Back problems among postmenopausal women taking estrogen replacement therapy: the study of osteoporotic fractures. *Spine* 2001;26:1606–1612.

10

Osteoporotic Vertebral Fractures

Neurological Complications

Michel Benoist

Paris Hospitals, University of Paris VII, 75116 Paris, France

Osteoporotic vertebral fractures (OVFs) are frequent complications of osteoporosis. They are usually benign and heal spontaneously in a few weeks or months. In general, the possibility of paraplegia or nerve root compression has long been excluded. In old major textbooks, spinal cord compression was not considered a possible complication of OVF. The dogma was that nontraumatic vertebral collapse implies tumoral pathology. However, since the first two cases described by Kempinsky (1) in 1958, an increasing number of observations of this devastating complication have been published.

In this chapter, clinical and imaging aspects of neurological complications are reviewed, as are their evolution under treatment. This presentation is based on four of the author's cases and on a review of the literature.

EPIDEMIOLOGY

The frequency of neurological complications of OVF is not known. Estimations by authors are largely variable. For example, in a 3-year period, eight such cases were disclosed among 138 French patients hospitalized for an OVF (2) and in ten (2%) of 497 Chinese patients hospitalized in Hong Kong from 1989 to 1994 (3). Shikata et al. (4) reported seven cases (12%) among 58 patients hospitalized for OVF. In contrast, among 673 patients, only 2 cases were encountered in another study (5). Aging of the population as well as the progress in imaging will probably increase the frequency in diagnoses of such cases in the future.

PATHOLOGY

Neurological symptoms are caused by a posterior bone fragment's impinging on the spinal canal. In most OVFs, the posterior wall of the vertebral body remains normal. The trabecular structure of the vertebral body is organized in three networks: one is vertical, and two are oblique. Intersection of the three networks creates a maximal zone of resistance at the level of the posterior wall. Bursting of the posterior wall in an OVF implies major osteopenia, both trabecular and cortical. Increase of the load on the posterior wall after a collapse of the anterior part of the vertebral body may also lead to a progressive disruption of the posterior border of the vertebra (2).

Fractures complicated by paraplegia are either burst or wedge fractures. In the case of burst fractures, the entire vertebral body is damaged. Cord compression is caused by projection of a bone fragment into the spinal canal. Wedge fractures involve only the anterior part of the vertebral body. Compression of the cord is located at the upper or lower part of the vertebral body with angulation and kyphosis. Additional factors in compression, such as discal herniation and a narrow spinal canal, have also been encountered. Moreover, disruption of the middle and posterior columns of the vertebral column as defined by Denis (6) is a source of instability. In addition to the mechanical compression, ischemia of the neural elements caused by compression of the vascular supply may be an aggravating factor (7).

Fractures usually occur at the thoracolumbar junction. In the review by Koeger et al. (2), of the 30 OVFs responsible for neurological complications, 25 were located between T-11 and L-2. Three patients had an involvement of two vertebrae. Similarly, in the series reported by Baba et al. (8), a single vertebra collapsed in 23 of 27 patients, and four had involvement of two vertebrae. Of the 29 OVFs, 27 were located between T-11 and L-2, one at L-4, and one at L-5. According to Denis's (6) classification, three patients had an unstable wedge fracture, and 24 had a burst fracture. One of the four cases of Salomon et al. (7) involved a single wedge fracture at the T-5 level. A burst fracture at the thoracolumbar junction was seen in the other three patients.

CLINICAL DESCRIPTION

Patients are predominantly elderly women with a severe senile or postmenopausal osteoporosis; for example, in the series of Baba et al. (8), only four of the 27 patients were men. The severity of osteoporosis can now be documented by measurement of bone density. An additional risk factor such as steroid therapy or alcoholism is associated in a few cases (1,9,10). The vertebral collapse may be spontaneous or may follow a minor trauma, usually a fall from the standing position on level ground (3–7). Most patients with vertebral fractures experience a period of acute back pain at the site of the collapse. Symptoms of pain are usually controlled by analgesics and physiotherapy and subside in a few weeks or months. An increase in dorsal kyphosis is often observed at the physical examination.

NEUROLOGICAL EXAMINATION

A small number of patients have spinal cord compression resulting from the fracture. These patients seek medical help primarily for back pain. In only a few cases, the neuro-

TABLE 10.1. *Level of compression in 37 patients*

Level	No. of patients
Spinal cord	18
Conus	5
Cauda equina	13
Nerve root	1
Total	37

From Koeger AC, Bourgeois P. Compressions nerveuses par tassement vertébral ostéoporotique. In: de Sèze S, Ryckewaert A, Kahn MF, et al., eds. *L'actualité rhumatologique.* Paris: Expansion Scientifique Française, 1992:112–122.

TABLE 10.2. *Neurological signs in 33 patients*

Sign	No. of patients
Complete paraplegia, vesicorectal dysfunction	12
Incomplete spastic ambulatory paraparesis	10
Femoral or sciatic neuralgia with major motor deficit	8
Neurogenic claudication (spinal cord or radicular)	3

From Koeger AC, Bourgeois P. Compressions nerveuses par tassement vertébral ostéoporotique. In: de Sèze S, Ryckewaert A, Kahn MF, et al., eds. *L'actualité rhumatologique.* Paris: Expansion Scientifique Française, 1992:112–122.

logical symptoms appear immediately or a few days after the OVF (2). In most patients, neurological complications are delayed, appearing a few weeks or months after the fracture. For example, in a review of 164 cases reported in Japan since 1974, the average onset of paraplegia was 5 to 7 months after fracture (11). In the series of Baba et al. (8), paraplegia developed 1 month to 1.5 years after significant spinal fractures. In the review by Koeger et al., the onset of symptoms was progressive, beginning from 10 days to a few months after OVF in 25 of 30 cases (2). Neurological symptoms and signs depend on the level of the OVF; Table 10.1 shows the level of the compression in 37 patients reviewed by Koeger et al. (2). Table 10.2 lists the neurological symptoms present in 33 patients of the same series. Spinal cord and cauda equina symptoms and signs are variable, including muscle weakness, sensory disturbances, hyperactive tendon reflex, Babinski's reflex, and rectal and bladder incontinence. Repeat neurological examination is mandatory because of the risk of neurological compromise, which is often delayed. Complete paraplegia may develop in 1 or 2 weeks or progressively, with bouts of aggravation occurring over 1 month to 1 year (7–12). Late and progressive paralysis follow the gradual retropulsion of the unstable fracture fragments into the spinal canal.

DIAGNOSIS

On conventional radiographs, the collapsed vertebra is usually seen at the site of the acute angle of the kyphosis. The retropulsed fragment is not always visible but can be suspected from disruption of the posterior vertebral body line, as described by Daffner et al. (13).

Myelography, which was used before the advent of computed tomographic (CT) scanner and magnetic resonance imaging (MRI), was able to confirm and localize the compression by showing a complete or partial block at the level of the compression. Since 1986, a less aggressive radiological examination has progressively replaced myelography (4,9,14,15). CT scanning is able to demonstrate the bursting of the vertebral body with encroachment of the retropulsed fragment in the spinal canal. According to McAfee et al. (16), bone disruption of all three columns is clearly visible on CT scans, which is a criterion for instability.

MRI is a most valuable alternative. First, the parasagittal image shows the compressed vertebral body as well as the retropulsed fragment and displacement of the cord (4,9,12,14). Second, MRI is a powerful tool for differentiating an OVF from vertebral fractures caused by malignancy, including lymphoma, myeloma, and metastasis. Fractures caused by malignancy are the main cause of neurological complications. MRI demonstrates the integrity of the bone marrow by showing a high signal intensity on T1-weighted images, whereas metastatic tumoral tissue replacing the bone marrow has a low signal intensity on these images. A normal fatty marrow is demonstrated by a low signal intensity on T2-weighted images, in contrast to the intense signal observed when metastatic tissue replaces the normal bone marrow. In the case of recent vertebral fracture, the compressed bone tissue of the collapsed body may have a low signal intensity on both T1- and T2-weighted images. Normalization after injection of gadolinium strongly suggests benignity (17,18,19) as well as the normal aspect of the epidural space and of the paraspinal soft tissues.

HISTOLOGICAL EXAMINATION

The osteoporotic nature of the collapse is usually recognized on CT scan and MRI. Postoperatively, osteoporosis is confirmed by the histological examination (2,4,7,8). Before the advent of MRI, preoperative transpedicular biopsy was necessary to differentiate osteoporosis from a malignant tumoral pathology; this is still true in doubtful cases (8,9,17,18).

EVOLUTION AND TREATMENT

Conservative therapy includes bed rest, neurological reeducation, and symptomatic therapy for sphincteric dysfunction. These measures have been used in a few cases in the literature, primarily when the general condition or the long duration of the paresis was considered a contraindication to major surgery. Medical treatment yields poor results. For example, of 37 patients reviewed by Koeger et al. (2) in 1992, 11 were treated conservatively; only four had an incomplete recovery and no improvement was observed in the remaining 7 cases (2).

Surgical cases achieve much better results. The surgical methods include laminectomy, laminectomy with posterior fusion, anterior decompression with posterior fusion, and anterior decompression with anterior fusion. Laminectomy without stabilization has been used in the past with mediocre results (2). In more recent reports, different types of surgery with the technical advances of instrumentation have been performed.

In this author's experience, four patients have been treated by Cotrel-Dubousset instrumentation and anterior fusion; all four have experienced good neurological recovery. Anterior decompression is logical, because the pathological process is located anteriorly. This procedure has been used by a few authors (3,4,8). Lee and Kevin (3) reported the results of 10 patients who underwent anterior decompression and fusion. Neurological recovery was incomplete, but sphincteric recovery was satisfactory, and although lower limb strength was never totally normal, all patients were able to walk with a cane or a frame. Kaneda et al. (20) developed an anterior decompression procedure that included a bioactive ceramic vertebral prosthesis replacement and special spinal implants. They obtained complete decompression with satisfactory results for the neurological deficits. However, the anterior approach entails serious risks in these old, frail patients. Probably for that reason, posterior decompression with various types of instrumentation has been used, in spite of the difficulties regarding the holding power of the implants on the fragile osteoporotic bone. In the series of Baba et al. (8), of 27 patients, 20 underwent posterior transpedicular decompression with Cotrel-Dubousset instrumentation; the other seven underwent anterior surgery, without instrumentation in two cases. Overall outcomes were satisfactory: 21 patients (78%) obtained good to excellent results. Interestingly, patients who underwent anterior surgery had an improvement rate of 58.6%, and those who underwent posterior surgery had an improvement rate of 64.5%; the difference is not significant. In the 20 patients with Cotrel-Dubousset instrumentation, there were

TABLE 10.3. *Correction of the kyphosis and neurological outcome*

		Kyphosis		Neurologic deficits (Frankel grades)		
Case	Region	Preoperative	Follow-up	Preoperative	Follow-up	Persistent local pain
1	T11–L2	50 degrees	18 degrees	C	E	(–)
2	T10–T12	30 degrees	9 degrees	B	E	(–)
3	T9–L1	38 degrees	26 degrees	C	D	(+/–)
4	T10–T12	33 degrees	12 degrees	C	E	(–)
5	T12–L2	28 degrees	15 degrees	B	D	(+/–)
6	T11–L1	33 degrees	11 degrees	C	E	(–)
7	L2–L5	20 degrees	0 degrees	C	E	(–)

From Shikata J, Yamamuro T, Ida H, et al. Surgical treatment for paraplegia resulting from vertebral fractures in senile osteoporosis. *Spine* 1990;15:485–489.

three minor instrumentation failures without instrument-related neurological problems during the average postoperative follow up of 3 to 7 years.

Seven patients were treated surgically by Shikata et al. (4). All but one experienced posterior decompression and stabilization. All patients had satisfactory results and were able to walk unassisted postoperatively. Table 10.3 shows the corrections of kyphosis and neurological outcomes of this series. Posterior decompression and stabilization with various devices have been performed by other authors (12,18,21). Analysis of the literature shows that the posterior approach has been used predominantly, most spine surgeons being more familiar with this approach.

CONCLUSIONS

Vertebral body collapse with neurological complications is not always tumoral. Osteoporosis must be remembered as a cause of paraplegia resulting from a compression fracture. The incidence of this complication of osteoporosis is low, but an increased number of cases have been reported coincidence with aging of the population. CT scanning and MRI are powerful diagnostic tools, usually able to distinguish osteoporosis from tumor. Development of paraplegia is usually delayed, and this necessitates a careful neurological observation in the weeks or months after an OVF.

Conservative treatment yields poor results and is indicated only when surgery is absolutely contraindicated in elderly patients who are in poor general condition with comorbidity. In contrast, surgical decompression with stabilization with the anterior or posterior approach yields better recovery of walking ability and of sphinteric function.

Therefore, and whatever the age of the patient, early surgery is strongly recommended.

REFERENCES

1. Kempinsky WH. Osteoporotic kyphosis with paraplegia. *Neurology* 1958;8:181–185.
2. Koeger AC, Bourgeois P: Compressions nerveuses par tassement vertébral ostéoporotique. In: de Sèze S, Ryckewaert A, Kahn MF, et al., eds. *L'actualité rhumatologique.* Paris: Expansion Scientifique Française, 1992: 112–122.
3. Lee YL, Kevin MH: The osteoporotic spine. *Clin Orthop* 1996;323:91–97.
4. Shikata J, Yamamuro T, Ida H, et al. Surgical treatment for paraplegia resulting from vertebral fractures in senile osteoporosis. *Spine* 1990;15:485–489.
5. Alcalay M, Debiais F. Ostéoporose et compression nerveuse. *Presse Med* 1988;17:1495–1496.

6. Denis F. The three column spine and its significance in the classification of acute thoracolumbar spinal injuries. *Spine* 1983;8:817–832.
7. Salomon C, Chopin D, Benoist M. Spinal cord compression: an exceptional complication of osteoporosis. *Spine* 1988;13:222–224.
8. Baba H, Maezawa Y, Kamitani K, et al. Osteoporotic vertebral fractures with late neurological complications. *Paraplegia* 1995;33:281–289.
9. Chazerain P, Marion MH, Metreau R, et al. Les compressions médullaires au cours des tassements ostéoporotiques. A propos de deux cas. *Rev Rhum Mal Osteoartic* 1989;56:791–794.
10. Quennec JY, De Bray JM, Andran M, et al. Osteonécrose vertébrale. A propos de 3 cas dont un compliqué d'une compression médullaire et 2 associés à une autre localisation nécrotique. *Rev Rhum Mal Osteoartic* 1985;52:1–5.
11. Mori S, Norimatsu H, Oka S. Burst fracture: osteoporotic vertebral compression fracture associated with paraplegia [In Japanese]. *Nippon Rinsho* 1994;52:2435–2441.
12. Tudeso N, Lafage MH, Leroux JL, et al. Fractures tassements vertébrales d'origine ostéoporotique avec compression nerveuse. *Rhumatologie* 1990;42:223–227.
13. Daffner H, Deel ZL, Rothfus WE. The posterior body line: importance in the detection of burst fractures. *AJR Am J Roentgenol* 1987;148:93–96.
14. Kaplan PA, Orton DF, Asleson RJ. Osteoporosis with vertebral compression fractures, retropulsed fragments and neurologic compromise. *Radiology* 1987;165:533–535.
15. Arciero RA, Leung KYK, Pierce JH. Spontaneous unstable burst fracture of the thoraco lumbar spine in osteoporosis. *Spine* 1989;14:114–117.
16. McAfee PC, Yuan HA, Lasda NA. The unstable burst fracture. *Spine* 1982;7:365–373.
17. Chevalier X, Wrona N, Avouac B, et al. Thigh pain and multiple vertebral osteonecrosis: value of magnetic resonance imaging. *J Rheumatol* 1991;18:1627–1630.
18. Laforgue P, Daumen-Legre V, Schiano A, et al. Les complications neurologiques des tassements vertébraux ostéoporotiques. *Rev Rhum Mal Osteoartic* 1990;57:619–625.
19. Laredo JD, Chicheportice V, Bondeville JM, et al. Diagnostic des tassements vertébraux non traumatiques bénins et malins. Apport de l'imagerie moderne. In: de Sèze S, Ryckewaert A, Kahn MF, eds. *L'actualité rhumatologique 1990.* Paris: Expansion Scientifique Française, 1990:219–230.
20. Kaneda K, Abumi K, Fujiya M. Burst fractures with neurologic deficits of the thoracolumbar spine: results of anterior decompression and stabilization with anterior instrumentation. *Spine* 1984;9:788–795.
21. Mazel C, Roy-Camille R, Lazennec JY, et al. Fractures ostéoporotiques du rachis avec signes neurologiques. Problèmes diagnostiques et thérapeutiques. A propos de deux cas. *Rachis* 1989;1:163–167.

11

Assessment of Vertebral Osteoporosis

*John A. Kanis, †Anders Odén, ‡Olof Johnell, and §Chris De Laet

*World Health Organisation Collaborating Centre for Metabolic Bone Diseases, University of Sheffield Medical School, Sheffield, United Kingdom; †Göteborg University, Göteborg, Sweden ‡Department of Orthopaedics, Malmö General Hospital, Malmö, Sweden; §Institute for Public Health, Erasmus, MC, Rotterdam, The Netherlands

Vertebral fractures form an integral component of the osteoporotic syndrome. Indeed, the majority of intervention studies have focused on the effectiveness of pharmacological agents to reduce the burden of vertebral fractures. There are a number of problems to consider in the assessment of vertebral fracture. Most fractures in general are clinically obvious and give rise to morbidity, but in the case of vertebral fractures, a proportion may not come to clinical attention. The uncertainty arises in defining the presence or absence of fractures. There is no general agreement on the criteria for the radiographic definition of vertebral fracture, and it is generally diagnosed through a change in vertebral shape. Thus, the incidence and prevalence of vertebral fracture depend critically on the methodology used. The incidence of symptomatic fractures is markedly lower than that judged from radiographic criteria alone. Furthermore, the major clinical manifestation of established vertebral osteoporosis is back pain, but this is nonspecific. Indeed, back pain is so common that, at least up to old age, it is more likely when present to have other causes (1).

The assessment of vertebral osteoporosis includes making an accurate diagnosis and a consideration of the differential diagnosis, which are dealt with elsewhere in this volume. A further consideration is the prognosis or risk assessment. Where the risk of further fractures is high, intervention should be considered. The prognostic assessment in established vertebral osteoporosis is reviewed briefly.

ESTABLISHED OSTEOPOROSIS

The internationally agreed definition of osteoporosis is a systemic skeletal disease characterized by low bone mass and microarchitectural deterioration of bone tissue, with a consequent increase in bone fragility and susceptibility to fracture (2). This definition acknowledges that low bone mass is an important component of the risk of fracture but that other abnormalities occur in the skeleton and that nonskeletal factors such as falls are also important. Nevertheless, only bone mass, measured as bone mineral density (BMD), can currently be measured with precision and accuracy, and its measurement forms the basis for the diagnosis of osteoporosis.

For diagnostic purposes, two thresholds of bone mineral density have been proposed for white women on the basis of the T-score (3,4). The first threshold defines the point at which the risk of a fracture in the future is very high (osteoporosis); the second is a higher threshold that may be more appropriate for investigating the impact of strategies to prevent bone loss in women at the time of menopause (low bone mass; osteopenia). Osteoporosis, is defined by a value for bone mineral density that is 2.5 standard deviations (SD) or more below the mean value for young adults (T-score ≤– 2.5 SD). Low bone mass denotes a T-score that lies between –1 and –2.5 SD. Severe or "established" osteoporosis is as defined earlier in the presence of one or more documented fragility fractures, usually of the wrist, spine, or hip. The preferred site for diagnosis is the proximal femur with the use of dual energy X-ray absorptiometry (5). The BMD threshold calculated for women can be used for men as well.

This does not mean that other techniques and other sites cannot be used for risk assessment. However, their prognostic significance differs from that provided from BMD measurements made at the proximal femur.

RISK OF VERTEBRAL FRACTURE

A large number of risk factors for vertebral osteoporotic fractures have been identified. Strong risk factors include age, body mass index, a maternal history of fracture, prior fragility fractures, and, in particular, low BMD. Many prospective studies have shown that BMD measurements provide prognostic information on vertebral fracture risk (3,6). One meta-analysis estimated that the risk of vertebral fracture is increased 1.8-fold for each standard deviation decrease in BMD at the femoral neck. Prognostic assessment is improved by measuring the site of biological relevance (the spine). Spine BMD measurements are associated with a 2.3-fold increase in risk for each standard deviation decrease in bone mineral density (6). BMD measurements are at least as good for predicting hip fracture as blood pressure measurements are for predicting stroke and are considerably better than cholesterol measurements for predicting myocardial infarction in men (3,6).

The risk of future vertebral fractures is optimally expressed as absolute risk—that is, probability. For example, to calculate the probabilities that an individual under given circumstances will sustain a fragility fracture in the future, the incidence of first fracture and, for long-term prediction, the mortality risk must be known. Such data are available for Sweden. For example, at the age of 50 years, the remaining lifetime risk of a clinical spine fracture was found to be 15.1% for women and 8.3% for men (7). The lifetime risk of other common osteoporotic fractures is shown in Table 11.1. Lifetime risk decreases progressively with age because, although the incidence rises with age, the increase in incidence does not compensate for the shorter life expectancy with age (Fig. 11.1).

TABLE 11.1. *Remaining lifetime risk of fracture (percentage) in men and women from Malmö, Sweden at the ages shown*

	Risk at 50 years			Risk at 80 years		
Type of fracture	Men	Women	Ratio	Men	Women	Ratio
Forearm	4.6	20.8	4.5	1.6	8.9	5.6
Hip	10.7	22.9	2.1	9.1	19.3	2.1
Spine	8.3	15.1	1.8	4.7	8.7	1.9
Proximal humerus	4.1	12.9	3.1	2.5	7.7	3.1
Any of these	22.4	46.4	2.1	15.3	31.7	2.1

From Kanis JA, Glüer CC. For the Committee of Scientific Advisors, International Osteoporosis Foundation. An update on the diagnosis and assessment of osteoporosis with densitometry. *Osteoporosis Int* 2000;11:192–202.

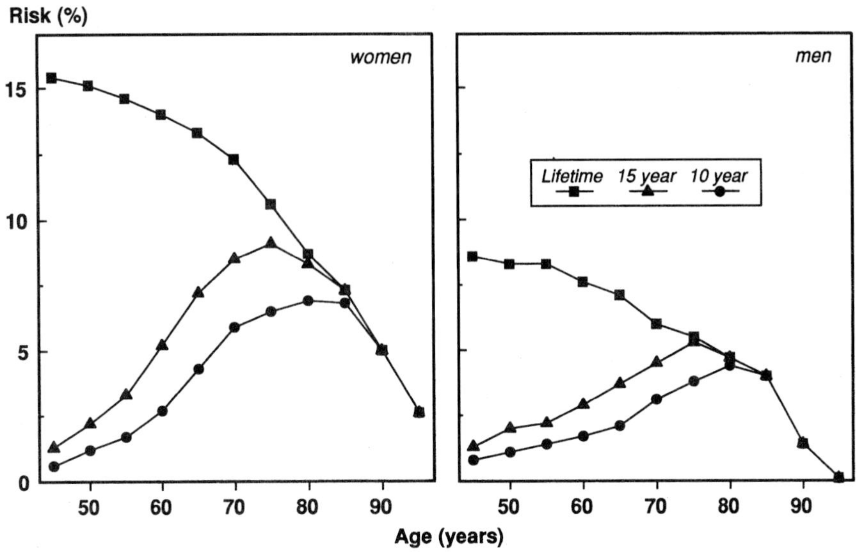

FIG. 11.1. Risk of a first vertebral fracture in men and women by age. Risks are shown as lifetime, 15-year or 10-year risk (5).

Estimates for lifetime risk are of value in considering the future burden of osteoporosis in the community and the effects of intervention strategies. They are less important for assessing risk to patients in whom treatment might be envisioned. This is because treatments are not currently given for a lifetime, as a result of side effects of continued treatment (as with hormone replacement therapy) or low continuance (most treatments). Moreover, the feasibility of lifelong interventions has never been tested with high-risk or global strategies (8). For the purposes of assessment in patients, a ten-year time frame is more suitable. This covers the 3 to 5 years or so in which the effectiveness of treatments has been well tested and also accounts for the offset time, the duration of time that benefits continue when treatment is stopped. Ten-year probability of vertebral fracture increases with age in both men and women up to the age of approximately 80 years. Thereafter, these risks decline, inasmuch as in the elderly the 10-year mortality risk exceeds the fracture risk.

TEN-YEAR RISK AND BONE MINERAL DENSITY

Risk prediction can be more accurately quantified after assessment with BMD. Ten-year risks according to T-score are given in Table 11.2 (9). Of importance is that ten-year probability of vertebral fracture varies according to both age and T-score. Thus, for a given T-score, 10-year probability increases with age. This is one of the reasons why the T-score alone is unhelpful for risk assessment. Also of importance is that a population of osteoporotic patients would have a higher risk than would patients at the threshold for osteoporosis. In populations of osteoporotic patients, many patients would have a T-score of less than –2.5, and the risk of vertebral fracture would therefore be higher than that at the threshold (Table 11.3).

TABLE 11.2. *Ten-year probability of spine fracture in men and women by age and T-score, assessed at the femoral neck*

	T-score						
Age (years)	+1	0	−1	−2.0	−2.5	−3.0	−4.0
Men							
50	0.5	0.9	1.5	2.5	3.2	4.1	6.9
55	0.6	1.0	1.7	2.9	3.8	5.0	8.5
60	0.7	1.1	1.9	3.1	3.9	5.0	8.1
65	0.9	1.4	2.2	3.4	4.2	5.3	8.3
70	1.1	1.8	2.9	4.7	6.0	7.6	12.2
75	1.1	1.9	3.3	5.6	7.2	9.4	15.6
80	1.3	2.1	3.4	5.5	6.9	8.7	13.7
85	1.2	1.9	2.9	4.4	5.4	6.7	10.1
Women							
50	0.4	0.6	1.1	2.0	2.6	3.5	6.1
55	0.4	0.7	1.4	2.5	3.4	4.6	8.3
60	0.6	1.0	1.9	3.4	4.6	6.1	11.0
65	0.8	1.4	2.6	4.7	6.2	8.3	14.6
70	0.8	1.6	2.9	5.5	7.4	10.0	18.0
75	0.7	1.3	2.5	5.0	6.9	9.5	17.9
80	0.7	1.2	2.4	4.6	6.3	8.7	16.1
85	0.6	1.1	2.1	4.0	5.5	7.5	13.6

The same threshold value for bone mineral density is used for both sexes.

TABLE 11.3. *Ten-year probability of vertebral fracture in women by age and diagnostic category according to T-score assessed at the femoral neck*

	T-score		
Age (years)	<0	<−1	<−2.5
45	0.8	1.1	2.1
50	1.4	1.9	3.5
55	1.9	2.5	4.6
60	2.9	3.6	6.4
65	4.5	5.3	9.0
70	6.0	6.7	10.9
75	6.4	6.9	10.7
80	6.8	7.1	10.2
85	6.7	6.9	9.4

Probabilities are shown for each age for all individuals below the average value for BMD and the thresholds for osteopenia and osteoporosis.

TABLE 11.4. *Ten-year probability (percentage) of a first spine fracture in men and women according to population relative risk at the ages shown*

	Age (years)							
Relative risk	50	55	60	65	70	75	80	85
Men								
1.0	1.5	1.7	2.2	3.2	4.6	5.5	6.3	4.2
2.0	3.1	3.3	4.3	6.3	8.9	10.6	12.1	8.2
3.0	4.5	4.9	6.4	9.3	13.0	15.4	17.5	12.0
4.0	6.0	6.4	8.4	12.2	16.9	19.9	22.4	15.6
5.0	7.5	8.0	10.4	15.0	20.5	24.1	26.9	19.0
6.0	8.9	9.5	12.4	17.7	24.1	28.0	31.0	22.2
Women								
1.0	1.6	2.2	3.5	5.5	8.1	9.0	9.3	8.8
2.0	3.1	4.4	6.9	10.8	15.5	17.2	17.6	16.5
3.0	4.6	6.5	10.2	15.7	22.3	24.5	25.0	23.4
4.0	6.1	8.6	13.3	20.3	28.4	31.1	31.1	29.6
5.0	7.6	10.7	16.4	24.7	34.1	37.0	37.3	35.1
6.0	9.0	12.7	19.3	28.8	39.2	42.3	42.5	40.0

OTHER RISK FACTORS

In addition to age and BMD, a number of other factors contribute to the estimation of fracture risk. Examples include attenuation of ultrasound waves, biochemical estimates of skeletal turnover, prior fragility fractures, the use of corticosteroids, and low body mass index (3). For this reason, combinations of risk assessment are likely to be of value in improving the accuracy with which patients at high risk can be confidently identified (10). For example, patients with a prior vertebral fracture are five times more likely to sustain another vertebral fracture than are those who have never sustained such fractures. Patients with prior vertebral fractures are also approximately twice as likely to sustain other common osteoporotic fractures (11). Other factors include premature menopause, certain diseases such as dementia, and the use of drugs such as the corticosteroids and major tranquilizers.

The parallel assessment of a number of risk factors with or without BMD assessment enables the identification of groups or individuals at high risk. Of interest is that the combination of relatively few risk factors can yield relative risks of 5 or more. The relationship between relative risk and 10-year risk for vertebral fracture is shown in Table 11.4 (12).

The consideration of multiple risk factors is commonly used for other multifactorial disorders such as cardiovascular diseases (13). The consideration of smoking, blood pressure, diabetes, and serum cholesterol levels enable the identification of patients at high risk, much better than the use of serum cholesterol levels alone (6).

The level of risk that mandates intervention or further assessment depends on many factors, including the risks and benefits of intervention. If for the sake of argument a probability in excess of 10% were unacceptable, then women with a relative risk of 2 after the age of 65 years would be categorized as within the treatment threshold; for men, the age would be 75 years. In younger women at the age of 55 years, the threshold is not exceeded, except at very high relative risks (5.0 or more; see Table 11.4). The setting of such thresholds will in part depend on health economic considerations. Such studies will be important for optimizing the selection of patients for treatment and then in the development of screening strategies.

REFERENCES

1. Kanis, JA, McCloskey EV. Epidemiology of vertebral osteoporosis. *Bone* 1992;13:S1–S10.
2. Consensus development conference: Diagnosis, prophylaxis and treatment of osteoporosis. *Am J Med* 1991;90: 170–110.
3. World Health Organisation. Assessment of fracture risk and its application to screening for postmenopausal osteoporosis. Technical Report Series 843. Geneva: World Health Organisation, 1994
4. Kanis JA, Melton LJ, Christiansen C, et al. The diagnosis of osteoporosis. *J Bone Miner Res* 1994;9:17–1141.
5. Kanis JA, Glüer CC for the Committee of Scientific Advisors, International Osteoporosis Foundation. An update on the diagnosis and assessment of osteoporosis with densitometry. *Osteoporos Int* 2000;11:192–202.
6. Marshall D, Johnell O, Wedel H. Meta-analysis of how well measures of bone mineral density predict occurrence of osteoporotic fractures. *BMJ* 1996;312:1254–1259.
7. Kanis JA, Johnell O, Oden A, et al. Long-term risk of osteoporotic fracture in Malmo. *Osteoporos Int* 2000;11; 669–674.
8. Royal College of Physicians. Clinical guidelines for the prevention and treatment of osteoporosis. London: Royal College of Physicians, 1999.
9. Kanis JA, Johnell O, Oden A, et al. Ten year probabilities of osteoporotic fractures according to BMD and diagnostic thresholds. *Osteoporos Int* 2001;12:989–995.
10. Kanis JA, Johnell O, Oden A, et al. Risk of hip fracture in Sweden according to relative risk: An analysis applied to the population of Sweden. *Osteoporos Int* 2000;11:120–127.

11. Klotzbuecher CM, Ross PD, Landsman PB, et al. Patients with prior fractures have an increased risk of future fractures: a summary of the literature and statistical synthesis. *J Bone Miner Res* 2001;15:721–727.
12. Kanis JA, Johnell O, Oden A, De Laet C, Jonsson B, Dawson A. Ten year risk of osteoporotic fracture and the effect of risk factors on screening strategies. *Bone* 2002;30:251–258.
13. Dyslipidaemia Advisory Group on behalf of the National Heart Foundation of New Zealand. National Heart Foundation clinical guidelines for the assessment and management of dyslipidaemia. *N Z Med J* 1996;109: 224–232.

12

Imaging and Differential Diagnosis of Vertebral Compression Fractures

Jan T. Wilmink

Department of Radiology, University Hospital, Maastricht, The Netherlands

In osteoporosis, fractures of the spine, hip, and wrist are the most frequent complications. The most serious fractures are those of the hip, which contribute significantly to morbidity, mortality, and costs. Fractures of the spine may be asymptomatic when solitary but become associated with increasing morbidity as they increase in number and severity. Imaging studies play a limited role in the assessment of osteoporosis. Conventional radiographic films have a low sensitivity in detecting loss of bone mass. Vertebral collapse can usually be ascertained, but it is often not possible to determine the cause of such collapse, be it osteoporosis or tumor infiltration.

Radiographic imaging techniques produce areas of contrasting brightness in the image by registering variations in radiological density (electron density). In this way, dense cortical bone can be differentiated from trabecular bone and bone tissue from soft tissue and air.

Magnetic resonance (MR) imaging operates under a completely different imaging principle. Whereas dense cortical bone absorbs a large proportion of the x-rays passing through and thus produces a bright (underexposed) area on the x-ray film, this is not the case in an MR image. Cortical bone is distinguished by its lack of MR signal and appears in the MR image as a linear dark structure. It impossible to even guess at a decrease in bone mineral density on the basis of the MR image. MR imaging is, however, capable of providing a good assessment of the composition of the bone marrow. In the spine, it is possible to distinguish between red juvenile bone marrow and yellow adult bone marrow. In adults, MR imaging can be used to detect bone marrow changes caused by tumor infiltration.

RADIOGRAPHIC IMAGING

Loss of vertebral bone mass, as occurs in osteoporosis, can be demonstrated in advanced cases on plain radiographs, but it has been estimated that 30% to 80% of skeletal calcium must be lost before the first changes are seen in the routine film. Early changes in density are difficult to assess reliably. With increasing severity of osteoporosis, the central portion of the vertebral body becomes lucent in comparison with the more dense vertebral endplates. In addition, as trabeculae are lost or thinned, the vertically oriented load-bearing trabeculae are least affected; there is thus a vertically striated appearance, which may even resemble that of a vertebral hemangioma (1).

Changes in the shape of the vertebral body may also occur. Anterior wedging is said to have occurred when the anterior height of the vertebral body is less than the posterior height by 4 mm or more. Wedge-shaped vertebral bodies indicate that fracture of the anterior surface of the vertebral body (anterior column) has occurred, leaving the posterior vertebral surface (middle column) intact. Flattening of the entire vertebra (so-called pancake vertebra) indicates that the anterior and middle columns have collapsed, as often have the posterior column (articular processes) as well. Sometimes the vertebral endplates show marked ballooning caused by pressure of the intervertebral disc, whereas the anterior and posterior vertebral borders remain intact. This produces so-called fish vertebrae. More local disruption of the endplates can lead to formation of cartilaginous areas or Schmorl's nodes.

None of these morphological changes are specific for osteoporosis. Wedge-shaped vertebrae and pancake vertebrae are also seen after trauma and with vertebral metastasis. Fish vertebrae also occur in osteomalacia, Paget's disease, and hyperparathyroidism, and cartilaginous nodes are also seen in Scheuermann's disease, hyperparathyroidism, and osteochondrosis.

MAGNETIC RESONANCE IMAGING

Some basic principles must be understood in order to clarify nomenclature. In MR imaging, the protons or hydrogen nuclei present in the human body are caused to resonate, like a tuning fork, which starts to vibrate when exposed to sound waves of appropriate frequency. When a collection of protons such as the human body is placed in a magnetic field, the protons orient themselves longitudinally to the field axis, and this produces in the body a weak magnetization in the longitudinal direction. When a radiofrequency (RF) signal of appropriate strength and frequency is beamed into the body, the magnetic vector of the protons is flipped into the transverse direction and, rotating within the magnetic field, produces an RF signal emanating from the body itself. When the external RF signal has been switched off, it is possible to register the RF signals of the protons, which gradually fade out as the original conditions are restored. The latter process is known as *relaxation.* Relaxation for longitudinal magnetization vectors is different from that of transverse magnetization vectors and is influenced by the chemical composition of the tissues of which the protons are a part, as well as by interaction between protons (2).

By the correct selection of both the interval between external RF pulses [known as repetition time (TR)] and the interval between excitation and signal readout [known as echo time (TE)], various tissue characteristics can be used to produce contrast in an image. When image contrast is based on tissue differences in longitudinal relaxation, the images are called T1-weighted, and when image contrast depends on tissue differences in transverse relaxation, the images are referred to as T2-weighted.

Besides longitudinal and transverse relaxation, other tissue characteristics can be used to produce contrast in an MR image: for example, proton density, fluid movement or flow, magnetization transfer between bound and unbound protons, and molecular diffusion. This great versatility provides MR imaging with such a significant advantage over radiographic imaging techniques, which can use only a single tissue characteristic to produce image contrast: namely, electron density.

In order to localize the various groups of protons within the body and thus provide an image, local variations within the magnetic field are induced by accessory magnets or gradient coils in order to provide spatial encoding. The process of creating an MR image features a complex sequence of various types of RF pulses and gradient switches and is referred to as an MR imaging pulse sequence. A commonly used pulse sequence is the spin-echo (SE) sequence. Various additions can be made to the pulse sequence: for instance, so-called presaturation pulses can be added to selectively suppress the signal from protons in fat or in water.

MR imaging contrast media that are based on gadolinium chelates are used for various purposes, much in the same way that radiologic contrast media are applied in computed tomographic (CT) imaging. When used in combination with a T1-weighted pulse sequence, these contrast media have the effect of speeding up longitudinal relaxation, and tissues in which these contrast media accumulate take on a bright appearance in a T1-weighted image.

With regard to T1 and T2 weighting, the following characteristics can be recognized in the image:

- T1-weighted images demonstrate a bright signal from fat and a dark signal from fluids and are sometimes referred to as "fat images."
- T2-weighted images are characterized by a bright water signal and are therefore referred to as "water images."

MAGNETIC RESONANCE IMAGING OF THE SPINE

In comparison with the older radiographic examination techniques such as plain film studies, myelography, CT scanning, and CT myelography, MR imaging has proved to be a significant step forward in rapid, reliable, and noninvasive spinal imaging. The spinal cord is easily and clearly depicted, without the intradural injection of contrast media that is necessary for myelography and CT myelography. Normal and abnormal structures within the spinal cord can be distinguished by MR imaging, and this is not possible with radiographic imaging (3,4).

Aside from neuroradiological applications, MR imaging is also very effective in detecting bone marrow changes. Various features of spinal anatomy exhibit different MRI signal patterns. The spinal cord has a gray aspect and is surrounded by cerebrospinal fluid, which is dark (hypointense) on T1-weighted images and bright (hyperintense) on T2-weighted images. Nerve roots departing and entering the spinal cord pass through the fluid-filled arachnoid space and are best seen in T2-weighted images. Specialized MR myelographic sequences that are very heavily T2-weighted produce clear images of individual nerve roots. Epidural fat has a bright signal intensity in the T1-weighted image, whereas adult bone marrow, which contains up to 80% fat, is shaded light gray. Intervertebral discs are always darker than adult bone marrow in the T1-weighted image. Juvenile bone marrow, which contains only 40% fat and a higher proportion of water and protein, is much darker. In T2-weighted SE images, bone marrow is a dark gray shade. MR imaging is the most sensitive technique available for demonstrating tumor infiltration of the marrow. The fatty bone marrow is replaced by tumor tissue with a higher water content, thus producing a decrease in signal intensity in the T1-weighted image and an increase in the T2-weighted picture (Fig. 12.1).

These changes in bone marrow composition form the most sensitive sign of vertebral metastasis and are seen earlier than the increased uptake seen in spinal metastasis on the bone isotope scan. The increased isotope uptake reflects osteoblast activity—attempts to

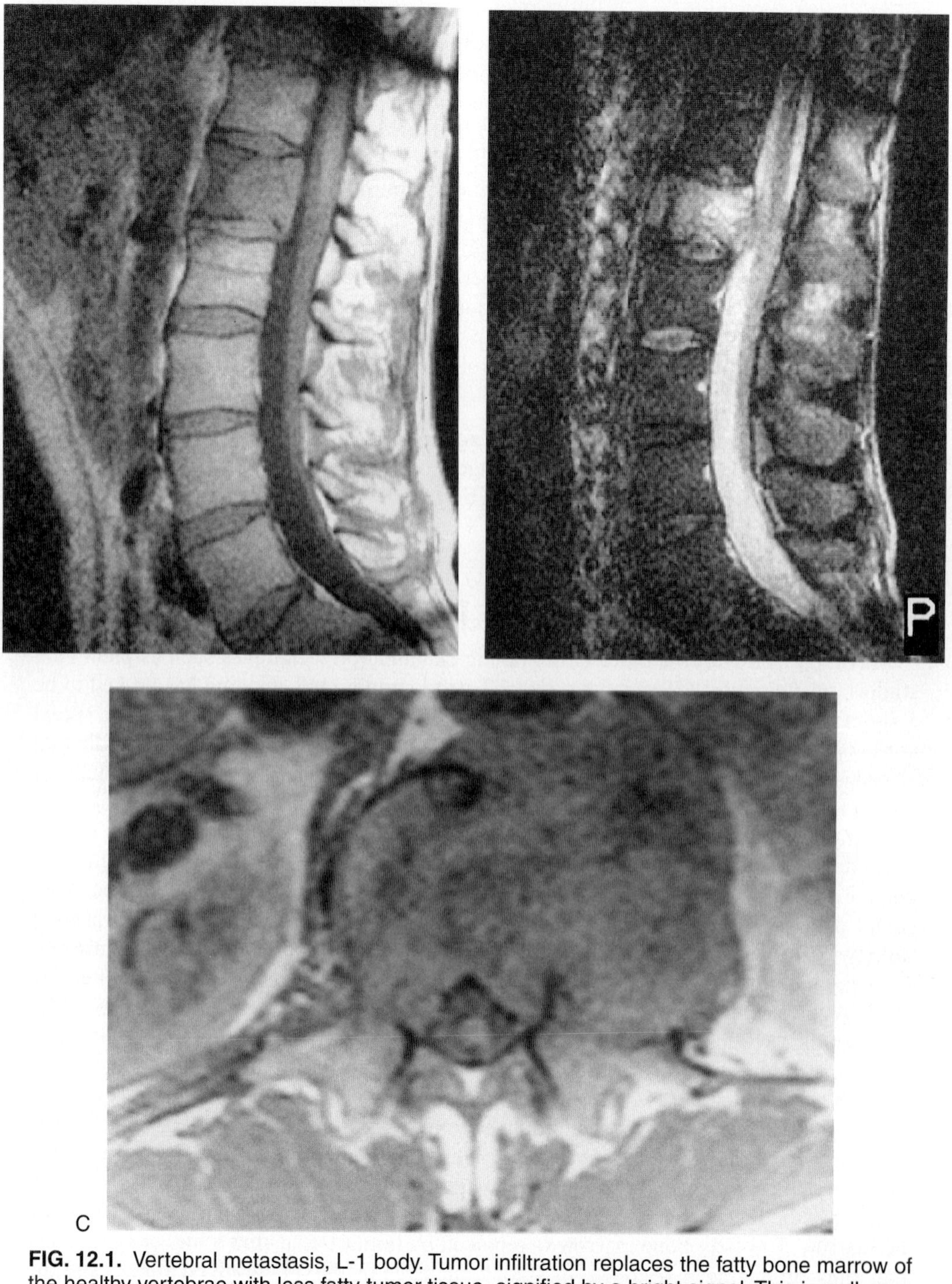

A B C

FIG. 12.1. Vertebral metastasis, L-1 body. Tumor infiltration replaces the fatty bone marrow of the healthy vertebrae with less fatty tumor tissue, signified by a bright signal. This is well seen in the T1-weighted image. **(A).** The T2-weighted image **(B)** shows that the water content of the metastatic tissue is greater than that of normal bone marrow. Note also bright water signal of cerebrospinal fluid in the dural sac and stationary blood in the basivertebral veins. T1-weighted axial image **(C)** shows "curtain sign," caused by bilateral encroachment of tumor from the vertebral body into the spinal canal. Midline encroachment is delayed by the posterior longitudinal ligament. Note also paravertebral expansion of tumor.

repair bone destruction by the tumor—which is seen only later in the course of the lesion than the subtle bone marrow changes demonstrated by MR imaging. Unfortunately, this high sensitivity for metastases is not matched by an equally high degree of specificity. The same pattern of signal change, with dark areas in the bone marrow on T1-weighted images and brighter areas in the T2-weighted pictures, is also seen in degenerative or inflammatory disease and in a fracture-hematoma.

Although the tumor can sometimes be seen to disrupt the normal anatomic confines of the vertebra, and thus reveals its presence, it is not always possible to distinguish with certainty between vertebral collapse caused by metastasis and a recent traumatic or osteoporotic vertebral fracture with a fracture-hematoma. In a later stage, when the hematoma has cleared, an osteoporotic fracture regains a normal bone marrow signal pattern on MR imaging (Fig. 12.2).

Some reports indicate that diffusion-weighted MR imaging can be useful in distinguishing between a fracture-hematoma and tumor infiltration (5). This is because diffusion characteristics of the free fluid in hematoma or edema are different from those of fluid in a collection of metastatic tumor cells.

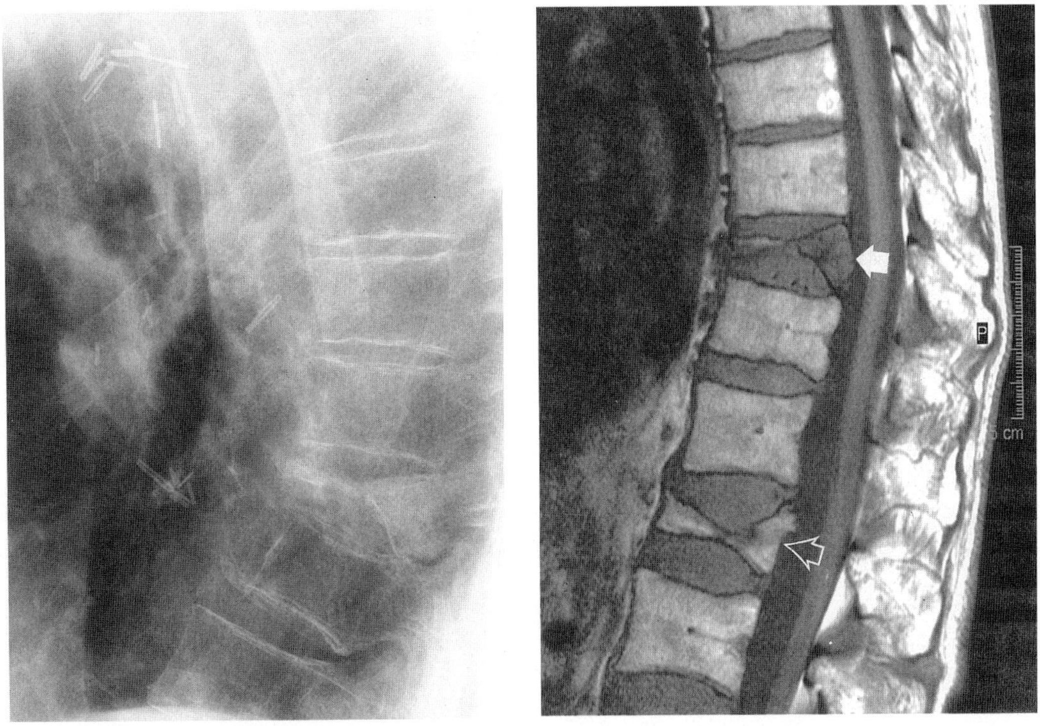

A B

FIG. 12.2. Osteoporotic or metastatic collapse? Plain film **(A)** in patient who has undergone pneumectomy for carcinoma shows a collapsed T-12 vertebra. The patient's history is indicative of metastasis, but other vertebrae show loss of bone mineral density and vertical striations, indicating osteoporosis. T1-weighted magnetic resonance image **(B)** shows loss of fat signal from the bone marrow of the collapsed T-12 vertebra (arrow). This could be caused by either metastasis or hematoma in recent osteoporotic collapse. The L-3 vertebra (open arrow) shows similar signs of collapse, probably of older date, because bone marrow has regained normal signal after dissipation of hematoma. The final diagnosis was osteoporotic collapse, confirmed by follow-up evaluation.

CONCLUSIONS

Diagnostic imaging has a limited role in patients with osteoporosis. Conventional radiographs are not useful for establishing the diagnosis of osteoporosis early in the course of the disease. Vertebral fractures can be demonstrated and monitored but not always classified with certainty as being caused by osteoporosis. MR imaging, although not useful in assessing the presence of osteoporosis, can be used in the differential diagnosis of a vertebral fracture that may be osteoporotic or caused by metastasis.

REFERENCES

1. Resnick D, Niwayama G. Osteoporosis. In: Resnick D, ed. *Diagnosis of bone and joint disorders,* 3rd ed. Philadelphia: WB Saunders, 1995.
2. Stark DD, Bradley WG. *Magnetic resonance imaging,* 2nd ed. St. Louis: Mosby—Year Book, 1992.
3. Manelfe C, ed. *Imaging of the spine and spinal cord.* New York: Raven Press, 1992.
4. Parizel PM, Wilmink JT. Imaging of the spine: techniques and indications. In: Algra PR, Valk J, Heimans JJ, eds. Diagnosis and therapy of spinal tumors. New York: Springer, 1998.
5. Baur A, Stabler A, Bruning R, et al. Diffusion-weighted MR imaging of bone marrow: differentiation of benign versus pathologic compression fractures. *Radiology* 1998;207:349–356.

13

Initial Assessment and Emergency Room Attitude in Osteoporotic Vertebral Fractures

Philippe Gillet

Orthopaedic Department, Centre Hospitalier Universitaire, B4000 Liège, Belgium

Most osteoporotic fractures of the spine are poorly symptomatic and lead to slow, progressive kyphosis of the thoracic spine and loss of lordosis of the lumbar spine, associated with progressive loss of trunk height. Episodes of pain may occur but are often tolerable, and few patients seek medical advice, especially emergency medical advice for this condition.

However, an acute pathological fracture of one or more vertebrae is accompanied by the sudden onset of disabling pain. The patient may then seek medical advice from a general practitioner or even visit an emergency department.

Vertebral osteoporotic fractures are not a benign condition; about one quarter of clinically diagnosed vertebral deformities result at one time or another in hospitalization (1). The emergency room is on occasion a starting point, through the diagnosis of a vertebral osteoporotic fracture, to initiate adequate assessment of the patient's status and adequate management of osteoporotic status, regardless of whether this condition is the prime cause of consultation. This is of particular importance to diminish the risk for further pathological fractures.

Vertebral fractures resulting from osteoporosis are not always adequately documented among hospitalized patients. In one study (2), the poor clinical recognition of this status and the inadequacy of treatment have been shown. To study the frequency with which vertebral osteoporotic fractures were effectively identified and treated by the clinicians when such a fracture was visible on radiographs, two radiologists retrospectively reviewed the chest radiographs of a group of 934 women aged 60 or older. It appeared that moderate or severe vertebral fracture could be identified in 132 patients (14.4% of the subjects) but that only 17 (1.8%) had a discharge diagnosis of vertebral fracture. For the 132 patients with a fracture, this fracture was documented in the medical record or discharge summary for only 17%, only 50% of the contemporaneous radiology reports identified the fracture, and the condition was found in only 23% of the contemporaneous radiologist's summary. The prescription of osteoporosis treatment was found in only 18% of the medical records of patients with vertebral fracture.

DIAGNOSIS: HISTORY AND CLINICAL SIGNS

Vertebral osteoporotic fracture is usually suspected in a postmenopausal woman in her 70s or older who suffers acute back pain after everyday activities or, at the most, a low-stress effort. If she has thoracic kyphosis, there is even greater suspicion of osteoporosis. Apart from this typical condition, vertebral osteoporotic fractures may occur in secondary osteoporosis, such as rheumatoid arthritis, liver disorders, steroid therapy, pregnancy, and breast-feeding (3–5). The front-line practitioner gathers early information through the patient's history and standard radiographs of the spine. Back pain is usually mid- or low-thoracic or upper lumbar. Pain may radiate anteriorly along the ribs. There may be a history of body height loss and previous back pain episodes, indicating probable earlier fractures that also led to kyphosis. A history of steroid therapy must always be sought. A history of smoking and heavy alcohol intake may indicate the risk for osteoporosis. Because a vertebral osteoporotic fracture is a fatigue or pathological fracture—that is, a fracture appearing during normal activities as a result of loss of normal bone resistance—the history usually does not include a discrete traumatic event.

Neurological symptoms are usually absent, but deficits caused by cord or root compression may exist (6).

DIAGNOSIS: IMAGING AND LABORATORY

Standard radiographs of the spine can be readily obtained. The most frequent aspects of osteoporotic spine fractures include central endplate fractures, anterior wedge fractures, and global body collapse. More life-threatening conditions must be considered for the differential diagnosis. Frequent diagnostic options are tumors, such as spinal metastasis or multiple myeloma, and spondylodiscitis. Specific standard radiographic aspects do not always exist. It is necessary to look for areas of bone destruction such as a missing pedicle on anteroposterior radiographs; this generally indicates a tumor, but ordinary central endplate fractures or wedge fractures may also occur in tumors. A complete collapse of a vertebral body and the existence of neurological signs indicate the greater probability of a tumor. In the case of spondylodiscitis, the classical image includes disc space narrowing and adjacent vertebral endplate destruction, but it must be remembered that in the initial stages, the standard radiograph often appears normal even though acute and disabling back pain may exist.

Computed tomography may be helpful for recognizing small fractures overlooked by conventional radiographs and may show areas of bone loss. Nuclear magnetic resonance (NMR) imaging is very helpful in spondylodiscitis, showing edema in the vertebral bodies adjacent to the involved disc space in the early stages and, later, any developing abscess; it may even precede signs on a technetium bone scan. NMR is also very helpful in the diagnosis of spinal tumors, especially to show the possible compromise of neurological structures.

However, for obvious reasons, computed tomography and NMR imaging are not front-line explorations, although NMR should be obtained if neurological signs are present and if the diagnosis of an infection or tumor is suspected. Such a neurological situation may decompensate fast and necessitate prompt treatment, sometimes emergency surgery.

Bone scans may be obtained to search for coexisting vertebral fractures not visible on standard radiographs; high uptake is, of course, not specific for benign fractures or lesions associated with a tumor or infection. The results must be evaluated according to the history, clinical signs, results of other imaging procedures, and laboratory findings.

Laboratory findings readily available in an emergency department are usually not specific in osteoporotic fractures. An elevated CRP level or erythrocyte sedimentation rate would be an indicator for a tumor or an infection instead, and an elevated leukocyte count would also suggest a spondylodiscitis.

THERAPEUTIC ATTITUDE ON THE FRONT LINE

Apart from pain, osteoporotic vertebral fractures rarely cause severe problems. Pain from vertebral osteoporotic fractures may be severe and last for days or weeks, but the natural history of the condition is favorable with regard to fracture healing and pain. The therapeutic challenge for the emergency practitioner or the family physician is to restore comfort. Avoidance of hospitalization is always desirable for elderly patients. Returning to their homes or to convalescent homes is usually possible with analgesics, bed rest, and sometimes a soft brace or a light Jewett corset. However, when bed rest seems unavoidable, an adequate family surrounding is necessary or, in the case of a convalescent home, the staff must be diligent in their care. Unfortunately, some convalescent homes for elderly people care for them only when they are healthy; they are not organized to take care of bedridden patients, which can lead to a multitude of everyday problems that are deleterious to the well-being of those fragile patients. Therefore, hospitalization is indicated if less than optimal condition for a safe return to the patient's usual surroundings may not be expected. If the patient with a vertebral fracture leaves the hospital, she or he and the family or nursing staff must be aware of possible complications. These include the unfavorable effect of analgesics on breathing, aside from the shallow breathing and fear of coughing that can lead to the pain itself. Such restrictions of breathing can lead to bronchial congestion and respiratory infection. Respiratory exercises should be prescribed. Analgesics may also cause urinary retention and constipation. Ileus may be the result of retroperitoneal bleeding, even in simple fractures; parenteral fluid therapy may be required, necessitating hospitalization.

Hospitalization must be also considered if the diagnosis is unclear, in order to schedule the aforementioned examinations.

If the patient leaves the hospital without a complete assessment of the osteoporotic condition, and if the disease was ignored by the patient, she or he should be urged to consult a general practitioner or, preferably, a rheumatologist or physiotherapist for adequate assessment and to initiate therapeutic measures. This is particularly important because of the risk of secondary spine fractures or hip fractures. Hip fractures in the elderly are associated with a survival rate of 15%; the excess mortality occurs mostly during the first 6 month after the fracture (1). This life-threatening condition can in some cases be avoided by the adequate management of osteoporosis, possibly recognized after a benign vertebral fracture. However, even benign spine fractures may become very badly tolerated, especially if multiple fractures occur over the time and lead the patient to a state of chronic debilitation (4,7,8).

CONCLUSIONS

Most osteoporotic vertebral spine fractures remain benign, but their effects may be largely underestimated, leading to discomfort or even debilitation. There is a risk in an overcrowded emergency department that such a condition may be overlooked; that setting, however, could be a privileged opportunity to recognize the disease and initiate proper assessment and treatment. Moreover, the emergency practitioner must not neglect the possibility of a more threatening condition such as metastasis and must be aware that secondary neurological compromise may be the result of an inadequate diagnosis. If there is doubt, hospitalization must be considered in order to obtain precise diagnosis. Hospitalization, which can be difficult in crowded wards, may also be necessary only to obtain adequate care for fragile patients with osteoporotic fracture.

REFERENCES

1. Dennison E, Cooper C. Epidemiology of osteoporotic fractures. *Hormone Res* 2000;54(Suppl 1):58–63.
2. Gehlbach SH, Bigelow C, Heimisdottir M, et al. Recognition of vertebral fracture in a clinical setting. *Osteoporos Int* 2000;11:577–582.
3. Anai T, Tomiyasu T, Arima K, et al. Pregnancy associated osteoporosis with elevated levels of circulating parathyroid hormone related protein: a report of two cases. *J Obstetr Gynaecol Res* 1999;25:63–67.
4. Hirano Y, Kishimoto H, Hagino H, et al. The change of bone mineral density in secondary osteoporosis and vertebral fracture incidence. *J Bone Joint Metab* 1999;17:119–124.
5. Smith R, Phillips AJ. Osteoporosis during pregnancy and its management. *Scand J Rheumatol Suppl* 1998;107: 66–67.
6. Heggeness MH. Spine fracture with neurological deficit in osteoporosis. *Osteoporos Int* 1993;3:215–221.
7. Lipps P. Epidemiology and predictors of fractures associated with osteoporosis. *Am J Med* 1997;103:3S–8S.
8. Nevitt MC, Ettinger B, Black DM, et al. The association of radiographically detected vertebral fractures with back pain and function: a prospective study. *Ann Intern Med* 1998;128:793–800.

14

Basis for Pharmacological Treatment

*Olof Johnell and †John A. Kanis

**Department of Orthopaedics, Malmö University Hospital, Malmö, Sweden, and †Centre for Metabolic Bone Diseases, University of Sheffield Medical School, Sheffield, United Kingdom*

Bone is a living tissue. Eighty percent of bone tissue is compact or cortical bone, as found in the diaphyses of long bones, and 20% trabecular bone as in the vertebral bodies and in long bones close to the joints. The composition of bone is 65% mineral, mainly in the form of hydroxyapatite, and 35% matrix. Of the dry weight, 90% is collagen. There are also other proteins and lipids that are important for the function of bone. The cells found in bone consist of osteoblasts, osteocytes, and osteoclasts. These cells are important because they govern the bone turnover, which occurs at a rate of 5% to 10% per year. Bone turnover is a special sequence that starts with a signal to the osteoblasts, which in turn give a signal to the osteoclasts to start resorbing bone. They resorb a pit on the surface of cancellous bone, and thereafter osteoblasts start to fill in the pit with matrix, which is later mineralized. The process is called *remodeling* and goes on throughout life. When there is an imbalance between resorption and formation, bone is lost, as in osteoporosis. This can be because resorption is increasing, as occurs in menopause, or formation is decreasing in relation to resorption, as in the very elderly. Three main hormones regulate bone resorption: parathyroid hormone (PTH), calcitriol (vitamin D), and calcitonin. Other hormones, however, are also involved. Several cytokines are involved in bone resorption, and a factor for osteoclast differentiation called receptor activator of nuclear factor κB ligand (RANKL) has been found. Another factor called osteoprotegerin has been discovered to act as a decoy receptor to RANKL, thereby inhibiting osteoclast formation. Thus, bone works as an organ. Furthermore, it can regulate plasma calcium by acting as a calcium reservoir. Bone architecture is under control of biomechanical systems that allow bone to adept its structure to function by changes in bone remodeling and fulfill its mechanical roles optimally. This explains why the trabeculae seen on radiographs are arranged according to the strain and stress put on the bone. Remodeling is thus needed to replace old bone, maybe at sites of fatigue damage by new bone with better biomechanical properties [additional reading: Kanis (1), Fleisch (2) and Official Publication of The American Society for Bone and Mineral Research (3)].

Because bone is a living tissue, it is possible for pharmacological intervention to reduce the number of fractures. The main mode of action of agents available today is to reduce resorption in bone, by affecting mainly the activity of the osteoclasts, and thereby reduce the loss of bone. Drugs that have this antiresorptive mode of action include bisphosphonates, estrogens, and selective estrogen receptor modulators (SERMs). Another potential mechanism of action is an anabolic approach, whereby agents increase the activity of osteoblasts. In the past, several drugs, including fluoride and anabolic steroids, have been tested, but there is no good evidence that treatment results in fracture reduction. The intermittent use of PTH has been shown to reduce the number of fractures in severely osteoporotic patients.

Both antiresorptive and anabolic treatments work on bone. Both treatments have interesting implications in the future for orthopedic surgeons, such as a biological approach to enhance bone incorporation in total hip and total knee replacements and maybe with spinal fusions, as well as a possibility to enhance fracture healing (4).

MEDICAL PREVENTION OF RECURRENCE OF FRACTURES

A patient with an osteoporotic fracture should be treated so as to avoid new fractures. This forms the basis for guidelines for orthopedic surgeons (5). Numerous studies have shown that patients who have sustained one osteoporotic fracture have a very high risk of sustaining another fracture. The risk has been summarized by Klotzbuecher et al. (6), who, in a meta-analysis of all studies, found that those with prevalent fractures have at least twice the risk of having a new fracture as the general population has. Furthermore, patients with osteoporotic fractures have also low bone mass, which increases the risk. Both low bone mass density (BMD) values and a history of previous fractures contribute to the risk of a new fracture.

The risk of having a new fracture is highest in the years immediately after a patient has had a fracture. This was shown by Johnell et al. (7) for clinical vertebral fracture and by Lindsay et al. (8) for vertebral deformities. Therefore, it is important to assess the fracture risk at the time of the fracture and after the acute fracture management has been provided, in order to prevent another fracture.

There are several ways to prevent recurrence of fractures. The first is life style changes, such as increased physical activities and adequate nutrition. These changes can be undertaken in large populations. However, there are very few and uncertain results from randomized controlled trials. Increased physical activity may have a moderate effect on bone mass but probably has a larger effect on muscle strength and balance. Other possibilities are training against falls and the use of hip protectors. In elderly patients, who have a notable tendency to fall, hip protectors have reduced the number of hip fractures in randomized controlled trials.

The patient with a fracture has been identified in several guidelines for treatment of osteoporosis. The American Academy of Orthopaedic Surgeons (AAOS) has started a program called "Bone up on bone loss" and has also authored an editorial on "when fracture treatment is not enough" (9). The European Foundation presented guidelines describing patients at high risk as patients with a previous fracture. The same has been done by the National Osteoporosis Foundation (NOF) in the United States (10). This organization has also highlighted fracture patients, emphasizing that patients with hip fracture and spine fracture have such a high risk for a new fracture that they could be treated independently of a BMD measurement. The Swedish Medical Product agency also recommends treating patients with osteoporotic fracture and who have a low bone density with a T score below –2.

For patients at high risk, pharmacological intervention to prevent new fractures is now possible. There are several large randomized trials with bisphosphonates, especially alendronate (11,12) and risedronate (13–15). Drug trials over 3 to 4 years have shown that bisphosphonates can reduce vertebral fractures by half and that this effect is partly a result of changes in BMD; thus, treating patients with low BMD yields a better effect than does treating patients with high BMD. In a few studies, bisphosphonates have also been shown to reduce the number of hip fractures by up to 50%. From the perspective of evidence-based medicine, the evidence that these drugs can prevent fracture in groups at high risk is strong.

In all these studies, the best cost-effective treatment—as judged by the number needed to treat (NNT)—has been in patients who in the randomized study have started with a previous vertebral fracture. In the study on alendronate by Liberman et al. (16), NNT was 18 if the patients had a previous vertebral fracture, in comparison with 100 without a previous fracture. [This was also found in the Fracture Intervention Trial (FIT) and in the study with SERMs (17).]

SERMs (17) are agents that work partly as antagonists against and partly as agonists for the estrogen receptor; they have effects similar to those of estrogen on bone and the cardiovascular system and effects opposite those of estrogen on the breast and uterus. One large study have shown that raloxifene can reduce the number of vertebral fractures by about 50% and can also reduce the incidence of breast cancer.

Estrogen (hormone replacement therapy): In randomized controlled trials, estrogen has had a good effect on bone mass. Most studies have been performed in women nearing menopause. There are few randomized controlled trials with fracture as the end point. A meta-analysis showed that there is approximately a 27% reduction of all fractures, especially in women younger than 60 years, who take estrogen (18).

Parathyroid hormone: The therapeutic use of PTH is, however, not yet approved by government agencies for the treatment of osteoporosis. One study has shown that intermittent daily PTH injections can reduce the number of vertebral fractures by more than 50%. It also decreases all nonvertebral fractures by about 50% (19).

Thus, there is good evidence that new fractures can be prevented cost effectively in patients who have already sustained vertebral fractures. This means that a patient with a vertebral fracture should, according to evidence-based medicine, also be assessed for osteoporosis after the fracture treatment has been started, to lower the risk of new fractures.

Orthopedic surgeons can start this assessment by measuring patients' BMD and then either treating the patients themselves or referring patients to a general practitioner or another physician interested in treating osteoporosis. Sevices should be organized to accomplish this, to ensure that the patients get the best treatment, not only for the fracture but also prevention of another fracture.

The pharmacological treatment to prevent osteoporosis does not compete with vertebral augmentation; instead, it should be the base treatment before the procedure.

BURDEN OF OSTEOPOROSIS

Because there is good evidence that orthopedic surgeons can assess fracture risk in osteoporosis with BMD measurements and that they can efficiently treat patients at high risk, it is important to estimate the size of the health care problem of osteoporotic fractures. The remaining lifetime risk in Malmö that a 50-year-old woman will sustain a hip fracture is 23%; a clinical spine fracture, 15%; a wrist fracture, 21%; and a shoulder fracture, 13%. The corresponding percentages for men are approximately half. These percentages are for the average population (20). The risk is at least twice as high for a patient who has already had a fracture. New osteoporotic fractures are associated with considerable mortality and morbidity. The loss of quality of life is severe in patients with hip fracture patients, especially during the first year after fracture. Sernbo and Johnell (21) found that only 50% regained their prefracture status.

Another fracture associated with high morbidity that has come to clinical attention is the clinical vertebral fracture, which reduces quality of life more extensively than previously recognized. Morphometric vertebral fractures, fractures identified on radiographs taken in a population, are also associated with reduction in quality of life, probably because affected patients have not been informed that they can be treated in the health care system and not getting any medical attention. Patients with wrist fractures have fewer problems, but about 10% have a long-standing problem with the affected arm.

The mortality rate is also increased after osteoporotic fractures (21,22). Patients with hip fractures have a very high rate of mortality after the fracture in comparison with the general population, especially after the first year. Patients with vertebral fractures also have an increased rate of mortality, whereas patients with wrist fracture do not have any increase in mortality in comparison with the general population.

COSTS

Apart from the morbidity and mortality, there is also a high cost to society for these fractures. A hip fracture is estimated to cost $15,000 to $20,000 the first year. Only a third of this cost is involved in the orthopedic care, and society has to pay a lot in the rehabilitation. New data have also shown that clinical vertebral fracture entails substantial costs. Such data can be used to calculate the cost effectiveness of treatment of osteoporosis. This chapter has shown that that it is cost effective to treat osteoporosis to prevent hip and vertebral fractures in patients at high risk, especially in those who have already had a fracture. Thus, it is important to set up programs to help patients with fractures prevent new fractures.

REFERENCES

1. Kanis JA. *Osteoporosis.* London: Blackwell Science, 1994.
2. Fleisch H. *Bisphosphonates in bone disease. From the laboratory to the patient,* 2nd ed. London: Parthenon Publishing, 1995.
3. Favus MJ, ed., for the American Society for Bone and Mineral Research. *Primer on the metabolic bone diseases and disorders of mineral metabolism,* 4th ed. Philadelphia: Lippincott Williams & Wilkins, 1999.
4. Johnell O. Orthopedic use of bisphosphonates. *Bone Depech* 2000;6:4–6.
5. Johnell O, Kannus P, Obrant KJ, et al. Management of the patient after an osteoporotic fracture. Guidelines for orthopedic surgeons—consensus conference on Treatment of Osteoporosis for Orthopedic Surgeons, Nordic Orthopedic Federation, Tampere, Finland 2000. *Acta Orthop Scand* 2001;72:325–330.
6. Klotzbuecher CM, Ross PD, Landsman PB, et al. Patients with prior fractures have an increased risk of future fractures: a summary of the literature and statistical synthesis. *J Bone Miner Res* 2000;15:721–739.
7. Johnell O, Odén A, Caulin F, et al. Acute and long-term increase in fracture risk after hospitalization for vertebral fracture. *Osteoporos Int* 2001;12:207–214.
8. Lindsay R, Silverman SL, Cooper C, et al. Risk of new vertebral fracture in the year following a fracture. *JAMA* 2001;285:320–323.
9. Tosi LL, Lane JM. Osteoporosis prevention and the orthopedic surgeon: when fracture care is not enough. *J Bone Joint Surg Am* 1998;80:1567–1569.
10. National Osteoporosis Foundation. *Physician's guide to prevention and treatment of osteoporosis.* Belle Mead, NJ: Excerpta Medica, 1998.
11. Black DM, Cummings SR, Karpf DB, et al. Randomised trial of effect of alendronate on risk of fracture in women with existing vertebral fracture. *Lancet* 1996;348:1535–1541.
12. Cummings SR, Black DM, Thompson DE, et al. Effect of alendronate on risk of fracture in women with low bone density but without vertebral fractures. *JAMA* 1998;280:2077–2082.
13. Harris ST, Wats NB, Genant HK, et al., for the VERT Study Group. Effects of risedronate treatment on vertebral and nonvertebral fractures in women with postmenopausal osteoporosis. A randomized controlled trial. *JAMA* 1999;282:1344–1352.

14. Reginster J-Y, Minne HW, Sörensen OH, et al., on behalf of the VERT Study Group. Randomized trail of the effects of risedronate on vertebral fractures in women with established postmenopausal osteoporosis. *Osteoporos Int* 2000;11:83–91.
15. McClung MR, Geusens P, Miller PD, et al., for the Hip Intervention Program Study Group. Effect of risedronate on the risk of hip fracture in elderly women. *N Engl J Med* 2001;344:333–340.
16. Liberman UA, Weiss SR, Bröll J, et al. Effect of oral alendronate on bone mineral density and the incidence of fractures in postmenopausal osteoporosis. *N Engl J Med* 1995;333:1437–1443.
17. Ettinger B, Black D, Mitlak BH, et al. Reduction of vertebral fracture risk in postmenopausal women with osteoporosis treated with raloxifene. *JAMA* 1999;282:637–645.
18. Torgerson DJ, Bell-Syer SE. Hormone replacement therapy and prevention of nonvertebral fractures: a meta-analysis of randomized trials. *JAMA* 2001;285:2909–2910.
19. Neer RM, Arnaud CD, Zanchetta JR, et al. Effect of parathyroid hormone (1-34) on fractures and bone mineral density in postmenopausal women with osteoporosis. *N Engl J Med* 2001;344:1434–1441.
20. Kanis JA, Johnell O, Odén A, et al. Long-term risk of osteoporotic fracture in Malmö. *Osteoporos Int* 2000;11:669–674.
21. Sernbo I, Johnell O. Consequences of a hip fracture: a prospective study over 1 year. *Osteoporos Int* 1993;3:148–153.
22. Center JR, Nguyen TV, Schneider D, et al. Mortality after all major types of osteoporotic fracture in men and women: an observational study. *Lancet* 1999;353:878–882.

15

Pharmacological Management of Osteoporosis

*Véronique Halkin and †Jean-Yves Reginster

**Unité d'Exploration du Métabolisme de l'Os et du Cartilage, Centre Hospitalier Universitaire de Liège, Liège, Belgium, and †Service de Santé Publique et d'Epidémiologie, Université de Liège; Centre Collaborateur Organisation Mondiale de la Santé pour les Aspects de Santé Publique des Maladies Rhumatismales, Liège; and Unité d'Exploration du Métabolisme de l'Os et du Cartilage, Centre Hospitalier Universitaire de Liège, Liège, Belgium*

Osteoporosis is characterized by a decrease in bone mass and a deterioration in skeletal microarchitecture, which lead to increased fragility and susceptibility to fractures (1). In treating established osteoporosis, the objectives are to prevent further skeletal deterioration and to improve bone mass, bone microarchitecture, or both to reduce the risk of vertebral and peripheral fractures (2).

One of the major determinants of skeletal weakness is bone loss that occurs after menopause as a consequence of an increased osteoclastic resorption, which is only partially compensated by a moderate rise in the rate of bone formation by osteoblasts (3).

Estrogens (4), selective estrogen receptor modulators (SERMs) (5), calcitonin (6,7), and bisphosphonates (8–10) are considered effective and well-tolerated agents for maintaining mineral density of trabecular and cortical bone at premenopausal levels by counteracting the exacerbated activity of osteoclasts induced by the sharp postmenopausal decrease in circulating endogenous estrogens. However, primary prevention of osteoporosis initiated in the immediate postmenopausal period is not yet considered a public health priority by specialists dealing with bone metabolic disorders, by primary care physicians, or by the general population (11). Subsequently, caregivers often face complicated situations when women consult them for the first time at later stages of the disease: namely, after the diagnosis of osteoporosis has already been made on the basis of random radiographs, densitometry measurements, or, even worse, a clinical fracture.

Promising results have been reported with inhibitors of bone resorption (12–16). Patients treated with these drugs usually achieve an increase in bone mass, which translates into a reduction in the incidence of incidental fractures in comparison with the rate observed in subjects receiving a placebo or treated with calcium alone.

None of the available medications has unequivocally demonstrated its ability to fully prevent the occurrence of new vertebral or peripheral osteoporotic fractures once the disease is established. Furthermore, some of these results are jeopardized by either potential severe toxicity (17–19) or exorbitant costs (20), both of which discourage widespread or prolonged use of these drugs. Therefore, new medications are developed in an effort to meet a better risk-to-benefit (efficacy versus tolerance) ratio in comparison with available medications.

After a review of the action of calcium, vitamin D, and hormone replacement therapy (HRT), this chapter focuses mainly on the new challenging drugs (SERMs and bisphosphonates) that contribute to a better preventive and therapeutic approach to postmenopausal osteoporosis and highlights some of the promising new agents (parathyroid peptides and strontium ranelate) for osteoporosis.

CALCIUM AND VITAMIN D

The role of calcium supplementation as a preventive measure or as a treatment for postmenopausal and senile osteoporosis has been one of the major controversies in this field since the mid-1970s (21).

Most of the discussions concerning the potential protective role of calcium on the aging skeleton were initiated by the demonstration that, in two rural communities with the same ethnic background, the incidence of hip fracture was significantly higher in a district in which calcium intake was low (around 450 mg per day) than in a district in which daily calcium intake averaged 1,200 mg per day (22). Several surveys of elderly people have shown that patients with osteoporosis took less calcium in their diet than those without osteoporosis (23,24). Some authors, in contrast, have reported that hip fractures are less common in population with low dietary intakes of calcium (25); however, there is evidence that an appropriate dietary calcium intake or a regular calcium supplementation leads to a substantial decrease in senile bone loss and fractures related to senile osteoporosis.

In a prospective study of a white population, including both genders, the age-adjusted risk of hip fracture was inversely associated with dietary calcium, whether considered as milligrams per day or as nutrient density. Men and women in the upper tertile of calcium intake (>700 mg/day) had a 60% lower hip fracture rate than did those in the lower tertile (<400 mg/day) (26). In several controlled trials, calcium supplements were used as placebo. In all these trials, bone loss was completely arrested when calcium supplements reached 1,500 mg per day. However, no formal data from controlled studies support the hypothesis that supplemental calcium alone reduces fracture rate (27).

Vitamin D levels vary with the seasons in the elderly and is lower during the winter in Europe than in both North America and Scandinavia. Oral vitamin D intake is lower in Europe that in both North America and Scandinavia. Hypovitaminosis D and related abnormalities in bone chemistry are most common in elderly residents in Europe but are reported in all elderly populations (28). The most convincing evidence of the usefulness of an association of calcium and vitamin D in prevention of hip fractures in elderly women was provided by a large prospective study that compared the effects of a daily supplementation of 800 IU of cholecalciferol and 1,200 mg of calcium on the frequency of hip fractures and other nonvertebral fractures in more than 3,000 healthy institutionalized women, whose mean age was 84 years. The number of hip fractures was 43% lower and the total number of nonvertebral fractures was 32% lower among the women treated with vitamin D_3 and calcium than among those who received a placebo (29). These results were later confirmed after an additional 18 months of treatment. At that time, the incidence of hip and nonvertebral fractures had been reduced by 27% and 28% in the women treated with calcium and vitamin D (30).

These results, however, were not confirmed by a prospective, double-blind study in which 1,916 women and 662 men, 70 years of age and older, were randomly assigned for a maximum of 3.5 years to 400 IU per day of vitamin D_3 or placebo, without calcium supplementation. The results of this study did not show a decrease in the incidence of hip and other peripheral fractures after vitamin D supplementation (31). More recently, 176 men and 213 women, aged 65 years and older, from the United States were treated for 3 years either with 500 mg of calcium and 700 IU of vitamin D_3 per day or with placebo. In this study, calcium and vitamin D moderately reduced bone loss in the femoral neck, spine, and total body and reduced the incidence of nonvertebral fractures (32).

HORMONE REPLACEMENT THERAPY

In 1941, Albright (33) reported the beneficial effects of estrogens in decreasing urinary calcium excretion and suggested that these hormones might be useful in preventing postmenopausal osteoporosis. Since then, estrogen replacement therapy (ERT) has been consistently regarded as the first choice for prevention of trabecular and cortical bone loss in postmenopausal women (34–37), notwithstanding serious controversies remaining about the cost effectiveness of treating every women at the time of menopause (38), the optimal timing for starting ERT (376), the minimal effective dose of ERT acting on bone (39), and the duration of ERT needed to prevent osteoporotic fractures (40). The effectiveness of ERT in preventing osteoporosis-related fractures is considered so indisputable that even regulatory authorities have lightened their requirement for granting marketing authorization to ERT products in postmenopausal osteoporosis, in comparison to what is currently requested for other therapeutic classes developed in this field (41,42). The demonstration of a skeletal benefit of ERT in terms of prevention of trabecular or cortical bone loss in postmenopausal women can be hardly challenged; however, in view of the numerous conclusive published studies dealing with this issue, the evidence that prolonged ERT use reduces the risk of hip fracture is somewhat equivocal. A review of all the prospective controlled trials evaluating the effect of estrogens in osteoporosis-related fractures (43) raised questions about the preferential treatment given to HRT products with regard to how much evidence is requested in order to claim antifracture efficacy at the level of the spine or the hip, in comparison with other currently developed medications. No systematic review has evaluated the effect of HRT on vertebral fracture rates. In one double-blind, randomized, controlled trial (44), 75 postmenopausal women, 47 to 75 years of age with one or more prevalent vertebral fractures, were randomly assigned to receive either transdermal HRT (17β estradiol and oral medroxyprogesterone acetate) or placebo. After 12 months, eight new fractures had occurred in seven women who received estrogen, whereas 20 had occurred in 12 women who received placebo; this finding meant a reduction of 61% of the vertebral fractures in the estrogen recipients. However, these results were based on the number of fractures per person-years (23 versus 58 per 100 person-years). When the results are expressed as the number of patients having experienced a new vertebral fracture, as recommended in regulatory guidelines (42), the difference between seven women experiencing fractures while taking HRT and 12 women who experienced fractures while taking placebo is no longer statistically significant.

In view of appropriate published studies that have demonstrated the antifracture efficacy of antiosteoporotic drugs, an open prospective, equivalence trial comparing HRT with these drugs, with spine or hip fracture reduction as the primary end point, would be valuable in scientifically validating the currently widespread dogma that HRT is to be used for life by postmenopausal women to prevent osteoporosis-related fractures.

SERMS

During the 1990s, a new family of compounds, the SERMs, emerged. SERMs are defined as compounds that produce estrogen agonism in one or more desired target tissues (e.g., bone, liver), together with estrogen antagonism and/or minimal (i.e., clinically insignificant) agonism in reproductive tissues, such as the breast or uterus (45). Raloxifene and its hydrochloride salt form are benzothiophene derivatives that were initially investigated as a treatment for advanced breast cancer (46,47). Raloxifene was also shown to inhibit the hypertrophy of the uterus in response to estrogens (48,49), to reduce serum cholesterol levels, and to increase bone mineral density (50). In light of this unique pharmacological profile, extensive investigations of raloxifene were promptly undertaken to evaluate its skeletal properties.

The Multiple Outcomes of Raloxifene Evaluation (MORE) (5) trial was designed to evaluate the effect of raloxifene on fracture incidence in 7,705 postmenopausal women with preexisting morphometric vertebral fractures or osteoporosis assessed by densitometry (T-scores >-2.5). In this 4-year randomized trial, 60 or 120 mg of raloxifene was compared with a placebo in women with a mean age of 60 years; all women received daily supplements of calcium (500 mg) and vitamin D (500 UI). In comparison with bone mineral density in the placebo recipients, bone mineral density increased after 36 months by 2.1% and 2.6% at the femoral neck and spine, respectively, in the women who took 60 mg of raloxifene and by 2.4% and 2.7% at the femoral neck and spine, respectively, in the women who took 120 mg of raloxifene ($p < 0.001$, all comparisons).

The risk for vertebral fractures detected clinically or radiographically was decreased by 30% to 50% among women treated with raloxifene for 48 months. The reduction, in comparison with findings for placebo, was statistically significant both for women with and for women without vertebral fractures at baseline. No significant reduction in non-spine fracture after 4 years was observed. Women receiving raloxifene had an increased incidence of venous thromboembolic events in comparison with the women receiving placebo, which was comparable to that reported for postmenopausal women receiving estrogen therapy or tamoxifen (51–54).

Breast cancer was significantly less frequent in the women receiving raloxifene. Raloxifene does not induce endometrial hyperplasia or endometrial carcinoma. Furthermore, it has been demonstrated that raloxifene has a rapid (after the first year) and sustained (during the fourth year) effect on bone and reduces the incidence of vertebral fractures both in women with and in women without prevalent vertebral fractures.

BISPHOSPHONATES

Bisphosphonates are potent inhibitors of bone resorption. They have been used in diseases characterized by an increase in bone turnover. Bisphosphonates may be divided in three classes. The simplest are etidronate and clodronate. Second-generation bisphosphonates are characterized by the presence of an amino group on the lateral chain; they include pamidronate, alendronate, and ibandronate. A third group is characterized by the presence of a cyclic structure on the side chain; it includes tiludronate and risedronate (55,56). This section focuses on the currently developed and marketed bisphosphonates for osteoporosis management.

Etidronate

Etidronate has been widely investigated as monotherapy for postmenopausal osteoporosis; it has been given either continuously (57) or intermittently (58). This bisphosphonate has already been used in several protocols on the basis of the concept of a "coherence therapy" of osteoporosis (59,60). Discrepant outcomes resulted from the various therapeutic regimens (57,60,61). In a multicenter North American trial (59), etidronate was administered at 400 mg per day for 14 days every 3 months for 2 years; participants were monitored for another year. The patients had sustained more than two prevalent fractures at the start of the trial, and the spinal bone mineral density (BMD) was below the 50th percentile of the distribution of BMD (17% of the population). Results revealed that the patients treated with etidronate experienced a significant reduction in the rate of vertebral fractures, in comparison with those treated with the placebo.

Alendronate

The effect of alendronate on the risk of both morphometric and clinically evident fractures was evaluated in the Fracture Intervention Trial (FIT) in postmenopausal women with (FIT1) or without (FIT2) prevalent fractures.

Two thousand twenty-seven women with at least one vertebral fracture at baseline (FIT1) were randomly assigned to receive either placebo (1005 women) or alendronate (1022 women). The initial 5-mg dose of alendronate was increased to 10 mg for each participant after 2 years for the remainder of the trial (11,62,63). Results of this 3-year trial showed a reduction in the incidence of women with new radiographic vertebral fractures by 47% and in the incidence of women with multiple (two or more) vertebral fractures by 90%, in comparison with those who received placebo (11). The incidence of hip fractures was reduced by 51%.

Reduction in fractures was also observed among the 4,432 women with low BMD but without preexisting radiographic evidence of vertebral fractures at baseline (FIT2) (63). There was a 44% reduction in the incidence of new radiographic vertebral fractures with alendronate, in comparison with placebo. In a subgroup of FIT2 concerning women with established osteoporosis (T-score < -2.5), a reduction of 56% in the incidence of hip fractures was observed.

These randomized placebo-controlled trials involving alendronate reported significant correlations between increase in BMD and reduction in new vertebral fractures (64). A further meta-analysis (65) confirmed the effects of alendronate on nonvertebral fractures and also demonstrated convincing evidence of its efficacy on hip fractures.

Esophageal erosion and ulcerative esophagitis were reported in association with the use of oral alendronate (66,67). However, careful adherence to the intake instructions, as explained in the SmPC, significantly reduces the risk of upper gastrointestinal lesions; among patients who took the drug properly, the incidence was down to the rate observed in the placebo-treated patients.

Risedronate

Risedronate was evaluated in two randomized placebo-controlled trials: called Vertebral Efficacy With Risedronate Therapy, one in North America (VERT-NA) (68) and one in Europe and Australia (VERT-MN) (69). These trials recruited women with either two or more radiographic vertebral fractures at baseline (69) or one radiographic vertebral fracture and low BMD (T-score < -2) (68). These women were randomly assigned to three groups for 3 years: in one, they received 2.5 mg of risedronate per day; in the second, 5 mg risedronate per day; and in the third, placebo. All patients also received a supplement of calcium (1 g per day) as well as vitamin D (≤500 IU daily), in case of low serum vitamin D levels at baseline.

In the U.S. trial (VERT-NA), 2,458 women were randomly assigned to these groups; the group receiving 2.5 mg of risedronate daily was discontinued after 12 months. The cumulative incidence of new radiographic vertebral fractures was 15% in the placebo group and 11% in the group taking 5 mg of risedronate per day; the latter corresponds to a 41% reduction. The cumulative incidence of nonvertebral fractures (wrist, hip, pelvis, humerus, leg, or clavicle) was reduced by 39% in the group receiving 5 mg per day (68).

In the trial conducted in Europe and Australia (VERT-MN), 1,226 women were randomly assigned to the three groups (69). The group receiving 2.5 mg/day risedronate was discontinued after 24 months. There was a 51% reduction of new vertebral fractures in the group receiving 5 mg of risedronate per day, in comparison with the placebo group. There was no significant reduction of the nonvertebral osteoporotic fractures ($p = 0.063$) (69).

The effect of risedronate on the risk of hip fracture in elderly women was studied by McClung et al. (70). Participants included (a) 5,445 women, 70 to 79 years old, who had osteoporosis and (b) 3,886 women, at least 80 years old, who had at least one nonskeletal risk factor for hip fracture or low BMD at the femoral neck. These women were randomly assigned to receive treatment with oral risedronate (2.5 or 5 mg daily) or placebo for 3 years.

Among the women aged 70 to 79 years who had a history of vertebral fracture at baseline, a 60% reduction of the risk of hip fracture associated with risedronate treatment was observed. In the other subgroups of the trial, no effect of risedronate on the reduction of hip fracture was demonstrated.

PROMISING NEW AGENTS

Parathyroid Peptides

Although secondary hyperparathyroidism resulting from decreased calcium absorption and subsequent increased bone resorption is considered a major determinant of hip fractures in the elderly, there has emerged strong evidence that parathyroid hormone (PTH) may also have an anabolic action on the skeleton (71,72).

In most studies performed with humans, the administration of PTH fragments increased axial trabecular bone mass, whereas cortical bone mass remained unchanged or even decreased (73). Studies claiming benefit with the 1-34 PTH fragment (hPTH 1-34) were conducted in the range of 400 to 800 U per day, and PTH stimulus given for a period exceeding 2 weeks resulted in increased bone mass (74,75).

Effects of hPTH 1-34 on fractures and BMD in postmenopausal women with osteoporosis have been investigated. In one study, 1,637 postmenopausal women with prior vertebral fracture received 20 or 40 μg daily of hPTH 1-34 or placebo, both administered subcutaneously. Median duration of the study was 21 months. Vertebral radiographs were obtained at baseline and at the end of the study, as were serial measurements of bone mass by dual energy x-ray absorptiometry. There was a reduction in incidental vertebral fractures of 65% and 69% in the groups of women treated with 20 and 40 μg of parathyroid hormone daily, respectively, in comparison with those receiving placebo. There was a diminution in nonvertebral fractures of 53% among the patients treated with 20 μg of parathyroid hormone daily, in comparison with those receiving placebo (76).

Strontium Ranelate

Strontium is a trace element proposed for the treatment of osteoporosis in the mid-1960s. The effects of stable strontium on bone metabolism are highly dependent on the dose used. Oral strontium administration in rats increases the amount of osteoid and the trabecular bone volume at low dosages that do not affect bone mineralization (77). Short-term treatment with low-dosage strontium transiently reduces osteoclastic activity, and longer term strontium supplementation induces a significant stimulation of bone formation and a positive trabecular balance (78). Strontium supplementation exhibits effects at both trabecular and cortical bone levels in rats supplemented with calcium. In these animals, treatment with a low dosage of strontium increased the number of bone-forming sites and vertebral bone volume but did not have a detectable adverse effect on the mineral profile, bone mineral chemistry, or bone matrix mineralization (79). In male monkeys, strontium administration did not induce major modifications of bone mineral at the crystal level (80); this result was supported by the demonstration of a positive correlation between vertebral bone mass and bone strength in rats treated for 2 years with strontium ranelate (81). Prolonged (2-year) administration of 2 g of strontium ranelate daily to postmenopausal osteoporotic women resulted in a decoupling between bone resorption (decrease in collagen crosslinks excretion) and bone formation (increase in bone-specific alkaline phosphatase), yielding a significant increase in the lumbar spine bone mineral density of treated subjects (82). During the second year of this study, the incidence of new vertebral fractures was significantly reduced in women receiving 2 g of strontium ranelate daily, in comparison with those receiving placebo (82).

In a double-blind, placebo-controlled, dose-finding study, 1 g of strontium ranelate per day was given to women in the early postmenopausal period who had no prevalent osteoporosis. This dosage induced a significant increase in spine and hip BMD. This effect was mediated by an increase in bone-specific serum alkaline phosphatase levels, which reflected a stimulatory action on bone formation. Frequency and distribution of adverse reactions were similar in strontium ranelate and placebo-treated patients (83).

CONCLUSIONS

Among the antiresorptive medications, the bisphosphonates (alendronate and risedronate) and the SERM raloxifene reduce incidental vertebral fractures rates. Alendronate and risedronate also show efficacy against nonvertebral fractures, but only alendronate has demonstrated consistent efficacy against hip fracture.

New agents, aiming at a fast increase in bone mineral content and a subsequent drastic reduction of incidental fractures, both at the spine and at the appendicular skeleton, focus on the stimulation of osteoblastic formation. hPTH 1-34, subcutaneous administrated, has a fast anabolic action on the skeleton and results in a significant reduction on spinal and paravertebral fractures. Strontium ranelate, with its ability to uncouple bone formation (which is stimulated) from bone resorption (which is decreased), is very promising. Long-term studies involving osteoporotic patients will assess its real value in comparison with that of currently marketed competitors.

REFERENCES

1. Reginster JY. *Osteoporose postménopausique: traitement prophylactique.* Paris: Masson, 1993.
2. Kaufman JM, Devogelaer JP, Raeman F, et al. Prevention and treatment of postmenopausal osteoporosis. National consensus of the "Belgian Bone Club," November 1996. *Clin Rheumatol* 1997;16:343–345.
3. Meunier PJ, Slosman D, Delmas PD, et al. The strontium salt S-12911: a new candidate for the treatment of osteoporosis. *Osteoporos Int* 1996;6:S241.
4. Christiansen C, Lindsay R. Estrogens, bone loss and preservation. *Osteoporos Int* 1991;1:714.
5. Ettinger B, Black D, Mitlak BH, et al. Reduction of vertebral fracture risk in postmenopausal women with osteoporosis treated with raloxifene. *JAMA* 1999;282:637–645.

6. Reginster JY, Denis D, Albert A, et al. 1-year controlled randomised trial of prevention of early postmenopausal bone loss by intranasal calcitonin. *Lancet* 1987;2:1481–1483.
7. Reginster JY, Jupsin I, Deroisy R, et al. Prevention of postmenopausal bone loss by rectal calcitonin. *Calcif Tissue Int* 1995;56:539–542.
8. Hosking DJ, McClung MR, Ravn P, et al. Alendronate in the prevention of osteoporosis: EPIC study two-year results. *J Bone Miner Res* 1996;11S1:133.
9. Mortensen L, Bekker P, Ouweland FVD, et al. Prevention of early postmenopausal bone loss by risedronate: a two-year study. *J Bone Miner Res* 1995;10S1:140.
10. Reginster JY, Lecart MP, Deroisy R, et al. Prevention of postmenopausal bone loss by tiludronate. *Lancet* 1989;2: 1469–1471.
11. Reginster JY, Deroisy R, Lecart MP, et al. Prévention de l'ostéoporose à Liège: le PIGEPS dix ans plus tard. *Santé Publique* 1996;2:139–150.
12. Black DM, Cummings SR, Karpf DB, et al. Randomised trial of effect of alendronate on risk of fracture in women with existing vertebral fractures. *Lancet* 1996;348:1535–1541.
13. Jensen GF, Christiansen C, Transbol I. Fracture frequency and bone preservation in postmenopausal women treated with estrogen. *Obstet Gynecol* 1982;60:493–496.
14. Liberman U, Weiss SR, Broll J, et al. Effect of oral alendronate on bone mineral density and the incidence of fractures in postmenopausal osteoporosis. *N Engl J Med* 1995;333:1437–1443.
15. Overgaard K, Hansen MA, Jensen SB, et al. Effect of salcatonin given intranasally on bone mass and fracture rates in established osteoporosis: a dose-response study. *BMJ* 1992;305:556–561.
16. Watts NB, Harris ST, Genant HK, et al. Intermittent cyclical etidronate treatment of postmenopausal osteoporosis. *N Engl J Med* 1990;323:73–79.
17. Axelrod DW, Teitelbaum SL. Results of long-term cyclical etidronate therapy: bone histomorphometry and clinical correlates. *J Bone Miner Res* 1994;9S1:136.
18. Beresford SA, Weiss NS, Voigt F, et al. Risk of endometrial cancer in relation to use of oestrogen combined with cyclic progestagen therapy in postmenopausal women. *Lancet* 1997;349:458–461.
19. Bergkvist L, Adami HO, Persson I, et al. The risk of breast cancer after estrogen-progestin replacement. *N Engl J Med* 1989;321:293–297.
20. Reginster JY. Calcitonin for prevention and treatment of osteoporosis. *Am J Med* 1993;95:44–47.
21. Reginster JY. Treatment of bone in elderly subjects: calcium, vitamin D, fluor, bisphosphonates, calcitonin. *Horm Res* 1995;43:83–88.
22. Matkovic V, Kostial K, Simonovic I, et al. Bone status and fracture rates in two regions of Yugoslavia. *Am J Clin Nutr* 1979;32:540–549.
23. Nordin BEC. Calcium balance and calcium requirement in spinal osteoporosis. *Am J Clin Nutr* 1962;10: 384–390.
24. Riggs BL, Kelly PJ, Kinney VR, et al. Calcium deficiency and osteoporosis: observations in one hundred sixty six patients and critical review of the literature. *J Bone Joint Surg Am* 1967;49:915–924.
25. Kanis JA, Passmore R. Calcium and osteoporosis. *J Nutr* 1986;116:2316–2319.
26. Holbrook TL, Barett-Connor E, Wingard DL. Dietary calcium and risk of hip fracture: 14-year prospective population study. *Lancet* 1988;2:1046–1049.
27. Heaney RP. Calcium in the prevention and treatment of osteoporosis. *J Int Med* 1992;231:169–180.
28. Lester E, Skinner RK, Foo AY, et al. Serum 25-hydroxy-vitamin D levels and vitamin D intake in healthy young adults in Britain and Denmark. *Scand J Clin Lab Med Invest* 1980;40:145–150.
29. Chapuy M, Arlot M, Duboeuf F, et al. Vitamin D3 and calcium to prevent hip fractures in elderly women. *N Engl J Med* 1992;327:1637–1642.
30. Chapuy MC, Arlot ME, Delmas PD, et al. Effect of calcium and cholecalciferol treatment for three years on hip fractures in elderly women. *BMJ* 1994;308:1081–1082.
31. Lips P, Graafmans WC, Ooms ME, et al. Vitamin D supplementation and fracture incidence in elderly persons. *Ann Intern Med* 1996;124:400–406.
32. Dawson-Hugues B, Harris SS, Krall A, et al. Effect of calcium and vitamin D supplementation on bone density in men and women 65 years of age or older. *New Engl J Med* 1997;337:670–676.
33. Albright F. Postmenopausal osteoporosis. *JAMA* 1941;116:2465.
34. Rosen CJ, Kessenich CR. The pathophysiology and treatment of postmenopausal osteoporosis. An evidence-based approach to estrogen replacement therapy. *Endocrinol Metab Clin North Am* 1997;26:295–311.
35. Eastell R. Treatment of postmenopausal osteoporosis. *N Engl J Med* 1998;338:736–746.
36. Lindsay R. Estrogen therapy in the prevention and management of osteoporosis. *Am J Obstet Gynecol* 1987;156: 1347–1351.
37. Ott S. Estrogen therapy for osteoporosis—even in the elderly. *Ann Intern Med* 1992;117:85–86.
38. Tosteson ANA, Rosenthal DI, Melton LJ, et al. Cost effectiveness of screening perimenopausal white women for osteoporosis: bone densitometry and hormone replacement therapy. *Ann Intern Med* 1990;113:594–603.
39. Genant HK, Lucas J, Weiss S, et al. Low-dose esterified estrogen therapy. *Arch Intern Med* 1997;157:2609–2615.
40. Cauley JA, Seeley DG, Ensrud K, et al. Estrogen replacement therapy and fractures in older women. *Ann Intern Med* 1995;122:9–16.
41. Guidelines for preclinical and clinical evaluation of agents used in the prevention or treatment of postmenopausal osteoporosis, April, 1994. In Food and Drug Administration: *Good guidance practices.* February 1997.

42. Committee for Proprietary Medicinal Products. Note for guidance on involutional osteoporosis in women. (CPMP/EWP/552/95.) Released at the meeting of the European Agency for the Evaluation of Medicinal Products, Human Medicines Evaluation Unit, November 19–20, 1996.
43. Reginster JY, Bruyere O, Audran M, et al (On behalf of the Group for the Respect of Ethics and Excellence in Science—GREES). Do estrogens effectively prevent osteoporosis-related fractures? *Calcif Tissue Int* 2000;67: 191–194.
44. Lufkin E, Wahner H, O'Fallon W, et al. Treatment of postmenopausal osteoporosis with transdermal estrogen. *Ann Intern Med* 1992;117:1–9.
45. Kaufmann RF, Bryant HU. Effective therapeutic management of the postmenopausal state will be a cornerstone in strategies for preserving or improving women's health in the 21st century. Selective estrogen receptor modulators. *Drugs New Perspect* 1995;8:531–539.
46. Grady D, Gebretsadik T, Kerlikowske K, et al. Hormone replacement therapy and endometrial cancer risk: a meta-analysis. *Obstet Gynecol* 1995;85:304–313.
47. Hol T, Cox MB, Bryant HU, et al. Selective estrogen receptor modulators and postmenopausal women's health. *J Womens Health* 1997;6:523–530.
48. Black LJ, Sato M, Rowley ER, et al. Raloxifene (LY139481) prevents bone loss and reduces serum cholesterol without causing uterine hypertrophy in ovariectomized rats. *J Clin Invest* 1994;93:63–69.
49. Black LJ, Jones CD, Facone JR. Antagonism of estrogen action with a new benzothiophene derived antiestrogen. *Life Sci* 1993;32:1031–1036.
50. Delmas PD, Bjarnasson NH, Mitlak BH, et al. Effects of raloxifene on bone mineral density, serum cholesterol concentrations, and uterine endometrium in postmenopausal women. *N Engl J Med* 1997;337:1641–1647.
51. Hulley S, Grady D, Bush T, et al., for the Heart and Estrogen/Progestin Replacement Study (HERS) Research Group. Randomized trial of estrogen plus progestin for secondary prevention of coronary heart disease in postmenopausal women. *JAMA* 1998;280:605–613.
52. Daly E, Vessey MP, Hawkins MM, et al. Risk of venous thromboembolism in users of hormone replacement therapy. *Lancet* 1996;348:977–980.
53. Perez-Gutthann S, Garcia-Rodriguez LA, Castellisague J, et al. Hormone replacement therapy and risk of venous thromboembolism: a population based case control study. *BMJ* 1997;314:796–800.
54. Fischer B, Costantino JP, Wickerham DL, et al. Tamoxifen for prevention of breast cancer: report of the National Surgical Adjuvant Breast and Bowel Project P-1 Study. *J Natl Cancer Inst* 1998;90:1371–1388.
55. Reginster JY, Gosset C, Fraikin G. Bisphosphonates for the treatment of osteoporosis. In: Meunier PJ, ed. *Osteoporosis: diagnosis and management.* London: Martin Dunitz, Ltd., 1998.
56. Reginster JY, Halkin V, Gosset C, et al. The role of bisphosphonates in the treatment of osteoporosis. *Drugs Today* 1997;33:563–570.
57. Heaney RP, Saville PD. Etidronate disodium in postmenopausal osteoporosis. *Clin Pharmacol Ther* 1976;20: 593–604.
58. Storm T, Thamsborg G, Steinich T, et al. Effect of intermittent cyclical etidronate therapy on bone mass and fracture rate in women with postmenopausal osteoporosis. *N Engl J Med* 1990;322:1265–1271.
59. Watts NB, Harris ST, Genant HK, et al. Intermittent cyclical etidronate treatment of postmenopausal osteoporosis. *N Engl J Med* 1990;323:73–79.
60. Pacifici R, MacMurtry C, Vered I, et al. Coherence therapy does not prevent axial bone loss in osteoporotic women: a preliminary comparative study. *J Clin Endocrinol Metab* 1988;6:747–753.
61. Smith ML, Fogelman I, Hart DM, et al. Effect of etidronate disodium on bone turnover following surgical menopause. *Calcif Tissue Int* 1989;44:74–79.
62. Black DM, Reiss TF, Nevitt MC, et al. Design of the Fracture Intervention Trial. *Osteoporos Int* 1993;3(Suppl 3):S29–S39.
63. Cumming SR, Black DM, Thompson DE, et al. Effect of alendronate on risk of fracture in women with low bone density but without vertebral fractures: results from the Fracture Intervention Trial. *JAMA* 1998;280:2077–2082.
64. Hochberg MC, Ross PD, Black DM, et al. Larger increases in bone mineral density during alendronate therapy are associated with a lower risk of new vertebral fractures in women with postmenopausal osteoporosis. *Arthritis Rheum* 1999;42(6):1246–1254.
65. Karpf DB, Shapiro DR, Seeman E, et al. Prevention of non-vertebral fractures by alendronate: a meta-analysis. *JAMA* 1997;277:1159–1164.
66. De Groen PC, Lubbe DF, Hirsch LJ, et al. Esophagitis associated with the use of alendronate. *N Engl J Med* 1996;335:1016–1021.
67. Maconi G, Porro GB. Multiple ulcerative esophagitis caused by alendronate. *Am J Gastroenterol* 1995;90: 1889–1890.
68. Harris ST, Watts NB, Genant HK, et al. Effects of risedronate treatment on vertebral and nonvertebral fractures in women with postmenopausal osteoporosis. *JAMA* 1999;282:1344–1352.
69. Reginster JY, Minne HW, Sorensen OH, et al. Randomized trial of the effects of risedronate on vertebral fractures in women with established postmenopausal osteoporosis. *Osteoporos Int* 2000;11:83–91.
70. McClung MR, Geusens P, Miller PD, et al. Effect of risedronate on the risk of hip fracture in elderly women. *N Engl J Med* 2001;344:333–340.
71. Dempster DW, Cosman F, Parisien M, et al. Anabolic actions of parathyroid hormone on bone. *Endocrinol Rev* 1993;14:690–709.

72. Pugsley LI, Selye H. The histological changes in the bone responsible for the action of parathyroid hormone on the calcium metabolism of the rat. *J Physiol (Lond)* 1993;79:113–117.
73. Eriksen EF, Melsen F, Mosekilde L. Drug therapy: formation-stimulating regimens. In: Riggs BL, Melton LJ III, eds. *Osteoporosis: etiology, diagnosis and management.* Philadelphia: Lippincott-Raven, 1995:403–434.
74. Reeve J, Arlot ME, Price TR, et al. Periodic courses of human 1-34 parathyroid peptide alternating with calcitriol paradoxically reduce bone remodeling in spinal osteoporosis. *Eur J Clin Invest* 1987;17:421–428.
75. Slovick DM, Neer RM, Potts JT. Short-term effects of synthetic human parathyroid hormone (1-34) administration on bone mineral metabolism in osteoporotic patients. *J Clin Invest* 1981;68:1261–1271.
76. Neer RM, Arnaud CD, Zanchetta JR, et al. Effect of parathyroid hormone (1-34) on fractures and bone mineral density in postmenopausal women with osteoporosis. *N Engl J Med* 2001;344:1434–1441.
77. Marie PJ, Garbat MT, Hott M, et al. Effect of low doses of stable strontium on bone metabolism in rats. *Miner Electrolyte Metab* 1985;11:5–113.
78. Marie PJ, Hott M. Short-term effects of fluoride and strontium on bone formation and resorption in the mouse. *Metabolism* 1986;35:547–551.
79. Grynpas MD, Hamilton E, Cheung R, et al. Strontium increases vertebral bone volume in rats at a low dose that does not induce detectable mineralization defect. *Bone* 1996;18:253–259.
80. Boivin G, Deloffre P, Perrat B, et al. Strontium (Sr) distribution and interreactions with bone mineral in male monkey iliac bone after strontium salt (S12911) administration. *Osteoporos Int* 1996;6:251.
81. Amman P, Rizzoli R, Deloffre P, et al. The increase in vertebral bone mass induced in intact rats by long-term administration of the strontium salt S-12911 is directly correlated with vertebral bone strength. *Osteoporos Int* 1996;6:259.
82. Reginster JY, Slosman DO, Delmas PD, et al. Strontium ranelate: dose-dependent effects in postmenopausal osteoporosis: the STRATOS 2-year randomized trial. *Clin Rheumatol* 2001;20:427–428.
83. Reginster JY, Roux C, Tsouderos Y, et al. Role of the strontium ranelate in the prevention of early post-menopausal bone loss: a double-blind, prospective, randomized, placebo-controlled study. *Arthritis Rheum* 1998; 41(S):580.

16

Osteoporosis, Physical Activity, Exercise, and Recommendations

Angela Maria Lis and Margareta Nordin

Occupational and Industrial Orthopaedic Center (OIOC), Hospital for Joint Diseases, Mount Sinai New York University Health Program of Ergonomics and Biomechanics, Graduate School of Arts and Science, New York University, New York, New York

Osteoporosis is a skeletal disorder characterized by a reduction of bone strength, which predisposes a person to an increased risk of fracture (1). The consequent changes in bone mass density and the microarchitectural deterioration of the bone tissue results in an alteration of the biomechanical response, making the bone more susceptible to stress and strain and increasing the risk for fractures.

Osteoporosis can be classified as primary or secondary. Primary osteoporosis occurs indiscriminately, regardless of gender, race, or age. However, its prevalence is noticeably higher in white postmenopausal women. Secondary osteoporosis is a direct result of medications, various medical conditions, or disease processes (1).

Currently, osteoporosis is understood to be a major health problem worldwide. The incidence of osteoporotic fractures has increased in association with a prolonged life expectancy and indications for changes in either bone quality or lifestyle from generation to generation. The rates of bone loss in untreated postmenopausal women 3 to 5 years after menopause are 4.5% per year of spinal trabecular mineral density and approximately 1% per year of lumbar bone mineral density (BMD) (2,3). White non-Hispanic women's low bone density has been recognized as one of the most important risk factors for osteoporotic fractures, which lead to financial, physical, and psychosocial consequences that significantly affect the individual as well as the family and the community. Although osteoporosis also occurs in men, most cases are found in women (1,4).

Researchers have focused their attention primarily on finding risk factors associated with primary osteoporosis. However, early prevention with feasible and successful interventions is equally important. There is evidence that physical activity and exercise are beneficial for the skeleton. Exercise has been promoted largely as a successful intervention to preserve skeletal health. Exercise for patients with osteoporosis has been associated with the reduction of age-associated osteoporotic fractures. The mechanisms by which exercise may affect the osteoporotic process are not clearly understood. However, studies have shown that the effects of exercise slow the process of BMD loss (5–7).

There is evidence that genetic factors play a major role in the determination of the peak bone mass in young adults, accounting for up to 80% of the variance (8,9). However, 20% or more of the variance in peak bone mass may be accounted for by environmental factors such as physical activity, smoking, nutrition, and calcium intake, among others.

Välimäki et al. (10) completed a prospective study to determine several independent predictors of BMD in young adults at the femoral neck and lumbar spine. Their results suggested that regular exercise, optimal calcium intake, and avoidance of smoking were important factors in achieving maximal peak bone mass in young adults. Furthermore, peak bone mass in early adulthood has been found to be an important determinant of bone mass later in life (11).

Sufficient exercise during childhood and continuation during adolescence is more effective for increasing bone mass and strength than exercise during adulthood alone (12). Childhood represents a unique opportunity to increase bone density and to modify skeletal dimensions and architecture in response to mechanical loads. Vigorous exercise during growth years may increase the accumulation of bone (13).

Gravitational and/or mechanical loading of the skeleton has been recognized as essential for maintaining bone mass over time (14). The relationship between mechanical loading and bone mass is curvilinear, with a much steeper slope at low levels of loading (Fig. 16.1) (13). In fact, an absence of a mechanical load on the skeleton, as occurs with complete immobilization, lead to a rapid decrease in BMD (14–16). Immobilized patients may lose up to 40% of their original bone mass in 1 year. Studies of bed rest indicate that standing upright for as little as 30 minutes each day prevents bone loss (13). It is there-

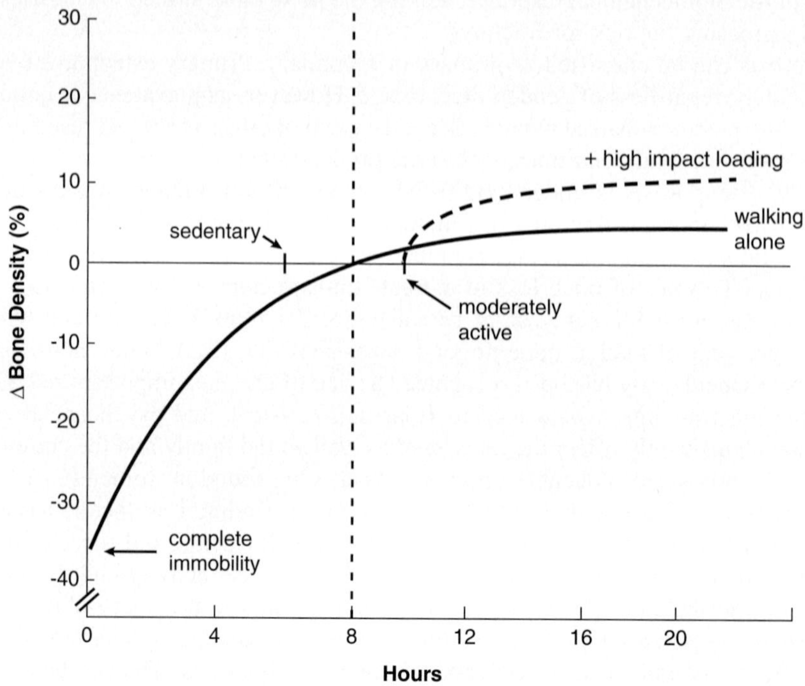

FIG. 16.1. The curvilinear nature of skeletal response. In an already ambulatory subject, the effect of immobility on bone mass is far greater than that of adding additional walking. Providing a higher intensity stimulus is more effective than simply extending the duration of ordinary loading activity. Ordinary activity, as shown by the region between sedentary and moderately active, is performed by most people and is characterized by a relatively modest dose-response slope. (From Marcus R. Role of exercises in preventing and treating osteoporosis. *Osteoporosis* 2000;27:135.)

fore logical to suggest that physical activity or exercise may be one way to prevent osteoporosis, aside from the multiple positive healthy effects that exercise confers.

THEORETICAL MODEL

The assumption that bone is capable of responding to changes to its mechanical loading environment by altering its density distribution is acknowledged (4). This mechanical adaptation is carried out primarily by cellular mechanisms of modeling and remodeling. In fact, movement and the mechanical loads that it produces presumably create a stimulus for bone adaptation, and yet this quantitative influence is still debated.

The response of bone to mechanical loading is immediate, is specific to the bone under load, and involves both cellular and tissue reactions. When a load is applied to the bone, it suffers a temporary deformation. The extent of that deformation is measured as strain. A cascade of cellular events occurs in response to changes in bone strain, reflecting an adaptation to the imposed loading environment.

Frost (17) proposed that bone appears to respond in different ways, depending on the relationship between the strain produced and the strain threshold of the bone under load. The strain model proposed by Frost suggests that bone has two separate strain ranges for its mechanically controlled modeling and remodeling. The strain level for mechanically controlled bone modeling is high (1500 to 3000 microstrain). Strain values higher than this threshold increase bone mass by increasing cortical bone apposition (causing an increase in cortical thickness and cross-sectional area). In contrast, the strain levels for the mechanically controlled bone remodeling are very low (100 to 300 microstrain). Stress levels over this threshold depress bone remodeling (activation frequency) and thereby preserve bone tissue; however, strain levels under this threshold increase activation frequency, and bone mass is lost, as occurs during prolonged bed rest (18). In conclusion, bone strains exceeding the minimum strain threshold for modeling result in a net increase of bone mass. Strains below the minimum effective threshold for remodeling result in an increase in remodeling and a net decrease in bone mass. At the same time, strain values between these thresholds result in no net change in bone mass.

Exercise intended to be osteogenic should therefore provide increased or unusual bone loading and should target specific areas that may suffer strain rates above the minimum threshold for modeling under physiological conditions. The evidence suggests that the bone-enhancing effect of exercise is through muscle contraction and mechanical loading, which cause strain or changes in the bone structure (16). However, the most effective exercise at different points of life in order to prevent and decrease the risk of osteoporotic fractures is still unclear. Greendale et al. (19) conducted a large study on an elderly population to find the relation between leisure time physical activity, BMD, and osteoporotic fractures. There was some bias in the results because they were based on self-reported activity levels at the time of questioning and three other periods in the past. The study clearly suggested a dose-response relationship between current levels of exercise and higher levels of BMD at the hip. It also indicated that the effects of exercise earlier in life may be sustained only if the exercise is maintained and that, on average, persons in higher tertiles of lifetime activity would have relatively higher consistent lifetime patterns of exercise.

The threshold of exercise level for benefit in BMD is still unclear. Results of cross-sectional and retrospective studies support the notion that elite athletes and other people who perform habitual exercises have increased bone density in relation to age-matched sedentary people (20,21). Athletes may have 10% to 40% greater bone mass or bone density than do sedentary persons of the same age, although the magnitude of this difference probably depends on the type and intensity of exercise; on the age, sex, and hormonal status of the individual; and on the number of years spent training (4,20). Bone sites that undergo mechanical loading during exercise are likely to show the greatest gains in bone density. Nevertheless, cross-sectional comparisons and retrospective studies must be interpreted with caution. The evidence does not reflect a temporal relationship, and thus the causal relationship and dose-response cannot be well established.

Layne and Nelson (22) conducted a literature review to find the association between progressive resistance training and bone density. They carefully reviewed nine cross-sectional studies that suggested a positive association between strength training exercises and increased bone density. Their literature review proposed that mechanical load applied to the bone through muscle and tendons have a direct effect on bone formation and remodeling. Taafe et al. (21) compared the bone effects of swimming versus weight-bearing activities on BMD of eumenorrheic athletes. Three groups were compared: gymnasts, swimmers, and nonathletic controls. The results showed that intensive weight-bearing activities such as gymnastics are powerful osteogenic stimuli and that long-term, non–weight-bearing activities such as swimming confer no beneficial effect on bone mass. In fact, for activities that did not involve weight bearing, such as swimming, even if they included muscle resistance, there was a reduction in bone mass, despite a higher level of activity, in comparison to the control group.

Kelley (23), however, found different implications in 1998 in a meta-analytic review of randomized trials to examine the effects of exercise in postmenopausal women. After subgroup and correlation analysis, the author concluded that exercise may slow the rate of bone loss in postmenopausal women. Up until then, there had been strong evidence that physical activity early in life contributes to higher peak bone mass. Evidence indicates that resistance and high-impact exercises are likely to produce a site-specific effect in BMD (23). However, there are no clear age-related recommendations in terms of type of exercise, or their intensity, duration, and frequency.

This chapter reviews current evidence regarding exercise for the maximization and maintenance of bone strength and provides recommendations of exercise for skeletal health for patients with or without bone fragility.

METHOD

A literature search of the Internet was performed through MEDLINE. The following keywords were used either alone or in various combinations for computer searches: "osteoporosis," "bone mineral density," "bone," "exercise," and "physical activity." Studies that include exercise as the primary intervention were included. Abstracts were reviewed, and only randomized controlled trials or prospective studies conducted after 1990 were included. Those that did not report BMD measures were excluded, as were those that did not have a comparison control group. Meta-analyses and review papers were also included for the presentation of the results and discussion session.

RESULTS

Fourteen studies were included and carefully reviewed (2,5–7,24–33). They are presented in Table 16.1 and Table 16.2. Table 16.1 includes only those with randomized control trial (RCT) design, and Table 16.2 includes nonrandomized prospective studies.

TABLE 16.1. *Randomized controlled trials*

Authors	Sample study groups	Follow-up	Inclusion criteria	Outcomes measured	Training program	Compliance	Results
Prince et al., 1991[7]	Exercise (*n* = 41) Exercise + calcium (*n* = 39) Exercise + estrogen replacement (*n* = 40) Control (*n* = 42)	2 years	Women 1–10 years postmenopause No smokers No hormone replacement therapy Bone density ≥290 mg/cm^2 (exercise groups) Bone density <290 mg/cm^2 (control group)	BMD: Vertebral Forearm: distal, medial, proximal	Supervised 1-hour weekly low-impact aerobic exercise class and 30 minutes of brisk walking twice per week (minimum: 10 classes in a 12-week period)	<50%	Increased BMD in all measures (slowing bone loss) in exercise + calcium and exercise + estrogen groups in comparison with control and exercise group*
Grove and Londeree, 1992[27]	High-impact exercise (*n* = 5) Low-impact exercise (*n* = 5) Control group (*n* = 5)	6 months/1 year	Early-postmenopausal women with hormone estrogen replacement therapy	BMD: Region of L-2 to L-4	Supervised strengthening/flexibility program three times per week	90%	Control group: linear decrease in BMD*
Nelson et al., 1994[6]	Exercise (*n* = 20) Control (*n* = 10)	1 year	Postmenopausal women without medication that affects bone metabolism	BMD: Region of L-2 to L-4 Femoral neck Total body mineral content	Exercise group: high-intensity strength training (machines, three sets eight rep) 2 days per week, 52 weeks	85.5% ± 1.8%	Increased BMD at FN and LS* in the exercise group in comparison with controls. Total body mineral content was preserved in the exercise group Decreased BMD in control group*
Hatori et al., 1993[28]	Moderate exercise level (*n* = 9) High exercise level (*n* = 12) Control (*n* = 12)	7 months	Postmenopausal women with no hormone replacement therapy or calcium supplementation	BMD: L-2 to L-4 vertebrae	30 minutes three times per week High level: walking above anaerobic threshold Moderate level: walking below anaerobic threshold	94%	Increased BMD at L-2 to L-4 level for the high exercise level group* No significant differences* between control and moderate exercise groups
Prince et al., 1995[31]	Placebo (*n* = 42) Milk powder (*n* = 42) Calcium tablets (*n* = 42) Calcium tablets and exercise (*n* = 42)	2 years	Women 10 or more years postmenopause without any hormone replacement therapy	BMD: Region of L-1 to L-4 Distal tibia/fibula Femor: neck, trochanter, intertrochanter	Supervised weight-bearing exercise, 4 hours per week	39%	Increased BMD at trochanter, intertrochanter, and ultradistal ankle site of all groups in relation to placebo group* Increased BMD at FN for the calcium + exercise group in relation to only calcium tablets group*

Continued on next page

TABLE 16.1. *Continued*

Authors	Sample study groups	Follow-up	Inclusion criteria	Outcomes measured	Training program	Compliance	Results
Bassey & Ramsdale, 1995[24]	High-impact exercise (*n* = 20) Control: low-impact exercise (*n* = 24)	12 months	Postmenopausal healthy women without any hormone replacement therapy	BMD: Distal radius Femur: neck, Ward's triangle, trochanter Region of L-2 to L-3	High impact: "heal drop" + weekly class of mixed exercises Low impact: weekly low-impact exercise + daily flexibility home exercises	84% ± 10% for exercise group 82% ± 9% control group	No increase in BMD at any place, and no significant differences in BMD between groups
Kerr et al., 1996[5]	Strength training (*n* = 25) Endurance training (*n* = 21) Control (contralateral limb of each subject)	12 months	Healthy postmenopausal women No hormone replacement therapy No calcium supplementation No high-intensity exercise	BMD: Femur: femoral neck, Ward's triangle, intertrochanteric site Radius: middistal and ultradistal zones	Three times per week: Strength training: high-load, low-repetition, weight-resistance training Endurance training: group: low-load, high-repetition, weight-resistance training	87%	Strength-training group: increased BMD (baseline vs. follow-up) at all sites* except FN Increased BMD in comparison with control limb, which showed decrease in BMD* No significant increase* in BMD for endurance group except in distal radius
Brooke-Wavell et al., 1997[25]	Exercise: Brisk walking (*n* = 38) Control (*n* = 40)	12 months	Healthy postmenopausal women without hormone replacement therapy	BMD: Femoral neck Calcaneus Lumbar spine	Supervised continuous daily brisk walking for 20–50 min	Not reported	Increased BMD at FN for exercise group (baseline vs. follow-up)* Decreased BMD at calcaneus in control group in relation to exercise group*
Snow Harter et al., 1992[33]	Progressive training: Jogging (*n* = 10) Weightlifting (*n* = 12) Control (*n* = 18)	8 months	Healthy premenopausal women	BMD: Region of L-2 to L-4 Femur: neck, trochanter, Ward's triangle	Jogging: speed to elevate HR at 0%–80% of age-predicted maximum Weightlifting: three times per week, three sets, one repetition 0%–85% RM	97% runners 92% weight training	Jogging as well as weightlifting increased BMD in region of L-2 l to L-4*
Heinonen et al., 1999[29]	Exercise to maintain effect of previous high-impact activity (*n* = 30) Control (*n* = 19)	8 months	Sedentary premenopausal women from previous RCT	BMD: Lumbar spine Femoral neck Distal femur Patella Proximal tibia Calcaneus Proximal radius	Unsupervised regular aerobic and step classes three times per week	Not reported	BMD at FN of exercise group continued significantly increasing* BMD was maintained at the distal femur, patella, proximal tibia, and calcaneus*

*$p < 0.05$.
BMD, bone mineral density; FN, femoral neck; HR, heart rate; LS, lumbar spine; RCT, randomized controlled trial; RM, resistance maximum.

TABLE 16.2. *Prospective nonrandomized studies*

Authors	Sample study groups	Follow-up	Inclusion criteria	Outcomes measured	Training program	Compliance	Results
Pruitt et al., 1992[32]	Exercise ($n = 17$) Control ($n = 9$)	9 months	Early postmenopausal women without hormone replacement or any medications or diseases that affect bone metabolism No vigorous exercise within 6 months before the study	BMD: Region of L-2 to L-4 Femoral neck BMC: Radius and ulna of nondominant forearm	Progressive resistive weight-training program (site-specific)	96%	Increased BMD at LS, reducing decline in lumbar BMD in exercise group*
Caplan & Ward, 1993[26]	Exercised ($n = 19$) Control ($n = 11$)	2 years	Postmenopausal women without hormone replacement or any medications that affect bone metabolism	BMD: Femur: neck, Ward's triangle, trochanter area Lumbar vertebrae	Twice per week, 60 minutes of aerobic weight-bearing exercises	Not reported	Exercise group: Consistent (but nonsignificant) increase in all femoral measures Protective effect in BMD at LS (change in BMD = –0.8, vs. –3.8 for controls, $p = 0.03$) Increased BMD at trochanter*
Kohrt et al., 1997[30]	Group exercise 1: joint reaction force (JRF)–oriented exercises ($n = 13$) Group exercise 2: ground reaction force (GRF)–oriented exercises ($n = 14$) Control group ($n = 12$)	11 months	Postmenopausal sedentary women No smokers	BMD: Region of L-2 to L-4 Femur: neck, trochanter, Ward's triangle Wrist: ultradistal and one-third distal radius region Total body Bone turnover	3.5 sessions per week GRF: walking, jogging, or stair climbing JRF: Weight lifting, rowing	81%	Increased BMD of whole body in relation to controls Increased BMD at femur (neck and Ward's triangle) for GRF group* All exercise groups showed inverse relationship between BMD and fat mass*
Iwamato et al., 1998[2]	Exercise + calcium + Control + calcium + Vitamin D ($n = 20$) Vitamin D ($n = 15$)	1 year	Postmenopausal women without hormone replacement or any medications that affect bone metabolism	BMD: Region of L-2 to L-4	Daily walking (step count) and gymnastic training program (at least 5 days per week)	Not reported	BMD at region of L-2 to L-4 increased over time for the exercise group*

*$p < 0.05$.
BMC, bone mineral content; BMD, bone mineral density; FN, femoral neck; LS, lumbar spine.

Exercise in Postmenopausal Women

The reviewed evidence supports the positive relationship between exercise and BMD. In fact, the results suggest an increase in BMD in postmenopausal women after they performed continuous supervised high-impact training (5,6,25,26,28,31). Researchers have found that high-intensity strength-training exercises with high loads at low repetitions produced a bone site-specific effect (5,6). Nelson et al. (6) conducted an RCT in postmenopausal women, comparing a high-intensity exercise training group with a control group. They found that the total body bone mineral content was preserved in strength-trained women but tended to decrease in the control group. These results were similar in site-specific measures, in which BMD decreased at the femoral neck and lumbar spine of the control group and increased in the exercise group. The purpose of the study was to measure the impact of exercise in the prevention of osteoporotic fractures. Nelson et al. concluded that there was a positive association between exercise and an increase in muscle mass, muscle strength, dynamic balance, and overall physical activity level, which demonstrated the simultaneous multifactorial effect of exercise in the prevention of osteoporotic fractures.

Kerr et al. (5) compared two randomly assigned groups of healthy postmenopausal women. A strength-training group (with high loads and low repetition) and an endurance-training group (with low loads and high repetition) were compared with the "nondominant" limb of each subject in the study. After 1 year of follow-up, the strength-training group had a significant increase in all the measured sites except the femoral neck in comparison with the baseline measures and the control group (Table 16.2). The endurance-training group did not show any significant increase in bone density. Pruitt et al. (32) also conducted a longitudinal nonrandomized trial, comparing one group undergoing a resistance weight-training program with a control group. Similar results were found; there was a significant increase in BMD at the lumbar spine and no differences at the femoral neck.

Whereas site-specific resistive exercises appear to have a consistent effect on bone mineralization, weight-bearing exercises such as walking are still controversial. Kohrt et al. (30) studied the effect of joint reaction force (JRF) exercises in comparison with ground reaction force (GRF) exercises. They hypothesized that the way forces act on the skeleton affects the bone turnover and, therefore, bone mass. Both exercise groups experienced significant increases in BMD of the whole body, lumbar spine, and Ward's triangle region of the femur. However, at the femoral neck, which is the site with the highest fracture incidence in the elderly, only GRF exercises such as walking, jogging, or stair climbing increased BMD ($p < 0.05$). The JRF exercises such as weightlifting and rowing, however, prevented faster mineral lost at the femoral neck. Other studies such as that conducted by Caplan and Ward (26) also found a protective effect from aerobic weight-bearing exercises at the lumbar spine and femur but no significant increase of BMD except at the trochanteric level.

Observational studies have shown that regular walkers experienced a reduced risk of fracture at the hip (34). This association, however, can be due to better health status or lifestyle in these people. The quantity and intensity of walking that are sufficient to produce significant bone changes are still unclear. Intervention studies in postmenopausal women who used walking as a form of exercise were reviewed. Brooke-Wavell et al. (25) examined the influence of brisk walking on the BMDs of postmenopausal women. They found that walking slowed the bone loss rate at the calcaneus, which, in fact, is the site that suffers highest mechanical strain and stress during the heel strike while walking. The lumbar spine BMD decreased over the year of follow-up in the control group but not in the walking group. Moreover, the amount of walking was correlated with changes in BMD at the femoral neck, which suggests a dose-response relationship. Hatori et al. (28) compared a control group with two groups that used different exercise intensities, determined by the anaerobic threshold reached while walking. A high-intensity exercise level corresponded to walking above the anaerobic threshold, and a moderate-intensity level corresponded to walking below the anaerobic threshold. A significant increase ($p < 0.05$) was found in BMD at the region of L-2 to -L-4 in the high-intensity exercise group after 7 months, whereas no significant differences were found between the control group and the moderate-intensity exercise group.

Low-impact exercises do not appear to be beneficial for increasing BMD (5,24,27,28, 32). In fact, researchers who compared high- versus low-impact exercises found that people who performed low-impact exercises (low loads, purely aerobic exercises) did not show any significant increase in BMD at specific sites or a significant difference in BMD in comparison with the control groups (5,24,28). In addition, in the majority of the studies, the control group showed a significant linear decrease in the BMD of the site measured at follow-up (6,25,27).

Exercise in Premenopausal Women

Studies in premenopausal women have yielded controversial results. Snow-Harter et al. (33) compared two different training groups (jogging versus weightlifting) with a nonexercise control group. After 8 months of training, both exercise groups showed a positive effect of the BMD at the lumbar spine (in the region of L-2 to -L-4; $p < 0.05$) but no effect on the femoral measures. These results did not show significant differences between the strength training with high load and low repetition and the jogging, which involved low load and high repetition. Non-RCTs such as those conducted by Gleeson et al. (35) and Rockwell et al. (36), however, do not support these results. In fact, Gleeson et al. (35) reported no significant effect of weightlifting on BMD, whereas Rockwell et al. (36) reported that weight training was associated with bone loss at the lumbar spine.

The strongest limitation for both studies is the lack of randomization and the difference in the population age, which affects not only the power of the studies but also the bone mass and level of activity before and during the study protocol (35,36). However, all the studies concluded the lack of effect of exercise training in BMD at the femoral neck. It is possible that the greater abundance of cortical bone at this site may require more training for a detectable response, because remodeling occurs on bone surfaces and the surface-to-volume ratio of cortical bone at this site is considerably less than that of trabecular bone (33). Researchers have suggested that perhaps longer training periods are needed to further increase bone mass (20,33). The maintenance of the exercise level also seems to be important. Previous studies have shown that the cessation of training is associated with decreases of the BMD gained (37). Heinonen et al. (29) conducted a second-part study from an RCT that showed significant BMD increase at the lumbar spine and several lower limb sites, to determine the effectiveness of self-controlled aerobic and step exercises in bone density maintenance in healthy premenopausal women. The intervention group from the previous RCT continued with unsupervised regular aerobic and step exercises three times per week for 8 months. Femoral neck BMD was maintained and continuously increased in the exercise group, in comparison with the nonexercised group, and it was maintained at the other measured lower limb sites (see Table 16.2). BMD measures were significantly different from those of the control group after 26 months ($p = 0.004$). Although the level of compliance with the unsupervised exercise training was not reported, the authors suggested that the increase in BMD induced by supervised high-impact training can be maintained with subsequent continuous, less demanding aerobic step classes. However, these results have not been reproduced in research with postmenopausal women.

Exercise and Calcium and/or Estrogen Supplementation

Calcium supplementation and hormone replacement therapy have been recognized as effective interventions for bone mass maintenance. The combined effect of these interventions with exercise has been the focus of several different studies (2,7,31). Prince et al. (7) completed a double-blind RCT with 120 postmenopausal women with low forearm bone density (<290 mg/cm^2). The women were randomly assigned to four groups: a control group, those performing exercise alone, those performing exercise and receiving dietary calcium supplementation, and those performing exercise and receiving estrogen replacement. The exercise regimen consisted of supervised low-impact aerobic exercise and brisk walking. Similar results in bone density and rate of bone loss were found in the control group and the group performing low-impact exercise without any supplementation. The low-impact exercise program alone was ineffective in preventing bone loss. In general, BMD significantly increased at the forearm only in the group performing exercise and receiving estrogen. The rate of bone loss was slowed or maintained low for the women at risk of osteoporotic fracture in the exercise groups with either calcium or estrogen supplementation. The results suggested a possible synergic action between exercise and calcium supplementation, in which the combination of dietary calcium supplementation and an exercise regimen prevented bone loss, whereas the exercise regimen alone did not. However, of importance is that the exercise was performed at low intensity, and compliance with the regimen was poor. No side effects were reported with the use of calcium supplementation, whereas there were some with the estrogen supplementation (7). Under these circumstances and considering the feasibility of the use of calcium supplementation without strong supervision, this protocol was suggested as a good intervention for bone loss prevention.

Prince et al. (31) in 1995 published another RCT with 2 years of follow-up. They compared the effects of several different approaches on bone density in postmenopausal women: calcium as a tablet, calcium as a tablet plus an exercise program, calcium as a milk powder supplement, and nontreatment (placebo). The exercise regimen that accompanied the calcium supplementation was 4 hours per week of a supervised weight-bearing exercise. Results suggested that both types of calcium supplementation provided in the study prevented age-related bone loss at the hip. Women in the exercise and calcium regimen showed an extra protective effect at the femoral neck in relation to the groups with a calcium-only regimen. Although it is still unclear how much the exercise enhances the calcium effectiveness, these results demonstrated a clear relationship between calcium intake and exercise. In fact, they suggested an increase in dietary intake of calcium to approximately 1.8 g of calcium per day plus an increase in exercise by 10% on the average to significantly decrease bone loss at the hip site (31). Iwamoto et al. (2) supported these results after conducting a nonrandomized trial in which they compared a group that performed exercise and received calcium supplementation with another that only received calcium supplementation (Table 16.2). The results revealed an association between calcium supplementation and bone mass maintenance, as well as an association between low- to moderate-intensity exercise plus calcium supplementation and an increase in BMD at the lumbar spine.

TABLE 16.3. *Exercise characteristics necessary to produce an osteogenic effect*

Loading: site specific, weight bearing, inducing muscle resistance
Intensity: exceeding normal daily loading with peak forces; consider strain thresholds
Frequency: progressive (as biomechanical tolerable); cessation of exercise results in return to pre-exercise bone mass
Type: diverse, vigorous, nonrepetitive, and enjoyable

DISCUSSION

After a review of different studies that suggest an association between exercise and bone mass density, some statements can be made. It has been shown that immobilization and nonskeletal loading results in a significant reduction in bone mass. The bone-enhancing effects of physical activity and exercise are achieved through muscle contraction and mechanical loading, which causes strain stimulus in the bone structure. The effect of exercise is site-specific, and its mechanical loads stimulate bone cells within the region through the deformation of surrounding tissue. Those loading exercises must be exertional in order to reach the peak forces needed to produce an osteogenic effect. In fact, high-impact loading sports, as well as resistive exercise training and vigorous weight-bearing activities, have shown an important effect in slowing the process of decreasing BMD. Some reports have presented bone mineral responses that are clearly different between groups performing high-impact exercise and those performing low-impact exercise (5,24,27,28). The bone remodeling response of groups performing low-impact exercise has not been significantly different from that of the control group that has not been subjected to any specific form of training (5,24,28). There is substantial evidence that bone mass and BMD are greater particularly at sites that undergo mechanical loading during the exercise, whereas other sites, such as the nondominant limb of the athlete, do not show the same changes (5,25,28,32).

The efficacy of exercise also depends on the type of exercise. When weight-bearing and loading exercises are chosen, the frequency and duration of application of the load play a significant role in the maintenance or increase of BMD (16). High-resistance weightlifting exercises or weight-bearing activities with low repetition are recommended for the sustenance of bone mass (38). Compliance with the activity is important. In fact, cessation of exercise prompts rapid metabolic bone changes inducing bone loss, and bone mass gradually returns to the pre-exercise level (16). High-impact training–induced significant BMD increases among premenopausal women can be effectively maintained with subsequent less demanding exercises (29).

Specific exercise characteristics must be indicated to produce an osteogenic effect (Table 16.3). Drinkwater et al. (15) suggested basic principles that must be applied for the purposes of training and research:

Principle of specificity: The primary effect of mechanical stress is localized to the site where it is applied (22). Thus, the exercise program chosen to prevent osteoporotic fractures should include activities that increase stress and strain levels at areas where osteoporotic fractures occur most frequently (the spine, femoral neck, and distal radius). At the same time, to assess the impact of exercise in BMD, it should be measured at the areas that are to be overloaded.

Principle of overload: The mechanical stress placed on the bone by the assigned activity must exceed the normal loading and reach the strain threshold needed to increase BMD.

Principle of reversibility: The increase in BMD during childhood and early adult years is an investment that will remain as long as a high level of physical activity is maintained. In fact, the positive effect of a bone remodeling training program in the elderly is lost if the program is discontinued.

Principle of initial values: People with the lowest levels of BMD have the greatest capacity for percentage improvement; those with average or above-average bone mass have the least.

Principle of diminishing returns: Each person has an individual biological ceiling that determines the extent of a possible training effect. As this ceiling is approached, gains in bone mass slow and eventually plateau.

Exercise in the prevention of osteoporosis plays a unique role at different ages. The skeletal response to exercise differs among children, young adults, and elderly people. Childhood represents the sole opportunity to gain bone density and modify skeletal architecture. The resultant exercise-related geometric adaptations offer mechanical advantages that in the future may reduce the risk of bone fracture (13). In active young adults, the primary effect of exercise is bone conservation more than acquisition (12,33). The percentage of improvement apparently occurs at a lower rate than in childhood, and it reaches a plateau that in fact is needed for bone mass maintenance (4,13–15). However, in elderly persons, exercise produces an important effect not only in the maintenance of BMD but also in the reduction of the rate of bone loss (7,12).

The type of exercise suggested at different ages must differ not only in the skeletal response but also in the age-related individual characteristics. In childhood, recreation must be the main factor to improve skeletal strength, socialization, early active lifestyle patterns, and motor development. In healthy young adults, vigorous exercise programs and resistance training of moderate to high intensity can preserve bone density or result in modest (1% to 3%) increases in mineral content at clinically relevant sites (7,12,29). Weight-bearing physical activity is also important for bone mass maintenance. An exercise program aimed at increasing muscle strength, fitness, balance, coordination, and stability is recommended for bone maintenance in adults. Although the frequency necessary to produce beneficial skeletal results is still controversial, two to three times per week is suggested by different authors (5–7,28,33). Training intensities higher than 70% of the resistance maximum (RM) have shown a beneficial effect on preserving bone density (5,6,33). Low-intensity exercises such as walking have a minimal effect on BMD (39). Nevertheless, some studies have proposed that women who walk more than 7.5 miles per week have a higher mean bone density of the whole body than do women who walk less than one mile per week (40). In adults, exercise in combination with calcium intake seems to produce an extra protective effect for BMD.

Exercises targeted at an elderly population should be carefully planned not only to produce a site-specific effect at areas where the osteoporotic fracture occurs most frequently but also to decrease the predisposition to fall (12). Although the evidence shows a moderate exercise effect in BMD, its effect on muscle strength is well recognized. In fact, low muscle strength, which has emerged as a risk factor for falls, responds dramatically to resistance exercise. A combination of aerobic and strength training exercise in conjunction with programs oriented toward stability and coordination is a safety measure for preventing falls and, consequently, osteoporotic fractures. In older men and women, differences in strength gain are not highly dependent on training frequency (13). However, in order to accomplish neuromuscular benefits, a modest intensity of exercise must be performed once or twice each week. The exercise program should emphasize safe and dynamic activities that engage this population in a more active and healthier lifestyle. For an exercise program to succeed, the patient must adhere to it. In the case of postmenopausal women, it is not possible to conclude that exercise alone is a preventive strategy for osteoporotic fractures. Supplemental interventions such as hormone therapy and increased calcium intake with exercise seem to be the most effective preventive strategies (28,31,41).

Lifestyle factors can clearly affect bone metabolism and thus bone mass (16). Suggestions must be made not only in terms of level of physical activity but also in terms of lifestyle modifications. The multifactorial characteristics of the risk factors associated with osteoporosis allow us to suggest different interventions that are oriented mainly toward early lifestyle modifications (Table 16.4).

Even in the absence of a significant, recognizable effect in the increase of BMD, any type of exercise and physical activity may be beneficial in many other ways. Regular exercise has been recognized to have an advantageous effect in various physiological and psychological aspects. It is well recognized to have a favorable effect on people's general sense of well-being (42). To decrease the risk of osteoporotic fractures, exercise also has an important effect on balance, muscle strength, flexibility, and coordination (42). At the same time, it has been found that with time and compliance, exercise allows people to progress in intensity, which suggests that after continuous training, they will be able to engage in more vigorous and energetic activities and greatly improve their quality of life.

TABLE 16.4. *Positive and negative lifestyle factors associated with bone metabolism*

Activity	Effect
Exercise*	
Jogging, continuous brisk walking (+)	Good for maintenance of bone mass
Swimming (+/–)	Good for maintenance of cardiovascular capacity; >1 hr/day/may decrease bone mass in women
Weight lifting and resistance exercise (+)	Increases bone mass (site specific)
Gymnastics (+)	Increases total body bone mass
Aerobic exercises (+)	Good for maintenance of bone mass
Stair climbing (+)	Good for maintenance of bone mass
Rowing (+)	Good for maintenance of bone mass
Nutrition	
Calcium (+)	Good for maintenance of bone mass, accompanied by exercise; decreases bone loss in postmenopausal women and is associated with increase in bone mass
Vitamin D (+)	Good for maintenance of bone mass; indirectly decreases bone resorption
High Protein (–)	Decreases bone mineral density
Caffeine (–)	High intake increases urinary calcium loss
Alcohol (–)	High intake accelerates bone loss
Sodium (–)	High intake increases urinary calcium loss
Anorexia	Increases bone loss
Mood	
Stress, depression, and sedentary occupation	Decrease physical activity, which is associated with faster bone loss
Others:	
Smoking	Predictor of low bone mineral density

Adapted from Sinaki M. Effects of physical activity in bone mass. *Curr Opin Rheumatol* 1996;8:376–383.

*No continuous exercise program and lack of compliance may adversely affect the positive results of earlier exercise program.

SUMMARY

1. Immobilization and nonskeletal loading results in a significant reduction in bone mass.
2. The bone-enhancing effect of physical activity and/or exercise occurs through muscle contraction and mechanical loading, which causes strain stimulus in the bone structure.
3. High-impact loading sports as well as resistive exercise training and vigorous weight-bearing activities have been shown to have an important effect in slowing the process of decreasing BMD.
4. There is substantial evidence that bone mass and BMD are greater particularly at sites that undergo mechanical loading during exercise.
5. Cessation of exercise prompts rapid metabolic bone changes that induce bone loss, and bone mass gradually returns to the pre-exercise level.
6. The skeletal response to exercise differs among children, young adults, and elderly people.
7. The type of exercise suggested at different ages must differ not only in the skeletal response but also in the age-related individual characteristics.
8. Exercise programs should emphasize safe and dynamic activities that engage people in a more active and healthier lifestyle.
9. Even in the absence of a significant recognizable effect in the increase of BMD, regular exercise has been recognized to have an advantageous effect on various physiological and psychological aspects.

REFERENCES

1. NIH Consensus Development Panel on Osteoporosis Prevention, Diagnosis, and Therapy. Osteoporosis prevention, diagnosis, and therapy. *JAMA* 2000;285:785–795.
2. Iwamoto I, Takeda T, Otani T, et al. Effect of increased physical activity on bone mineral density in postmenopausal osteoporotic women. *Keio J Med* 1998;47:157–161.
3. Ettinger B, Genant HK, Cann CE. Postmenopausal bone loss is prevented by treatment with low-dosage estrogen with calcium. *Ann Intern Med* 1987;106:40–45.
4. Bouxsein ML, Marcus R. Overview of exercise and bone mass. *Osteoporosis* 1994;20:787–801.
5. Kerr D, Morton A, Dick I, et al. Exercise effects on bone mass in postmenopausal women are site-specific and load-dependent. *J Bone Miner Res* 1996;11:218–255.
6. Nelson M, Fiatarone M, Morganti C, et al. Effects of high intensity strength training on multiple risk factors for osteoporotic fractures. A randomized controlled trial. *JAMA* 1994;272:1909–1914.
7. Prince R, Smith M, Roger D, et al. Prevention of postmenopausal osteoporosis. A comparative study of exercise, calcium supplementation, and hormone-replacement therapy. *N Engl J Med* 1991;325:1189–1195.
8. Pollitzer W, Anderson J. Ethnic and genetic differences in bone mass: a review with a hereditary vs. environmental perspective. *Am J Clin Nutr* 1989;50:1244–1259.
9. Slemenda CW, Christian JC, Williams CJ, et al. Genetic determinants of bone mass in adult women: a reevaluation of the twin model and the potential importance of gene interaction on heritability estimates. *J Bone Miner Res* 1991;6:561–567.
10. Välimäki M, Kärkkäinen M, Lamber-Allardt C, et al. Exercise, smoking, and calcium intake during adolescence and early adulthood as determinants of peak bone mass. *BMJ* 1994;309:230–235.
11. Hui SL, Slemenda CW, Johnston CC Jr. The contribution of bone loss to post-menopausal osteoporosis. *Osteoporos Int* 1990;1:30–34.
12. Forwood M, Larsen J. Exercise recommendations for osteoporosis. A position statement of the Australian and New Zealand Bone and Mineral Society. *Aust Fam Physician* 2000;29:761–764.
13. Marcus R. Role of exercises in preventing and treating osteoporosis. *Osteoporosis* 2000;27:131–141.
14. Drinkwater BL. 1994 C.H. McCloy Research Lecture: does physical activity play a role in preventing osteoporosis? *Res Q Exerc Sport* 1994;65:197–206.
15. Drinkwater BL, Grimston SK, Raab-Cullen DM, et al. American College of Sport Medicine Position Stand on osteoporosis and exercise. *Med Sci Sports Exerc* 1995;27:i–vii.
16. Sinaki M. Effects of physical activity in bone mass. *Curr Opin Rheumatol* 1996;8:376–383.

17. Frost H. Skeletal structural adaptations to mechanical usage (SATMU)–1. Redefining Wolff's law: the bone modeling problem. *Anat Rec* 1990;56:403–413.
18. Mosekilde L. Osteoporosis and exercise. *Bone* 1995;17:193–195.
19. Greendale G, Barrett-Connor E, Edelstein S, et al. Lifetime leisure exercise and osteoporosis. The Rancho Bernardo Study. *Am J Epidemiol* 1995;141:951–959.
20. Etherington J, Harris PA, Nandra D, et al. The effect of weight-bearing exercise on bone mineral density: a study of female ex-elite athletes and the general population. *J Bone Miner Res* 1996;11:1333–1338.
21. Taafe D, Snow-Harter C, Connolly D, et al. Differential effects of swimming versus weight-bearing activity on bone mineral status of eumenorrheic athletes. *J Bone Miner Res* 1995;10:586–593.
22. Layne J, Nelson M. The effects of progressive resistance training on bone density: a review. *Med Sci Sports Exerc* 1999;31:25–30.
23. Kelley G. Exercise and regional bone mineral density in postmenopausal women. A meta-analytic review of randomized trials. *Am J Phys Med Rehabil* 1998;77:76–87.
24. Bassey EJ, Ramsdale SJ. Weight-bearing exercise and ground reaction forces: 12 month randomized controlled trial of effects on bone mineral density in healthy postmenopausal women. *Bone* 1995;16:469–476.
25. Brooke-Wavell K, Jones PR, Hardman AE. Brisk walking reduces calcaneal bone loss in post-menopausal women. *Clin Sci (Lond)* 1997;92:75–80.
26. Caplan GA, Ward JA. The benefits of exercise in postmenopausal women. *Aust Journal Public Health* 1993;17:23–26.
27. Grove KA, Londeree BR. Bone density in post-menopausal women: high impact vs. low impact exercise. *Med Sci Sports Exerc* 1992;24:1190–1194.
28. Hatori M, Hasegawa A, Adachi H, et al. The effects of walking at the anaerobic threshold level on vertebral bone loss in postmenopausal women. *Calcif Tissue Int* 1993;52:411–414.
29. Heinonen A, Kannus P, Sievanen H, et al. Good maintenance of high-impact activity-induced bone gain by voluntary, unsupervised exercises: an 8 month follow-up of a randomized controlled trial. *J Bone Miner Res* 1999; 14:125–128.
30. Kohrt W, Ehsani A, Birge S. Effects of exercise involving predominantly either joint-reaction or ground-reaction forces on bone mineral density in older women. *J Bone Miner Res* 1997;12:1253–1261.
31. Prince R, Devine A, Dick I, et al. The effects of calcium supplementation (milk powder or tablets) and exercise on bone density in postmenopausal women. *J Bone Miner Res* 1995;10:1068–1075.
32. Pruitt L, Jackson R, Bartels R, et al. Weight training effects on bone mineral density in early postmenopausal women. *J Bone Miner Res* 1992;7:179–185.
33. Snow-Harter C, Bouxsein M, Lewis B, et al. Effects of resistance and endurance exercise on bone mineral status of young women: a randomized exercise intervention trial. *J Bone Miner Res* 1992:7:761–769.
34. Cummings SR, Nevitt MC, Browner WS, et al. Risk factors for hip fracture in white women. *N Engl J Med* 1995;332:767–773.
35. Gleeson PB, Protas EJ, LeBlanc AD, et al. Effects of weight lifting on bone mineral density in premenopausal women. *J Bone Miner Res* 1990;5:153–158.
36. Rockwell JC, Sorenson AM, Baker S, et al. Weight training decreases vertebral bone density in pre-menopausal: a prospective study. *J Clin Endocrinol Metab* 1990;71:988–993.
37. Vuori I, Heinonen S, Sievanen H, et al. Effects of unilateral strength training and detraining on bone mineral density and content in young women: a study of mechanical loading and de-loading on human bones. *Calcif Tissue Int* 1994;55:59–67.
38. Ernst E. Can exercise prevent postmenopausal osteoporosis? *Br J Sports Med* 1994;28:5–6.
39. Swezey R. Exercise for osteoporosis—is walking enough? The case for site specificity and resistive exercise. *Spine* 1996:21:2809–2813.
40. Krall E, Dawson-Hughes B. Walking is related to bone density and rates of bone loss. *Am J Med* 1994;96:20–26.
41. Hoidrup S, Gronbaek M, Pedersen AT, et al. Hormone replacement therapy and hip fracture risk: effect modification by tobacco smoking, alcohol intake, physical activity, and body mass index. *Am J Epidemiol* 1999;150: 1085–1093.
42. Walker M, Klentrou P, Chow R, et al. Longitudinal evaluation of supervised versus unsupervised exercise programs for the treatment of osteoporosis. *Eur J Applied Physiol* 2000;83:349–355.

17

Vertebral Compression Fractures and Orthoses[1]

Bart W. Koes

Department of General Practice, Erasmus University Rotterdam, Rotterdam, The Netherlands

OSTEOPOROSIS

Osteoporosis is characterized by low bone mineral density and a loss of structure of the bone with a related higher risk of fractures. About 30% of postmenopausal white woman suffer from osteoporosis. There is a strong relation to increasing age; the incidence of osteoporosis increases from 15% among women aged 50 to 59 years to 70% among women aged 80 years and older. In The Netherlands, the Osteoporosis Society estimates that of a total population of 16 million people, 800,000 persons have osteoporosis. In the United States, osteoporosis is reported to be the most common metabolic bone disease. Because of an increasing mean age of the population in the coming years, the incidence and prevalence of osteoporosis and related fractures are expected to increase in various western countries.

VERTEBRAL DEFORMITY AND FRACTURES

The prevalence of vertebral deformity, which is often associated with osteoporosis in the elderly, is reported in the range of 6% to 25% among people older than 50 years, depending on the definitions used. Pluijm et al. (1), in a study with 527 people older than 65 years, showed that 39% had at least one vertebral deformity. They also found that, even if vertebral deformities are not clinically manifested, people with this condition reported having functional limitations and poorer self-perceived health (1).

Most osteoporotic fractures occur in woman. The fracture rate increases with age. Most fractures involve the hip, the wrist, and the spine. The exact incidence and prevalence of vertebral fractures are difficult to estimate. Partly because vertebral fractures may occur without symptoms (such as pain or decreased function), they may therefore not be diagnosed. In addition, there are currently various classification systems and measurement instruments in use, which hampers clear insight into the actual numbers.

It is estimated that 30% of vertebral fractures lead to clinical symptoms. A compression fracture could, however, be accompanied by severe, acute low back pain, lasting for

[1]Presented at the Brussels International Spine Symposium Vertebral Osteoporotic Compression Fractures, November 16–17, 2001.

3 to 4 weeks. In most cases, the fractures stabilize after a few weeks, but in a small percentage of patients, the pain persists (2).

Vertebral fractures may lead to a loss of height. Other possible consequences include the development of thoracic kyphosis and possibly less "long volume."

PREVENTIVE AND THERAPEUTIC MEASURES

There are many preventive and therapeutic interventions for the management of vertebral compression fractures. These include patient education and counseling, dietary advice, physical exercises, and medication. One of the therapeutic options is the prescription of orthoses. In the literature, various synonyms, such as *braces, corsets,* and *belts,* are in use. Levine (3) made a distinction between corsets and braces; lumbar corsets are designed to increase the intraabdominal pressure without immobilizing the back. He stated that "women with spinal osteoporosis may need to wear a lumbar corset continuously." Braces and belts reduce the lumbar motion and are recommended for short-term use in acute low back pain.

SIDE EFFECTS

In the literature, there have been warnings about the potential harm related to the wearing of orthoses. For example, "in general, braces and corsets should not be prescribed for a long period, because of potential side-effects such as psychological and physiologic dependence, abdominal and lumbar muscle atrophy (with an increased risk of re-injury)" (3). Other authors have reported contraindications such as skin lesions or gastrointestinal disorders (4).

This chapter focuses on what is known about the rationale and efficacy of orthoses for patients with vertebral compression fractures.

RATIONALE

Immobilization

The rationale behind the prescription of orthoses is that they are able to immobilize the spine to some extent. Calmels and Fayolle-Minon (4) distinguished between restriction of intervertebral mobility and restriction of overall spinal mobility.

With regard to intervertebral mobility, they found various studies that suggested that immobilization was better at the upper lumbar spine than at the level of L-4 to -L-5 or L-5 to -S-1. They also found wide interindividual variation and that stiff corsets were associated with greater motion restriction than were flexible supports (4).

With regard to overall spinal mobility, they concluded that orthoses may restrict only extreme motions and may be more effective on lateral bending than on flexion and extension. The more stiff orthoses appear better able to reduce mobility than the flexible ones (4).

In a review, van Poppel et al. (5) also investigated the potential of lumbar supports in relation to restriction of trunk motion. They found evidence that lumbar supports reduce trunk motion for flexion-extension and lateral bending. In the same study, they found that there was no evidence that lumbar supports reduce electromyographic activity of the erector spinae muscles or increase abdominal pressure (5).

Pain Reduction

Tanner et al. (6) reported that pain relief is the most common reason for application of spinal orthoses, especially in the acute phase. The acute pain may be sharp, localized to the affected vertebrae, aggravated with spine loading activity and with flexion, and relieved in a neutral position. After 2 to 3 months, a compression fracture should have healed, and so it is no longer a source of local pain (6).

EFFICACY

In Osteoporosis

No systematic review, meta-analysis, or any randomized clinical trial evaluating the efficacy of orthoses for vertebral compression fractures could be identified. A few descriptive studies describing various types of orthoses and their potential value for the management of vertebral fractures were found.

In a pilot study, Kaplan et al. (7) investigated the effect of back supports on back strength in patients with osteoporosis. Forty-five woman aged 40 years and older with osteoporosis were randomly assigned to three groups. Group 1 received only instruction in postural exercises, group 2 received instruction in postural exercises and a conventional thoracolumbar support, and group 3 received instruction in postural exercises and a weighted kyphoorthosis (a posture training support). There was wide variation in compliance with the intervention. Only 5 of 15 subjects in group 2 (thoracolumbar support) completed the study. In group 1 (exercises only), 11 subjects completed the study, and in group 3 (posture training support), all 15 completed the study.

Back strength increased in all three groups, but significant differences could not be detected, possibly because of the small sample size. The authors recommended further studies in order to evaluate the effects of posture training support and of postural exercises.

Of Orthoses for Low Back Pain

Although as yet no randomized clinical trials evaluating orthoses for vertebral compression fractures could be identified, such trials have been conducted for low back pain. In a systematic review of the literature, Van Tulder et al. (8) summarized the available evidence on the efficacy of lumbar supports for the prevention and treatment of low back pain.

Prevention

Five randomized clinical trials and two nonrandomized clinical trials focused on the primary prevention (preventing the onset of lower back pain or on secondary prevention (preventing recurrent episodes of low back pain). Unfortunately, the overall methodological quality of the trials was rated low. In the four randomized clinical trials in which lumbar supports were compared with no intervention, there appeared to be no difference in the incidence of back pain for up to 12 months of follow-up. Also, in comparison with the results of other preventive interventions (two randomized clinical trials), no differences between intervention and lumbar supports were found in incidence rates.

Therapy

One low-quality randomized clinical trial compared the effect of lumbar support with that of no intervention and reported a significant effect of the pain index used in favor of lumbar support. Lumbar supports were compared with other interventions in four other randomized clinical trials. Three of these found no difference in effect for pain outcomes, whereas one study did report an effect in pain outcome in favor of lumbar supports. Overall, the reviewers concluded that there is conflicting evidence about the efficacy of lumbar supports in the treatment of low back pain.

Compliance

Only a few studies reported data regarding compliance of wearing lumbar supports. Of the preventive studies, three randomized clinical trials had compliance rates varying from 43% of the subjects who wore the support at least half of the time (5) to 80% of the subjects who wore the support most of the time (9). Of the therapeutic trials, only one presented compliance data. This trial reported that 56% of the patients wore the support more than 7 hours a day (10).

Prescription of Orthoses

In the absence of evidence from sound randomized clinical trials or even nonrandomized clinical studies evaluating the effects of orthoses for vertebral compression fractures, the prescription of orthoses, if any, may depend largely on personal experiences and preferences of clinicians.

Once the decision has been made that an orthoses may be helpful for a patient, other available interventions such as advice, pain medication, and exercise factors (such as extent of immobilization of thoracic or lumber spine, compliance, and costs) will be considered. In addition, skin tolerance, obesity, and respiratory diseases may interfere with the wearing of a (type of) orthoses.

Tanner et al. (6) proposed orthosis selection on the basis of the level of fracture and premorbid functional level. The recommendation included rigid, semirigid cervicosacral and thoracolumbosacral orthoses, with or without stays and shoulder straps and whether or not custom molded. The validity of this prescription scheme has, however, not yet been investigated.

CONCLUSIONS

Orthoses have long been prescribed for the management of vertebral compression fractures. The proposed rationale varies from pain management in the acute phase to prevention of the development of kyphosis. Surprisingly, no randomized clinical trials and, therefore, no systematic reviews of these trials could be identified. Consequently, there is at present no support for or argument against the efficacy of orthoses for vertebral compression fractures. In addition, there is a wide variation in opinions and beliefs regarding the efficacy of orthoses, and prescription rates among health care professionals are consequently quite variable.

Although orthoses have been available for a very long time, they should still be considered an experimental intervention for vertebral compression fractures. Prescription of orthoses should therefore be carried out only within the framework of evaluation studies.

This framework could include case studies, case series, nonrandomized clinical trials, and well-designed and well-executed randomized clinical trials. In view of the current use of orthoses and their potential value for subgroups of patients with vertebral compression fractures, such studies should be initiated.

REFERENCES

1. Pluijm SMF, Tromp AM, Smit JH, et al. Consequences of vertebral deformaties in older men and women. *J Bone Miner Res* 2000;15:1564–1572.
2. Andersson GB, Bostrom MP, Eyre DR, et al. Consensus summary on the diagnosis and treatment of osteoporosis. *Spine* 1997;22(24 Suppl):63S–65S.
3. Levine AM. Spinal orthoses. *Am Fam Physician* 1984:29:277—280.
4. Calmels P, Fayolle-Minon I. An update on orthotic devices for the lumbar spine based on a review of the literature. *Rev Rhum Engl Ed* 1996;63:285–291.
5. van Poppel MNM, de Looze MP, Koes BW, et al. Mechanisms of action of lumbar supports: a systematic review. *Spine* 2000;25:2103–2113.
6. Tanner R, Mueller M, Osterman H. Spinal orthotics: selective use in rehabilitation of vertebral osteoporosis. *J Back Musculoskel Rehabil* 1993;3:44–56.
7. Kaplan RS, Sinaki M, Hameister MD. Effect of back supports on back strength in patients with osteoporosis: a pilot study. *Mayo Clin Proc* 1996;71:235–241.
8. van Tulder MW, Jellema P, van Poppel NMN, et al. Lumbar supports for prevention and treatment of low back pain. Cochrane Database Syst Rev 2000;(3):CD001823.
9. Anderson CK, Morris TL, Del Vechio DC. *The effectiveness of using a lumbar support belt.* Dallas: Advanced Ergonomics, Inc., 1993.
10. Hsieh CJ, Phillips RB, Adams AH, et al. Functional outcomes of low back pain: comparison of four treatment groups in a randomized controlled trial. *J Manipulative Physiol Ther* 1992;15:4–9.

18
Pain Clinic Treatments

Charles E. Pither

Pain Management Department and Pain Input Unit, St. Thomas's Hospital, London, United Kingdom

Pain that has a sudden onset is usually related to tissue damage of some form. Treatment proceeds in a traditional manner with a medical assessment, including investigations to reach a diagnosis, and the use of appropriate therapy to treat the cause. As the problem resolves, the pain subsides, and treatment can be withdrawn. Healing or resolution of the lesion results in diminution of the nociceptive signals, with cessation of the pain experience. The pain may need treating in its own right; treatment most likely involves the administration of effective analgesics in appropriate dosages.

Unfortunately, according to clinical experience, problems do not always resolve in this way. Frequently, pain does persist even after adequate healing of the original injury. The presence of persistent, chronic pain mandates a broader range of treatment than simple analgesics. In fact, affected patients can be as complex, demanding, and difficult to treat as any found in hospital waiting rooms. This, at least in part, is because of the whole-person nature of their difficulties. Many such patients are clinically depressed and disabled. To be effective, treatment must address these aspects of their difficulties alongside the pain sensation.

It is clear that such patients are best treated in an interdisciplinary pain clinic. Although for some scientists the notion of a clinic devoted to a symptom, rather than a disease entity or process, is a regressive step, single disciplines often have little to offer the patient with chronic pain.

The prediction of long-term problems after an episode of acute back pain is dependent not on any measurable level of tissue abnormality or clinical findings but rather on a number of psychosocial variables (1). For this reason, it is of paramount importance to view the pain complaints in the context of the individual's psychological state, the environment, and other relevant variables affecting the patient, such as issues relating to work, litigation, or the benefits system. If such variables are to be taken into account, a thorough and broad assessment of the sufferer is crucial.

This chapter focuses on the assessment and treatment of patients who have had pain for many months without resolution and for whom the pain is intrusive and limits function. Such patients benefit from being referred to a pain center.

ASSESSMENT OF THE PATIENT WITH PAIN

Pain is always a subjective perception experienced only by the individual. There are always limits on the ability of the sufferer to convey exactly the nature of this experience.

In a traditional medical setting, the interpretation of the patient's symptoms leads to a diagnosis and the delivery of appropriate and curative treatment. However, for pain in the presence of vertebral collapse, therapy must be guided not only by the history, the examination, and the results of diagnostic tests but also by the effect the pain has on the patient and the presence of external influences. If all this is to be assessed properly, it is important that sufficient time is allowed and that appropriate disciplines are incorporated into the process. These disciplines include psychology, physiotherapy, and various medical specialties. In addition, it is frequently helpful to use standard psychometric or other questionnaires, which can provide supportive information for the decision-making process (2).

Assessment should focus on the following parameters:

- The nature of the symptoms (the illness).
- The nature and extent of the pathological process (the disease).
- The degree of psychological distress (depression and anxiety).
- The patient's perceived decrement of function (disability).
- The presence or absence of social reinforcement

It is important to make a distinction between the level of disability experienced by the patient and the level of impairment as assessed by medical examination (3).

PAIN CLINIC TREATMENTS

Pain is a multidimensional experience influenced by processes at all levels within the central nervous system. Seldom if ever is chronic pain relieved completely by manipulation of peripheral nociceptive inputs. For this reason, pain clinic therapy is usually multimodal and is aimed at symptom relief rather than disease management. Treatment is pragmatic in that the therapy with the greatest likelihood of relieving pain is initiated first. If this fails to provide benefit, other therapies are tried. The aim is not simply to cure the condition—pain clinic treatment seldom if ever provides a complete cure—but rather to improve the quality of life for the sufferer.

In general, four treatment modalities are available:

1. Drugs
2. Stimulation analgesia [transcutaneous electrical nerve stimulation (TENS) and acupuncture].
3. Nerve blocks and injections (particularly epidural and paravertebral techniques).
4. Psychological techniques

Drugs

The drug management of the pain of osteoporosis is the same among many specialists. Because this chapter focuses on the pain clinic, it does not go into detail of the general management of osteoporosis, although it is acknowledged that some such treatments (e.g., bisphosphonates) do have an effect on pain (4).

For a similar reason, the acute pain associated with a proven fracture is not addressed in depth because it is not the province of the pain clinic. Most patients referred to a pain clinic have pain that has persisted for at least 6 months and normally have experienced a failure of simple analgesic management.

Nonsteroidal Antiinflammatory Drugs

The use of nonsteroidal antiinflammatory drugs (NSAIDs) is logical for the pain of osteoporosis, inasmuch as prostaglandins are implicated in the genesis of the condition (5). However, recommendations for longer term use must be balanced against the significant risk of side effects. A small number of patients claim ongoing long-term benefit from NSAIDs but seldom to the extent that they no longer consider themselves to have a pain problem or are able to function normally. In this situation, there is a theoretical argument for switching to a more modern cyclooxygenase-2 (COX-2) preparation, such as rofecoxib or celecoxib.

For longer term management, NSAIDs do not have a significant role.

Opioids

The use of opioid analgesics is logical for persistent pain in which there is a continued nociceptive source of pain, as is the case in crush fracture (6). For many patients, compound analgesics, such as coproxamol, are prescribed by their primary physicians. If such drugs fail to control the pain, the use of more powerful analgesics can be beneficial. Drugs of intermediate strength such as tramadol or dihydrocodeine can enhance pain relief, especially when given in slow-release preparations. These drugs can cause mild sedation and unwelcome central side effects. These are less troublesome when given in a nighttime dose for nocturnal pain, when such effects can be beneficial. Tramadol, with its mixed mode of action, seems to be more effective in neuropathic pain states.

The decision to use the full-strength agonists such as morphine requires more thought. It must be remembered that opioids are not effective as treatment for distress, but distress is frequently what sends the patient to the physician and provokes the decision to increase the strength of the medication. This is illogical but difficult to avoid. Modest doses of slow-release morphine preparations can be of benefit in a selected group of patients, who seemingly can get benefit from a stable dosage over a prolonged period of time. It is, however, difficult to predict who will obtain worthwhile effects; thus, a trial is appropriate, starting at a dosage of 10 to 20 mg of slow-release morphine twice daily. Frequently, such dosages are more effective than the array of less potent analgesics that the sufferer is taking, and they cause no serious side effects.

A small number of patients with pain at night often benefit considerably from a dose taken at bedtime. In this situation, of course, any sedative effects are generally welcome, because they aid sleep.

Tricyclic Antidepressants

Tricyclic antidepressants are much appreciated by pain specialists. They are a class of drugs that frequently have a beneficial effect in chronic pain states, although they are often associated with unwelcome side effects. Tricyclic antidepressants have been shown to produce pain relief in neuropathic pain states (7) but are often of benefit in mixed or nociceptive pain problems. The three main effects that can be expected are improved sleep, improvement of mood, and reduction of pain. Prescription of a tricyclic antidepressant is appropriate when the pain is starting to cause depression, general dysthymia, or secondary problems with sleep. Amitriptyline is the standard drug but does have many unwanted effects, and some patients find that they cannot tolerate even a small dose.

Trimipramine and imipramine are better in this regard. Sensitive patients should commence on 10 mg at night and try to increase the dosage to 20 or 30 mg. Others who less frequently experience side effects from medications start with 25 mg. There is no point in increasing doses to higher levels unless the patient is clinically depressed.

The role for more modern antidepressants such as selective serotonin reuptake inhibitors is less clear. Patients can certainly benefit from these medications, and a beneficial effect on pain is occasionally seen. In most cases, however, the profile of effects is less useful for the treatment of chronic pain.

Anticonvulsants

Historically, this group of drugs has been used extensively for chronic pain, largely in neuropathic pain states (8). In the case of osteoporotic vertebral collapse, their most greatest use is in cases in which there is clearly a radicular component to the pain. Historically, carbamazepine has been the drug of first choice, but it often has unacceptable side effects. Other drugs such as phenytoin and sodium valproate have less efficacy. Without a doubt, the most effective drug in the whole arena of neuropathic pain is gabapentin. Although its mechanisms of action are uncertain, this drug has helped a great many patients with problems that had not previously responded to drug therapy. The dose is increased slowly from an initial dose of 300 mg/day to a maximum of 2800 mg/day.

Stimulation Analgesia

Transcutaneous Electrical Nerve Stimulation

There is no doubt that TENS has a useful role in the treatment of both acute and chronic pain from vertebral collapse, especially when there is a radicular component to the pain (8). More than 75% of patients find the device helpful initially. For this reason, a trial of TENS should be offered to those with persistent pain. It is usually necessary to explain and demonstrate the use of the device to patients in an educational visit. This service is carried out by an experienced nurse. Patients are then given a TENS device on loan to try at home for a 3-week period. They are instructed in electrode placement and given a suggested timetable to experiment with it. If they find the device helpful, they can then purchase a device for themselves.

Although TENS frequently produces effective analgesia, there are some problems with the technique. First, it is difficult to predict, on the basis of disease categorization, who will benefit. It is clear from the large amount of research on TENS that it can be effective in many conditions but not with a great deal of consistency. One patient with thoracic pain will find the device most helpful and use it as part of a multimodal treatment program, whereas another will find that it aggravates the pain.

The second problem is that the effectiveness of the technique decreases rapidly with time. By 3 months, the number gaining benefit has dropped from greater than 70% to less than 30%. However, some patients still use the machines either occasionally or regularly, claiming significant ongoing benefit.

Acupuncture

Acupuncture has been used for many thousands of years for the treatment of a variety of conditions, and, without a doubt, produces multiple effects within the sensory processing system (9). Pain can be modified by dry needling; the mechanisms of action are, however, unclear.

There are few outcome data relating to the treatment of the pain of vertebral collapse, but most pain clinicians see the technique as being a useful component of their armamentarium.

Nerve Blocks

Epidural Injection

Epidural injections have been used for many years as a treatment option for patients experiencing back pain. The rationale has been based on considerable anecdotal evidence of efficacy, a theoretical basis for expectation of benefit, and a lack of other more effective therapies. By injecting into the epidural space, many structures can be brought into contact with the injected substances. These structures include the internal facet capsule, the longitudinal ligament, the annulus of the disc, the nerve root itself, and other sensitive neural elements within the spinal canal. If, as is likely, the sources of pain in osteoporotic collapse are multiple (10) and related in part to the presence of inflammation secondary to the injury, the injection of antiinflammatory medications nearby is logical (11).

The author is of the opinion that steroid is a vital component of the injected substances and that this should be a depot preparation to prevent the rapid systemic absorption.

Most outcome data relate to the use of epidural injections in the lumbar region, for which there is undoubtedly there is a greater body of experience. However, because collapse is more common in the thoracic area, blocks are more frequently needed at this level. Because the lumbar epidural space is larger and the spinal cord terminates at the upper level, lumbar injection is safer, at least as far as the likelihood of penetration of the spinal cord is concerned. For this reason, many practitioners have been more reluctant to either perform or recommend thoracic epidural injection, on the grounds of safety. This is irrational, however, because the technique is safe, and with experience, the injection can be performed very simply and with minimal trauma or risk.

Technique

Thoracic epidural block can be performed by numerous techniques, and it is neither possible nor desirable to suggest that one approach is favored or safer than any other. There are, however, some theoretical considerations that confer advantages to certain techniques.

The block can be satisfactorily carried out as an outpatient procedure, without the use of sedation. In general, a single dose of local anesthetic and steroid is administered. A great many volumes and agents have been used with vigorous protagonists for differing regimens. Physicians who favor large volumes believe that the use of a greater volume can ensure that some of the drug does get to the affected segment. Others believe that a small volume delivered precisely to the problem area may be more effective. In general, this will entail an x-ray-guided procedure.

Blocks can be repeated if they are of benefit or thought to be technically deficient. With repeat injections, the dose of steroid must be monitored closely.

Risks

Inevitably, the risks that attend epidural injection are greater when it is performed above the lumbar region, but these risks are still very low. Spinal cord injury does occur (13).

Respiratory and cardiovascular effects of the block also occur but seem to be of no clinical significance. In general, the complications are the same for any entry to the epidural space: dural puncture, hematoma, nerve injury, and infection.

Efficacy

The use of epidural injections for back pain has been the subject of numerous studies but all too few well-controlled trials. No studies have specifically related to the treatment of chronic pain in patients with osteoporotic collapse. It is, however, fair to extrapolate from the metaanalyses that have been carried out.

Koes et al. (14), in a systematic review, examined the efficacy of epidural steroid injections for low back pain. Twelve randomized studies were identified; with only four scored more than 60 points on methodological assessment. Of these four studies, two reported positive benefit, and two reported negative outcomes. This pattern was repeated for the other eight studies; half indicated that the treatment was more effective than the reference condition, and half reported that it was no better or worse. Koes et al. concluded that there were flaws in the designs of most of the studies and that the efficacy of epidural steroid injection has not yet been established. Watts and Silagy (15) undertook a metaanalysis to assess the benefit of epidural corticosteroids in the treatment of sciatica, identifying 11 trials that included 907 patients. Their analysis showed that the use of epidural steroids increased the odds ratio of short-term pain relief (>75%) to 2.61 (95% confidence interval, 1.9 to 3.77). For longer term relief (up to 1 year), the odds ratio fell to 1.87 (95% confidence interval, 1.31 to 2.68). Their conclusion was that the epidural administration of corticosteroids is effective in the management of lumbosacral radicular pain.

It should be noted that these two studies adopted different methods and examined different aspects of outcome. It has long been clinical wisdom that epidural injections are more effective for radicular or limb pain than for back pain, and this picture emerges from these metaanalyses. Both studies also demonstrated the lack of serious side effects with no long-term adverse consequences.

Paravertebral or Foraminal Block

Pain from a collapsed vertebra frequently has a radicular pattern. It is likely that this is caused by irritation of the nerve root as it exits the intervertebral foramen. Pain is not simply caused by physical irritation of the root; it may well involve inflammation caused by the release of chemical mediators from the damaged tissues (16). Epidural injection can allow the injected material to reach the affected areas, but if the compression is significant, there may be a physical barrier to penetration. For this reason, the use of a paravertebral technique is logical.

Injection is made outside the spinal canal under radiographic guidance. A 22-gauge needle is inserted 3 to 4 cm from the midline and slid down the lateral border of the vertebral body toward the intervertebral foramen. Sometimes a paresthesia is elicited. Caution must be exercised in the thoracic region to avoid contact with the pleura. Contrast medium can be injected to ascertain the spread of the injected material. A dose of 3 to 6 mL of local anesthetic, combined with a steroid preparation, is injected. The procedure can be performed bilaterally at the same level and at more than one level.

Only a few studies have investigated the efficacy of paravertebral blocks in any situation, and none have in osteoporosis. Anecdotal evidence supports their use for persistent pain, especially when radicular pain is an issue.

Psychological Techniques

Interdisciplinary Treatment and Pain Management Programs

Spinal pain represents the largest category of patients referred to pain clinics in the United Kingdom. The epidemiology of back and neck pain and studies of the factors that affect the development of chronicity clearly demonstrate the importance of psychosocial factors (1). After an episode of acute back pain, the likelihood of the development of persistent pain and disability is not predicated by physical or disease related factors, but it is related to reported pain level in the initial attack, perception of damage and illness, and psychological distress as measured by depression inventories. The elucidation of this aspect of back pain has led to the description of so-called "yellow flags" or psychosocial risk factors (17).

Yellow flags cover such areas as attitudes and beliefs about pain, behaviors, compensation issues, diagnosis and treatment, emotions, family issues, and work. The assessment and treatment of low back pain are increasingly taking these factors into account, and the need to address them if effective treatment is to be provided is increasingly recognized. It therefore follows that for a great many spinal pain problems, treatment must encompass broader dimensions than the purely biological. It is not simply a case of substituting psychological or psychiatric therapy for ineffective medical treatment: These patients are not psychotic, and their pain problems cannot be cured by psychological treatment. Psychological therapies do have a role but only when combined with broader "medical" treatment. This has led to the provision of interdisciplinary therapy, in which various disciplines work together to provide therapy to address the patient's problems. Such disciplines include physiotherapy, psychology, medicine, nursing, occupational therapy, ergonomics, and fitness instruction. Many patients receive outpatient treatment in one or many of these disciplines, often with little benefit.

In general, the most commonly used psychological treatment approaches adopt cognitive-behavioral techniques. Cognitive-behavioral principles can be listed as follows:

- The way a person "feels" about issues, events, or bodily sensations depends on his or her evaluation of them.
- This internal evaluation is influenced by the person's knowledge and understanding of the causes, or meaning, of the symptom or event.
- The person's knowledge base is a complex repository of information (both correct and incorrect), views, beliefs, and experiences.
- When the person does not have hard facts or information, he or she makes inferences to fill in the gaps in his or her knowledge.
- Such inferences may not be correct.
- The conclusion that a person comes to about a symptom or issue, on the basis of both the available facts and the inferences that he or she makes, has an emotional loading. This conclusion is the same regardless of the truth of the inference. For example, if the discovery of a lump in a breast implies cancer, the emotional experience will be negative even before clinical confirmation of malignancy.

- Although such processes are normal and essentially human, the views that people take can at times, and about certain individuals, be too strongly held, too rigid, or erroneous. Because pain is usually a very negative experience, it is not surprising that it can often become associated with a series of negative emotions.
- Patterns of negative thinking tend to become stereotyped and automatic. Thus, sufferers report that the same negative series of thoughts occur several times a day, often provoked by everyday situations. This process has been termed *catastrophization.* These thoughts provoke negative emotions such as fear, low mood, anger, frustration, and despair.
- In the context of spinal pain, many people experiencing pain have a catalog of negative or catastrophic views as to the cause, implications, and prognosis of the illness.
- Such inferences are usually erroneous, but this does not prevent them from having a considerable influence on the sufferer in terms of negative emotional load.
- Inferences will also alter behavior.
- A belief that back pain represents crumbling of the bones is not compatible with activities that provoke pain because, to the sufferer, the increased pain signifies crumbling or worsening of the damage being done to the spine.
- This process has been termed *fear avoidance* and commonly accompanies chronic spinal pain.

The aim of cognitive-behavioral therapy is to teach patients ways to recognize these automatic negative thoughts when they occur and to challenge them with other perceptions in a more balanced and, it is hoped, accurate representation (18). Alternative, less catastrophic ways of viewing problems produce less negative emotions, enabling patients to feel better. These techniques are combined with practical approaches aimed at gradually reintroducing patients to feared activities, tasks, and movements. In practice, the undertaking of these techniques devolves to two areas: physiotherapy-led stretching and exercise in the gym and occupational therapist–led activity programming involving planning, goal setting, and pacing.

This form of treatment is usually delivered in a group setting for a fixed length, such as 3 or 4 weeks. Programs differ depending on the level of difficulties experienced by the patient and the goals of the therapy. The literature is replete with outcomes from various protocols, delivered by differing disciplines in a multitude of settings. There is no agreed nomenclature for such programs, but in general, *functional restoration* is the term given to a physically based rehabilitation program with some psychological input, aimed at returning patients to normal function, including work. Pain management programs are aimed at more disabled and distressed patients, for whom normal function may not be a realistic expectation. Such programs are more psychological in their emphasis.

Pain Management

The concept of pain management is validated by examination of patients who have chronic pain problems but manage to function normally and enjoy a good quality of life. Such people seem to do the following:

- Understand the likely cause of their pain and have overcome fears about it.
- Take as few medications as possible.
- Maintain physical fitness and keep as active as possible.
- Pace activities, avoid overexerting themselves, and avoid getting into overactivity/underactivity cycles.

- Have methods for coping with flareups and setbacks.
- Keep their mood positive and avoid catastrophizing.
- Use a relaxation technique.

The aims of a pain management program are thus to teach pain sufferers these skills while aiding them in improving physical performance with a stretching and exercise regimen. treatment is typically delivered in a group of eight to ten patients over a certain number of weeks. In the United Kingdom, this is organized either as an outpatient program of 6 to 8 weeks' duration or as a residential package of 3 or 4 weeks' duration (19).

Outcome data from such programs indicate that very significant changes can be made in a number of domains that cumulatively improve quality of life. There are very few outcome data specific to pain secondary to osteoporotic collapse. In a metaanalysis, Morley et al. (20) reported that, in comparison with control treatment conditions, cognitive-behavioral interventions showed clear superiority in reducing pain level, enhancing cognitive coping, and reducing behavioral expression of pain.

CONCLUSIONS

Chronic pain after osteoporotic vertebral collapse is common but is usually related to a complex series of interactions rather than a single source of pain. Once the pain becomes chronic, the chances that a simple treatment will be curative diminish, as secondary physical and psychological mechanisms intrude.

Pain clinics aim to provide pragmatic symptomatic relief with a focus on pain relief and function rather than disease modification. Treatment approaches utilize drug therapy, including the use of coanalgesics such as tricyclic antidepressants and antiepileptics; simulation analgesia, including TENS; and nerve blocks and injections. For patients who fail to respond to these physical or pharmacological maneuvers, treatment on a pain management program can be helpful.

REFERENCES

1. Burton AK, Tillotson M, Main CJ, et al. Psychosocial predictors of outcome in acute and sub-chronic low back trouble. *Spine* 1995;20:722–728.
2. Williams A. Measures of function and psychology. In: Wall PD, Melzack R, eds. *Textbook of pain,* 4th ed. Edinburgh: Churchill Livingstone, 1999:427–444.
3. Waddell G. *The back pain revolution.* Edinburgh: Churchill Livingstone, 1998:119–134.
4. Managing osteoporosis. *Drug Ther Bull* 1996;34:45–48.
5. Golde B. New clues to the etiology of osteoporosis: the effects of prostaglandins (E2 and F2 alpha) on bone. *Med Hypotheses* 1992;38(2):125–131.
6. Collett BJ. Chronic opioid therapy for non-cancer pain. *Br J Anaesth* 2001;87:133–143.
7. McQuay HJ, Moore RA. An evidence-based resource for pain relief. Oxford, UK: Oxford University Press, 1998.
8. Woolf CJ, Thompson JW. Stimulation induced analgesia, transcutaneous nerve stimulation (TENS) and vibration. In: Wall P, Melzack R, eds. *Textbook of pain,* 4th ed. Edinburgh: Churchill Livingstone, 1999:1191–1208.
9. Filshie J, White A. *Medical acupuncture, a western scientific approach.* Edinburgh: Churchill Livingstone, 1998.
10. Passeri M, Baroni MC, Pedrazzoni M, et al. Treatment experience with chronic spinal pain in involutions in osteoporosis. *Ann Ital Med Int* 1992;7:137–153.
11. Abram SE. Pain mechanisms in lumbar radiculopathy. *Anaesth Analg* 1988;67:1135–1137.
12. Manchikanti L. Cervical epidural steroid injection with intrinsic spinal cord damage. *Spine* 1999;24:1170–1172.
13. Hodges SD, Castleberg RL, Miller T, et al. Cervical epidural steroid injection with intrinsic spinal cord damage. Two case reports. *Spine* 1998;23:2137–2142.
14. Koes BW, Scholten RJ, Mens JM, et al. Efficacy of epidural steroid injections for low-back pain and sciatica: a systematic review of randomized clinical trials. *Pain* 1995;63:279–288.
15. Watts RW, Silagy CA. A meta-analysis on the efficacy of epidural corticosteroids in the treatment of sciatica. *Anaesth Intensive Care* 1995;23(5):564–569.
16. Olmarker K, Rydevik B. Selective inhibition of TNF alpha prevents nucleus pulposus induced thrombus formation. *Spine* 2001;26:863–869.

17. Kendall NA. Psychosocial approaches to the prevention of chronic pain: the low back paradigm. *Baillieres Best Pract Res Clin Rheumatol* 1999;13:545–554.
18. Turk DC, Meichenbaum D, Genest M. *Pain and behavioral medicine: a cognitive behavioral perspective.* New York: Guilford Press, 1983.
19. Turner JA. Efficacy of cognitive therapy for low back pain. *Pain* 1993;52:169–177.
20. Morley S, Eccleston C, Williams A. Systematic review and meta-analysis of randomized controlled trials of cognitive behavior therapy and behavior therapy for chronic pain in adults, excluding headache. *Pain* 1999;80:1–13.

19

The Clinical Use of Cortoss Synthetic Bone Void Filler in the Repair of Fractures in the Vertebral Body

*Jean Palussière, †Jérôme Berge, ‡Afshin Gangi, and §Hervé Deramond

**Institut Bergonie, Service de Radiologie, Bordeaux, France; †Service de Neuroradiologie, Diagnostique et Therapeutique Centre Hospitalier Pellegrin, Bordeaux, France; ‡Hôpitaux Universitaires de Strasbourg, Hospices Civiles, Strasbourg, France; §Service de Radiologie A, CHU Amiens-Hôpital Nord, Amiens, France*

The use of vertebroplasty with the instillation of polymethylmethacrylate (PMMA) as an alternative to the open surgical treatment of pathological vertebral compression fractures has previously been reported (1–4). Since the early 1990s, PMMA has been instilled in vertebral bodies under fluoroscopic guidance for the treatment of pain related to osteoporotic compression fractures or tumor invasion (5,6). The pathophysiological mechanism through which vertebroplasty is effective is not yet known. Theories that have been proposed have included the toxic effects of free monomers on the nerve endings and ablation of the nerve endings caused by the high temperatures resulting from the exothermic polymerization reaction. The explanation for the relief of pain is probably associated with reinforcement and subsequent strengthening (stabilization) of the partially collapsed and fractured osteoporotic vertebra (7–9). Articles dealing with the clinical effects of percutaneous vertebroplasty report good and rapid analgesic performance with low complication rates. All articles, including the only two prospective ones published to date (8,10), report success rates of 80% or higher. These prospective studies measured the effect at 24 and 72 hours, respectively, after treatment. All studies have highlighted the almost immediate onset of the analgesic effect.

The clinical goals of vertebroplasty are immediate reduction or complete relief of pain, improvement or at least maintenance of function, prevention of further vertebral collapse, and long-term stability. The interest in vertebroplasty has increased dramatically, both in patients and in physicians.

Clinical results with the use of PMMA in PVP have yielded high success rates in relieving pain while providing adequate intervertebral stability with few reported complications (11). However, safety concerns regarding the injection of PMMA into the spine have developed. To obtain ideal injection characteristics, surgeons have increased the monomer-to-powder ratio from the indicated composition, thus raising the concentration of toxic chemicals (12). In addition, poor visualization and a high temperature rise during the procedure can adversely affect material placement and preservation of surrounding spinal tissue. Another limitation of the PMMA system for percutaneous vertebroplasty includes the lack of dose flexibility, resulting in longer and more expensive procedures.

MATERIALS AND METHODS

A prospective clinical study, begun in the spring of 2001, is being conducted in Europe. The objective of this study is to demonstrate the safety and performance of the new cortical bone void filler in percutaneous vertebroplasty for the management of pain associated with documented acute osteoporotic vertebral fracture, metastatic osteolytic vertebral lesions, or angioma. To participate, patients have to have fracture-related pain measuring at least 50/100 on the Visual Analogue Scale (VAS), which also causes a change in lifestyle or disability. Patients are scheduled for follow-up 4 days, 1 week, and 1, 3, and 6 months after the procedure.

Cortoss cement is provided in a double-lumen cartridge with specially designed tips for mixing. After the composite is expressed through these tips, polymerization begins, and the material is ready for use. The delivery system with changeable mix tips allows the physician to prepare fresh material at any time it is needed during the procedure. Two metal trocars of 10 gauge diameter are introduced through the pedicles under fluoroscopic control. Metal catheters are then introduced in the trocars, and the composite is injected through them with 1-mL syringes. These catheters are replaced after delivery is interrupted.

RESULTS

At the time of writing, a total of 24 patients have been enrolled. Twenty-three suffered from osteoporotic fractures and one from metastatic collapse. The average pain scores in these patients were 69 (n = 24) before treatment, 38 (n = 24) at day 4, 33 (n = 24) at 1 week, 29 (n = 21) at 1 month, and 39 (n = 13) at 3 months. This represents a reduction of pain of 46% at day 4, 51% at 1 week, 58% at 1 month, and 43% at 3 months. Of the 24 patients, 21 (88%) had at least a 20% improvement in pain at 1 week (range, 20% to 100%). The quality of life of the patients is being evaluated with the Short Form 12 (SF-12) questionnaire and a mobility assessment; results from these tests are not yet available.

CASE REPORTS

Case 1

Three years earlier, an 89-year-old woman complained about acute and severe back pain related to a T-12 vertebral collapse (Fig. 19.1A), which necessitated complete bed rest for 3 months. Three weeks before the procedure, she had complained about severe and disabling back pain at the upper lumbar level. The patient was treated with morphinic drugs and bed rest; she moved with difficulty and exacerbation of the pain, which was evaluated at 90/100 on the VAS. Plain films (see Fig. 19.1B) and a computed tomographic (CT) scan (see Fig. 19.2A,B) showed an L-1 osteoporotic vertebral fracture with an osteonecrotic area in the inferior part of the vertebral body. Percutaneous vertebroplasty was indicated and performed 23 days after the bone event through a bilateral parapedicular approach (Fig. 19.3A,B) and injection of 4.5 mL of Cortoss cement without leakage (Fig. 19.4A,B). The patient's condition improved dramatically just after the procedure, and she was able to walk again with help and decreased pain (VAS score, 30/100). The day after the procedure, morphinic drugs were stopped. She was discharged 2 days later, walking without help (VAS score, 0/100) and no morphinic drugs.

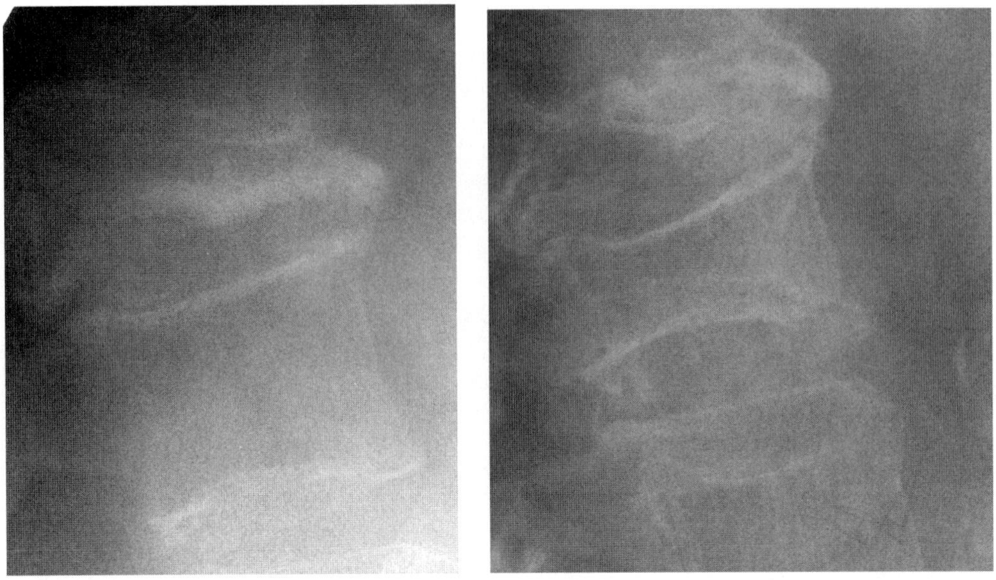

A B

FIG. 19.1. A: Lateral plain film 1 year before the onset of the recent back pain, showing T-12 osteoporotic vertebral collapse. **B:** Lateral plain film 2 weeks after the onset of the new severe back pain, showing L-1 osteoporotic compression fracture.

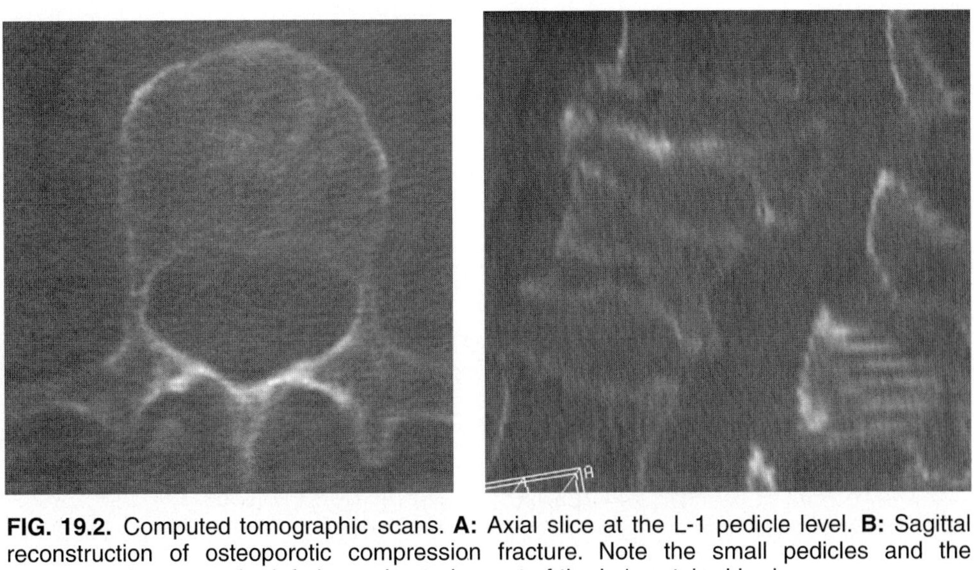

A B

FIG. 19.2. Computed tomographic scans. **A:** Axial slice at the L-1 pedicle level. **B:** Sagittal reconstruction of osteoporotic compression fracture. Note the small pedicles and the osteonecrotic area at the inferior and anterior part of the L-1 vertebral body.

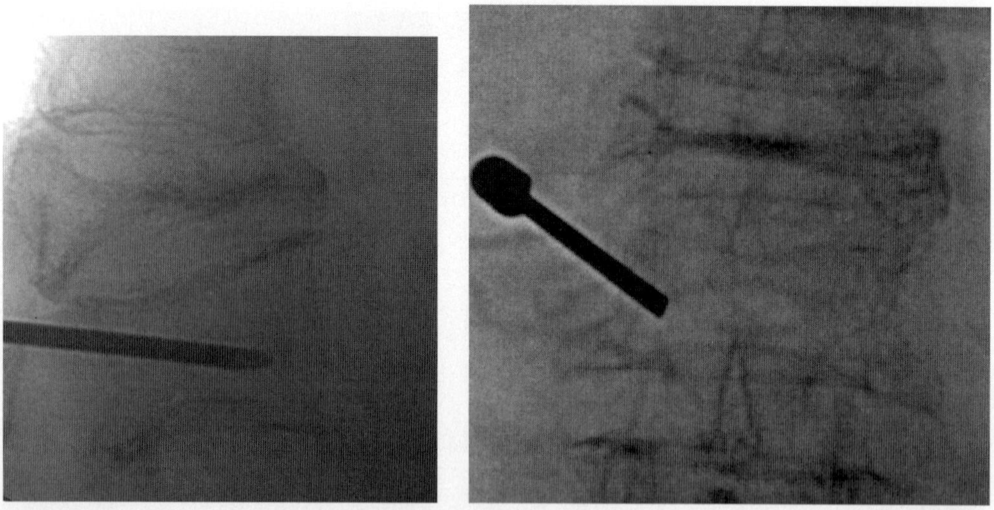

A B

FIG. 19.3. Percutaneous vertebroplasty. **A:** Lateral view. **B:** Frontal view. Parapedicle approach of the vertebral body because of the small pedicles

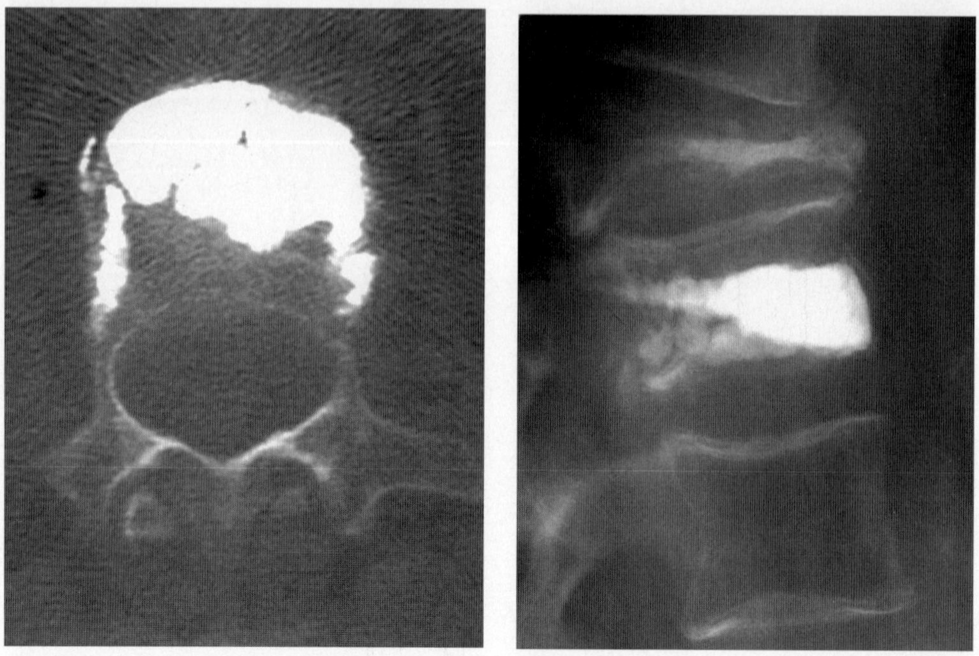

A B

FIG. 19.4. Percutaneous vertebroplasty. **A:** Computed tomographic scan control, axial slice. **B:** Plain film control, lateral view. Good distribution of the Cortoss cement without any leakage.

Case 2

A 73-year-old woman had radiological signs of possible vertebral collapse of T-5 to T-8 after radiation therapy for thymic cancer. She was eventually hospitalized with pain from simply lifting a pot of water, and compression fractures of T-5 to T-8 were diagnosed. It was decided to augment all four vertebral bodies with Cortoss cement (3 mL, 3 mL, 2 mL, and 4 mL, respectively) with general anesthesia, after which pain disappeared within 24 hours. There was minimal leakage of Cortoss cement into a foraminal vein at the T-6 level. In Fig. 19.5, preprocedural, periprocedural, and postprocedural radiographs show good filling of all four vertebral bodies and further description radiographs.

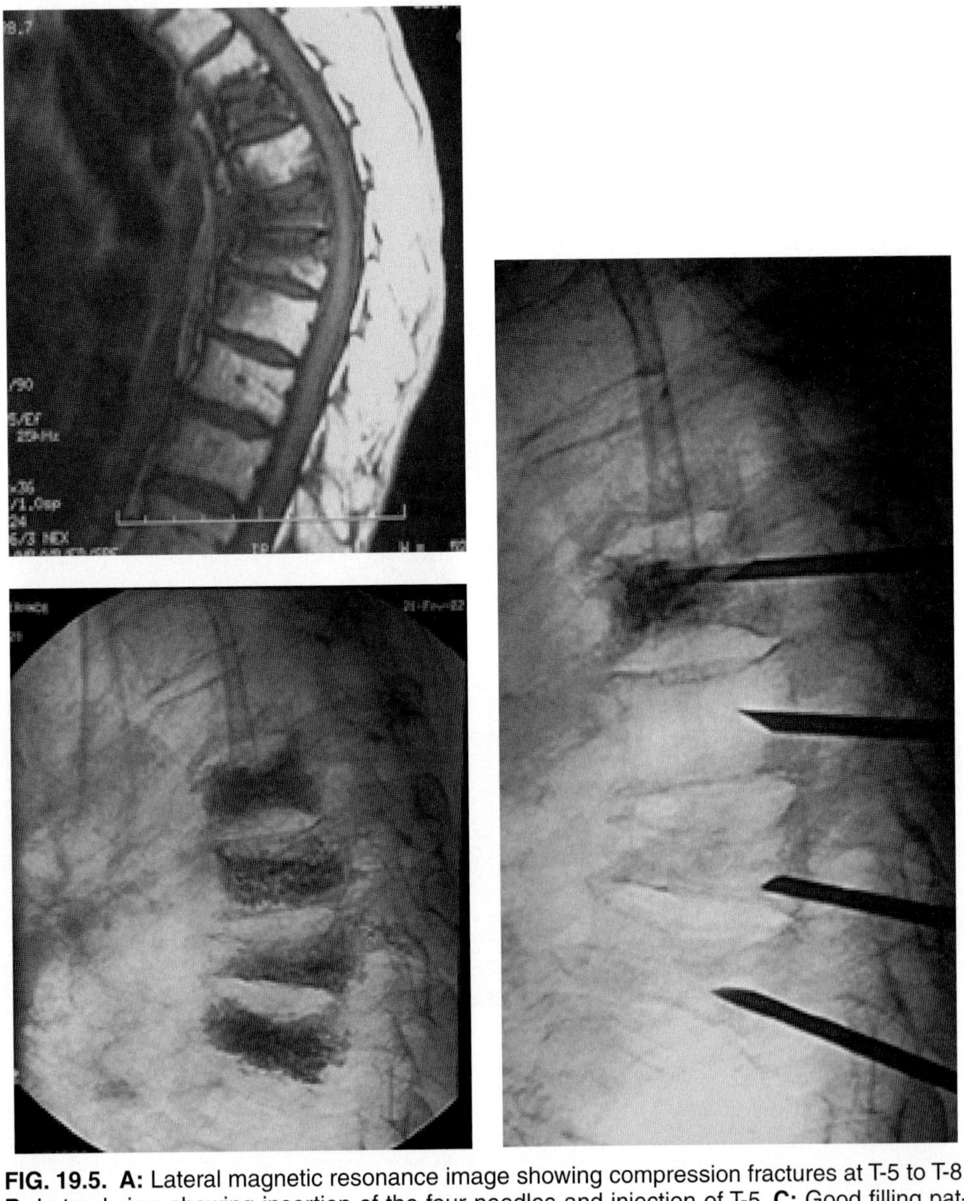

FIG. 19.5. A: Lateral magnetic resonance image showing compression fractures at T-5 to T-8. **B:** Lateral view showing insertion of the four needles and injection of T-5. **C:** Good filling pattern of augmented bodies.

Case 3

A 66-year-old man with a metastatic lesion in T-8 of unknown origin at time of diagnosis underwent percutaneous vertebroplasty with injection of 8 mL of Cortoss cement after a biopsy was taken. The procedure was uneventful (no leakages). Preintervention and postintervention CT scans are shown in Fig. 19.6.

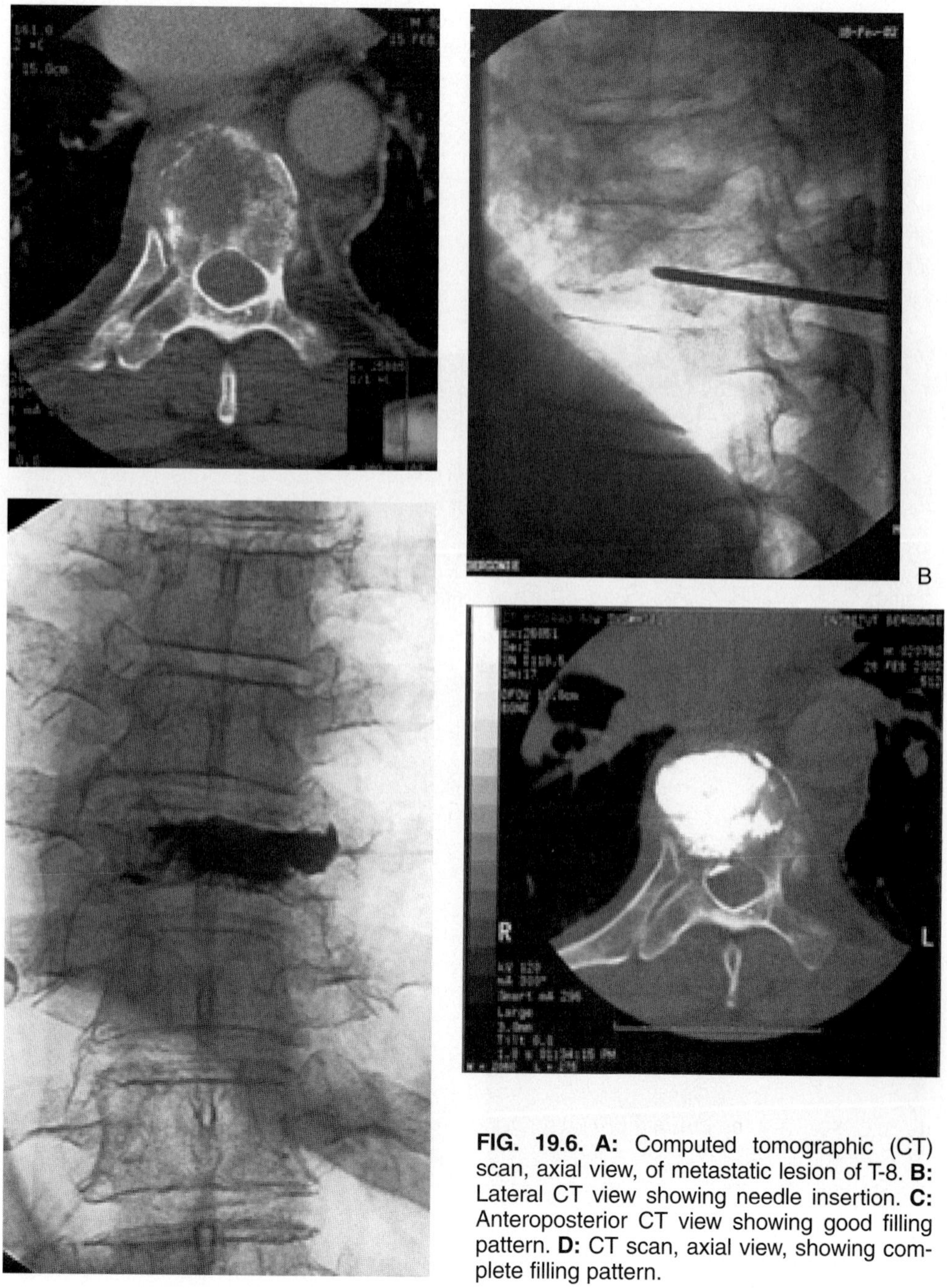

FIG. 19.6. A: Computed tomographic (CT) scan, axial view, of metastatic lesion of T-8. **B:** Lateral CT view showing needle insertion. **C:** Anteroposterior CT view showing good filling pattern. **D:** CT scan, axial view, showing complete filling pattern.

DISCUSSION

The delivery of the material through dedicated catheters and syringes works well. Because of the consistency of the material, little pressure is required to inject the material, and as soon as the pressure on the plunger is relieved, the flow of material halts immediately. The radiopacity of the material makes the detection of even small leakages relatively easy. In about half the patients, the injection was stopped once or multiple times because either a leakage appeared on fluoroscopy or the material was getting close to reaching the posterior wall, which can be considered an early warning for the development of leakages. After the injection was stopped, the catheter was removed and the material was left to set for the next 2 to 2.5 minutes. After that time, a new catheter-syringe combination was prepared, and the injection continued. In most cases, the previously injected material had set and formed a dam that protected against further leakages in the same arca. The amount of material injected per vertebra varied between 1 and 8 mL.

The most common procedure-related complications were small paravertebral and intradiscal leakages. None of these leakages had any clinical consequences. In four patients, the material polymerized inside the delivery catheter while it was still located in the vertebral body. In two cases, this was discovered only after the removal of the needle and catheter, and a small pipe of material was left in the soft tissue extending from the pedicle posteriorly. In one patient, the resulting local pain was treated through infiltration of the area with local anesthetics and steroids, with reasonable success. In the second patient, the procedure had to be stopped, and a second fractured vertebra was left untreated. In the other two patients, it proved easy to break the material loose inside the vertebra by turning the catheter and slightly tilting the needle. The catheter with the polymerized material was then retrieved without any adverse consequences. As a result of these experiences, the surgical technique has been emended to reduce the risk of this complication.

This was the first clinical experience with a new bioactive material, especially designed to replace and reinforce load-bearing bone, in vertebroplasty. Its differences in flow and polymerization characteristics in comparison to PMMA were not fully appreciated, and the first patients in the initial study were treated with the standard techniques used for PMMA. This led to unsatisfactory results, especially concerning the degree of fill that was achieved.

The development of the dedicated catheter–based delivery system has rendered the whole procedure more reliable and reproducible and allows the operator to obtain the desired degree of fill, without the need to hurry or the use of excessive amounts of force to complete the injection. In the future, further refinements to the delivery system are anticipated. The combination of this new bioactive material and its dedicated delivery system simplifies the procedure, enhances its safety, and creates a biologically and biomechanically superior construct.

Like patients in other clinical series, the majority of patients in this study appear to have benefited from the procedure; their pain was significant reduced almost immediately after treatment. In light of the characteristics of the bioactive material used, this observation makes it less likely that factors such as thermal necrosis or monomer toxicity play a role in the clinical effectiveness of vertebroplasty. Rather, the results lend further support to the theory that the immobilization and stabilization of the fracture itself are the main factors that underlie the beneficial effects of vertebroplasty. As reported in another article (5), we did not see a correlation between the amount of material injected and the clinical effect. One explanation could be that there appears to be a very wide radiographic variation in fracture patterns, often between fractured vertebrae within individual patients. Although there still is a need for data from prospective, randomized studies comparing vertebroplasty with other modes of treatment, the results obtained so far in this study support the conclusions of earlier studies that describe the effectiveness of vertebroplasty in treating pain caused by vertebral compression fractures.

Cortoss cement is well suited for use in the treatment of vertebral compression fractures. Results indicate that Cortoss cement addresses the shortcomings of PMMA for vertebral augmentation. Cortoss cement is stronger than PMMA when injected into the spine, results in easier radiographic visualization, and requires a lower peak cure temperature. The Aliquot™ delivery system allows for accurate doses of Cortoss cement to be injected directly to the region of interest.

Cortoss cement is a fixed composition material with less variability than current variations of PMMA and, in conjunction with the Aliquot delivery system, can be accurately delivered in incremental doses without excessive material waste.

REFERENCES

1. Cortet B, Cotten A, Deprez X. [Value of vertebroplasty combined with surgical decompression in the treatment of aggressive spinal angioma. 3 cases]. *Rev Rhum Ed Fr* 1994;61(1):16–22.
2. Cybulski GR. Methods of surgical stabilization for metastatic disease of the spine. *Neurosurgery* 1989;25(2): 240–252.
3. Harrington KD. Anterior decompression and stabilization of the spine as a treatment for vertebral collapse and spinal cord compression from metastatic malignancy. *Clin Orthop* 1988;233:177–197.
4. Nicola N, Lins E. Vertebral hemangioma: retrograde embolization-stabilization with methyl methacrylate. *Surg Neurol* 1987;27:481–486.
5. Deramond H, Depriester L, Galibert P, et al. Percutaneous vertebroplasty with PMMA. Technique, indications, and results. *Radiol Clin North Am* 1998;36(3):533–546.
6. Gangi A, Dietemann JL, Guth S, et al. CT & fluoroscopic VP: results & complications in 187 pts. *Sem Interven Radiol* 1999;16(2):137–142.
7. Chiras J, Depriester C, Weill A, et al. Percutaneous vertebral surgery. Technics and indications. *J Neuroradiol* 1997;24(1):45–59. (In French).
8. Cortet B, Cotten A, Boutry N, et al. Percutaneous vertebroplasty in the treatment of osteoporotic vertebral compression fracture: an open prospective study. *J Rheumatol* 1999;26:2222–2228.
9. Mathis JM, Barr JD, Belkoff SM, et al. Percutaneous vertebroplasty: a developing standard of care for vertebral compression fractures. *AJNR Am J Neuroradiol* 2001;22(2):373–381.
10. Heini PF, Wälchli B, Berlemann U. Percutaneous transpedicular PVP with PMMA: operative technique and early results. *Eur Spine J* 2000;9:445–450.
11. Belkoff SM, Mathis JM, Erbe EM, et al. Biomechanical evaluation of a new bone cement for use in vertebroplasty. *Spine* 2000;25:1061–1064.
12. Jasper LE, Deramond H, Mathis JM, et al. The effect of monomer-to powder ratio on the material properties of cranioplastic. *Bone* 1999;25(2 Suppl):27S–29S.

20

Vertebroplasty and Kyphoplasty in the Treatment of Osteoporotic Vertebral Compression Fractures

Isador H. Lieberman

Department of Orthopaedic Surgery, The Cleveland Clinic Foundation, Cleveland, Ohio

Osteoporosis is a systemic disease currently afflicting more than 24 million Americans; this number is likely to rise as the population ages. The disease results in progressive bone mineral loss and concurrent changes in bone architecture that leave bone vulnerable to fracture, often after minimal or no trauma. The spine is the most common site of osteoporotic fracture; vertebral compression fractures (VCFs) occur in up to 50% of women aged 80 years and older and in 25% of women aged 70 to 79 years (1,2). Overall, 700,000 people per year in the United States suffer a VCF, this frequency exceeds even that of hip fractures (3). Osteoporotic VCFs have been shown to be associated with up to a 30% age-adjusted increase in mortality (4). The cost to society of managing patients with osteoporotic VCF in the United States in 1995 was $746 million (5). Possible acute complications of vertebral fracture include cord compression, urinary retention, and ileus (6). Long-term consequences include considerable pain (reported in 35% of patients with detectable VCFs) (7), as well as pulmonary compromise (a 9% loss in predicted forced vital capacity with each vertebral fracture) (8). Other chronic sequelae include deconditioning, deformity, insomnia, and depression, resulting in substantial physical, functional, and psychosocial impairment (8,9).

NONOPERATIVE MANAGEMENT OF VERTEBRAL COMPRESSION FRACTURES

Two-thirds of patients with acute, painful VCFs experience improvement regardless of the treatment applied. Traditional, nonoperative management includes bed rest, analgesics, and bracing. This type of medical management however, fails to restore spinal alignment, and the lack of mobility itself can result in secondary complications, including worsening osteoporosis, atelectasis, pneumonia, deep vein thrombosis, decubitus ulcer, and pulmonary embolism. An alternative approach is ambulatory mobility supervised by a physiotherapist, plus hydrotherapy (10). In one third of patients, severe pain, limited mobility, and poor quality of life persist despite appropriate nonoperative management. No patient spontaneously achieves realignment of the spine, correction of sagittal contour, or restoration of vertebral height.

OPERATIVE MANAGEMENT OF VERTEBRAL COMPRESSION FRACTURES

Historically, the only alternative to nonoperative management for symptomatic vertebral fractures was open surgical decompression (anterior or posterior decompression and stabilization by internal fixation hardware and bone grafting), and this was usually reserved for patients with gross spinal deformity or neurological impairment (<0.5%) (6). The reason for this surgical caution was the adverse risk/benefit ratio in this elderly population, which is characterized by poor bone quality and multiple comorbid conditions.

Percutaneous vertebroplasty (PVP) is a minimally invasive method that involves the percutaneous injection of polymethylmethacrylate (PMMA) into a collapsed vertebral body to stabilize the vertebra. Originally developed for osteolytic metastasis, myeloma, and hemangioma, the procedure resulted in quick, effective pain relief, and complication rates were low (11–13). PVP is now also increasingly used for the treatment of osteoporotic vertebral fractures (14). However, PVP does not expand the collapsed vertebra, potentially locking the spine in a kyphotic posture. In addition, the PMMA bone filler is associated with certain problems (epidural leakage, thermal necrosis, inability to integrate with bone, handling difficulties, toxicity to patient and operator) (2,15).

Kyphoplasty is a newer, minimally invasive technique with a number of potential advantages over PVP, including lower risk of cement extravasation and better restoration of vertebral body height (16). A cannula is introduced into the vertebral body, followed by insertion of an inflatable bone tamp, which when deployed reduces the compression fracture and restores the vertebral body toward its original height, while creating a cavity to be filled with bone cement. The cement augmentation is therefore done with more control into the low-pressure environment of the preformed cavity with viscous, partially cured cement.

PERCUTANEOUS VERTEBROPLASTY

Background

Percutaneous vertebral augmentation, or PVP, was first devised by Galibert et al. (17) in 1984 and initially involved the augmentation of the vertebral body with PMMA during open procedures to allow stable fixation of internal hardware. PVP was first described in French literature in 1987 (17) but was not performed in the United States until 1994. Originally targeted toward osteolytic metastasis, myeloma, and hemangioma, PVP resulted in early appreciable pain relief, and complication rates were low (13,17). Its indications now include treatment of osteoporotic vertebral collapse with chronic pain, treatment of asymptomatic vertebral collapse, and even prophylactic intervention for at-risk vertebral bodies (18). Nevertheless, the treatment of acute fractures in ambulatory patients and prophylactic treatment remain controversial (19). In fact, vertebral augmentation itself is somewhat controversial; questions concern a lack of defined indications, expected complications, outcome measures, and the need for long-term follow-up data (2).

An unanswered question in PVP concerns the mechanism of pain relief. The most intuitive explanation involves simple mechanical stabilization of the fracture; the cement stabilizes vertebral bodies and offloads the facet joints. However, another possibility is that analgesia results from local chemical, vascular, or thermal effects of PMMA on nerve endings in surrounding tissue (14,20). Supporting this concept is the lack of correlation between cement volume and pain relief (21,22). Further evidence against an effect resulting solely from mechanical stabilization is the fact that PVP typically does not restore lost vertebral body height and therefore does not correct altered biomechanics (1,19).

Technique

Injection of opacified PMMA is performed via a transpedicle or paravertebral approach under continuous fluoroscopic guidance to obtain adequate filling and to avoid PMMA leakage. For complex or high-risk cases, computed tomographic and fluoroscopic guidance are sometimes combined (11,19). In routine cases, PVP can be performed with local anesthesia and slight sedation in less than an hour (1), although general anesthesia is sometimes required because pain may intensify during cement injection (14). Before PMMA injection, intraosseous venography is often used to determine the filling pattern and to identify sites of potential PMMA leakage (outlining the venous drainage pattern, confirming needle placement within the bony trabeculae, and delineating fractures in the bony cortex). However, some authors have dispensed with routine venography (1).

Contraindications to vertebroplasty include coagulopathy, absence of facilities to perform emergency decompressive surgery in the event of a complication, and extreme vertebral collapse (>65% to 70% reduction in vertebral height) (14). However, in experienced hands this last contraindication may be relative (19,23).

Results

The available clinical studies, mostly European, have reported pain relief in about 90% of cases treated for osteoporotic fracture, with only infrequent clinically significant complications (0% to 10%), most of them minor (13,19). In a series of 80 patients treated with PVP for osteoporotic vertebral collapse, 90% gained immediate pain relief (11). During follow-up period of 1 month to 10 years, only one complication was reported; intercostal neuralgia treated by local anesthetic infiltration. In another prospective study, 45 vertebral augmentations in 17 osteoporotic patients led to significant and lasting pain reduction during the 1-year follow-up (1). Although cement leakages occurred in 20% of vertebral bodies, none had clinical sequelae. In a retrospective review of 70 augmented vertebrae in 38 consecutive patients with osteoporosis, treatment resulted in pain relief within 48 hours in 36 (95%) of patients. The pain relief was durable in 34 (89%) of the patients during follow-up periods averaging 18 months. Twenty-four patients (63%) experienced marked to complete pain relief, 12 (32%) experienced moderate relief, and two (5%) experienced no significant change (19). Of eight patients with malignant neoplasm of the spinal column that was treated with vertebroplasty, four (50%) experienced pain relief in this series (19). Cortet et al. (24) studied 16 patients with 20 osteoporotic vertebral compression fractures who underwent PVP. They found a statistically significant decrease in pain with several standardized scoring systems at all observed time points during the 6-month follow-up period, along with concurrent, significant improvement in overall health status. No adverse events and no additional vertebral fractures occurred during the follow-up period. Another study of 29 patients with 47 painful osteoporotic vertebral fractures reported a 90% success rate in terms of significant pain relief immediately after treatment (13). Two patients sustained rib fractures during the procedure, which resulted in pain that subsequently resolved; otherwise, no clinically significant complications were noted.

Complications

The principal risk of PVP, which involves the forced injection of low-viscosity PMMA cement into the closed space of the collapsed vertebral body, is cement extravasation. Extravasation rates are as high as 40% when used to treat osteoporotic fractures (13). The likelihood is greater when cement with a liquid rather than paste consistency or a higher PMMA volume is used (25). However, in most settings, the majority of extravasations have no clinical relevance, at least in the short term (1).

The consequence of an extravasation depends on its location. In epidural or foraminal extravasation, nerve root compression and radiculopathy are the major risks, occurring in 11 of 274 patients (4%) treated by Deramond et al. (11). Three patients required surgical nerve root decompression, which has been described by other authors as well (6,21). Extravasation into perivertebral veins can cause cement embolism to the lungs; deaths attributed to cement embolism have been documented. However, the two deaths attributed to pulmonary embolism were reported to be unrelated to the procedure; no cement material was detected by chest radiograph of the first patient (14,26), and the second pulmonary embolism arose from deep vein thrombosis in the lower extremity (11). However, extravasation into adjacent discs or paravertebral tissue, although common, generally produces no symptoms and carries little clinical significance; many such extravasations can be avoided by careful needle positioning (11).

Other operative and long-term complications of PVP are specific to PMMA as a filler (1,18,27). The physician may work with PMMA in large batches in order to keep it liquid and to extend the working time for vertebroplasty. However, its high polymerization temperature (86°C to 107°C within the cement core) (28) can damage adjacent tissue, including the spinal cord and nerve roots; in nine cases, this led to an inflammatory reaction and transitory exacerbation of pain (14). When PMMA monomer is injected, vigilance and caution is required of the physician. Absorption of PMMA during the injection can induce hypotension by virtue of its cardiotoxic and arrhythmogenic properties (29). Because placing a material in the spine affords proximity and access to the chest and the heart, vertebral augmentation with PMMA mandates meticulous attention to technique.

Overall, the risk of complications that carry clinical significance after PVP for osteoporotic vertebral fracture is 1% to 3%, and most potential complications can be avoided with good technique (11).

KYPHOPLASTY

Background

Kyphoplasty is a new technique evolved from a marriage of vertebroplasty with balloon angioplasty. It has a number of potential advantages, including a lower risk of cement extravasation and better restoration of vertebral body height. A cannula is introduced into the vertebral body, via a transpedicle or extrapedicle route, and is followed by insertion of an inflatable bone tamp, which when deployed reduces the compression fracture and restores the vertebral body toward its original height. This then creates a cavity to be filled with bone cement. The cement augmentation can now be completed with more control into the low-pressure environment of the preformed cavity with viscous, partially cured cement. Use of a cannula for bone filler with a steel stylet as a plunger enables the operator to apply cement at considerably higher viscosity than is possible with injection through a 5-mL syringe and an 11-gauge needle. Both the higher cement viscosity and lower pressure injection reduce the risk of cement extravasation. Filling is performed under continuous lateral fluoroscopic guidance, as in vertebroplasty. The procedure can be performed with general anesthesia or local anesthesia with intravenous sedation; some patients are able to return home the same day of the procedure.

Technique

With the patient under general or local anesthesia in the prone position on a radiolucent spinal frame, two C-arms are positioned for anteroposterior and lateral fluoroscopic images. Once positioned, the C-arms or the patient is not moved, so as to ensure repeatable images throughout the case. Two 3-mm incisions are made at the vertebral level, parallel to the pedicles in both planes. Then a guide wire or biopsy needle is advanced into the vertebral body through a transpedicle or extrapedicle approach, depending on fracture configuration and the patient's anatomy. The guide wire is then exchanged for the working cannula through a series of obturators. Once the working cannula is positioned, the surgeon reams out a corridor to accommodate the inflatable bone tamp (IBT) and positions the IBT under the collapsed endplate. To deploy the IBT, inflation proceeds slowly under fluoroscopic guidance until maximum fracture reduction is achieved or the balloon reaches a cortical wall. At this point, the surgeon deflates and removes the IBT, mixes the cement, prefills the cement cannulae, and allows the cement to partially cure in the cement cannulae. Once partially cured, PMMA is slowly extruded into the vertebral body through each pedicle under continuous lateral fluoroscopic guidance. This technique permits low-pressure filling. In most instances, the volume of cement can slightly exceed that of the bone cavity to interdigitate filler from the central bolus with the surrounding bone. Once filling is complete and the cement has hardened, the surgeon removes the cannula and closes the 3-mm incisions.

Results

Kyphoplasty has been slowly advanced through a few surgical centers participating in a multicenter study begun in 1999. A phase I efficacy study of 70 consecutive kyphoplasty procedures in 30 patients with painful, progressive osteoporotic or osteolytic VCFs has been completed (16). The mean duration of symptoms was 5.9 months. Symptomatic levels were identified by correlating the clinical data with magnetic resonance imaging findings. Preoperative and postoperative radiographs were compared to calculate the percentage of height restored. Outcome was further assessed by comparing the preoperative and latest postoperative surveys of the patients' health status, self-reported on the 36-item Short Form Health Survey (SF-36) (30). In 70% of the vertebral bodies, kyphoplasty restored, on average, 47% of the lost vertebral height ($p = 0.001$). SF-36 scores for bodily pain ($p = .0001$), physical function ($p = .002$), and vitality ($p = .001$) were among the measures that showed substantial and significant improvement. Complications were infrequent. One patient experienced perioperative pulmonary edema and a myocardial infarction secondary to intraoperative fluid overload; two patients suffered rib fractures caused by positioning during the procedure. Cement leakage occurred at 6 (8.6%) of 70 treated levels; however, no complications were related directly to selection of this technique or to use of the IBT. In an ongoing evaluation, the results of this initial series have been maintained in the most recent follow-up of over 70 consecutive patients up to 14 months.

VERTEBROPLASTY VERSUS KYPHOPLASTY

Although both vertebroplasty and kyphoplasty provide excellent pain relief, kyphoplasty has the potential to improve spine biomechanics and decrease the risk of cement extravasation. PVP usually does not expand the vertebral body or restore normal spine alignment. Preliminary data indicate that kyphoplasty may restore near-normal height, preventing kyphosis, which leads to respiratory and digestive problems. Restoration of height and sagittal alignment may also work to protect vulnerable vertebral levels above or below the treated site or sites by minimizing force transfer.

PVP carries a higher risk of cement leakages because the PMMA is injected in a liquid state and will leak through any cracks in surrounding bone. In performing vertebroplasty, the operator injects the liquid cement, typically pausing or stopping once a leakage becomes evident. On the other hand, in kyphoplasty, the expanded balloon creates a cavity and pushes bone to the edges of the cavity, thus sealing off potential fissures and cracks. Greater placement control is possible in kyphoplasty, in which the operator can fill the cavity with a more viscous cement to the point at which the cement bolus reaches and interdigitates with the bony margins. The initial kyphoplasty findings show lower rates of cement extravasation than in published vertebroplasty series, which supports the hypothesis that injection of high-viscosity cement into a previously formed cavity may be an improvement over the injection of low-viscosity liquid cement into the unreduced vertebral body.

CONCLUSIONS

Osteoporotic VCFs pose significant clinical problems, including spinal deformity, pain, and reduced pulmonary function and mobility, as well as an overall increase in mortality among elderly patients. Traditional medical and surgical options prove inadequate in many cases.

PVP is a relatively noninvasive technique that has gained increased acceptance since the early 1990s in the treatment of symptomatic osteoporotic vertebral fractures. The available clinical studies describe pain relief achieved in more than 90% of patients with symptomatic osteoporotic fractures, with only infrequent, mostly minor complications. Some of the drawbacks of PVP stem from the use of PMMA because of its toxicity and poor handling characteristics, rather than from the procedure itself.

Kyphoplasty is a modification of PVP that is under study. It may add a margin of safety by virtue of a lower observed incidence of cement leakage. Kyphoplasty may be shown to be worthwhile in treating acute vertebral fracture in high-risk patients to predictably restore vertebral height and to facilitate a low-pressure filling procedure. Favorable outcomes in early trials include early mobilization, which has the potential for decreasing mortality. Considering the higher rates of mortality that is associated with osteoporotic compression fractures, early mobilization in these patients is of prime importance.

The next logical step beyond treatment of evident vertebral fractures is prophylactic augmentation. Prevention of osteoporotic vertebral fractures with a combination of pharmacological agents and timely reinforcement of at-risk osteoporotic vertebrae are the ultimate goals, aside from prevention of osteoporosis itself. For this step, new osteoconductive synthetic composites will figure more prominently as an emerging alternative to cement. Advances in minimally invasive surgical techniques, imaging, and synthetic engineering are rapidly changing the treatment protocols available for osteoporotic compression fracture.

REFERENCES

1. Heini PF, Wälchli B, Berlemann U. Percutaneous transpedicular vertebroplasty with PMMA: operative technique and early results. A prospective study for the treatment of osteoporotic compression fractures. *Eur Spine J* 2000; 9:445–450.
2. Einhorn TA. Vertebroplasty: an opportunity to do something really good for patients [Editorial]. *Spine* 2000;25: 1051–1052.
3. Riggs BL, Melton LJ III. The worldwide problem of osteoporosis: insights afforded by epidemiology. *Bone* 1995;17(Suppl 5):505S–511S.
4. Kado DM, Browner WS, Palermo L, et al., for the Study of Osteoporotic Fractures Research Group. Vertebral fractures and mortality in older women: a prospective study. *Arch Intern Med* 1999;159:1215–1220.
5. Ray NF, Chan JK, Thamer M, et al. Medical expenditures for the treatment of osteoporotic fractures in the United States in 1995: report from the National Osteoporosis Foundation. *J Bone Miner Res* 1997;12:24–35.
6. Bostrom MP, Lane JM. Future directions. Augmentation of osteoporotic vertebral bodies. *Spine* 1997;15(Suppl 24):38S–42S.
7. Cooper C, Atkinson EJ, O'Fallon WM, et al. Incidence of clinically diagnosed vertebral fractures: a population-based study in Rochester, Minnesota, 1985–1989. *J Bone Miner Res* 1992;7:221–227.
8. Leech JA, Dulberg C, Kellie S, et al. Relationship of lung function to severity of osteoporosis in women. *Am Rev Respir Dis* 1990;141:68–71.
9. Lyles KW, Gold DT, Shipp KM, et al. Association of osteoporotic vertebral compression fractures with impaired functional status. *Am J Med* 1993;94:595–601.
10. Patel U, Skingle S, Campbell GA, et al. Clinical profile of acute vertebral compression fractures in osteoporosis. *Br J Rheumatol* 1991;30:418–421.
11. Deramond H, Depriester C, Galibert P, et al. Percutaneous vertebroplasty with polymethylmethacrylate. Technique, indications, and results. *Radiol Clin North Am* 1998;36:533–546.
12. Chiras J, Depriester C, Weill A, et al. [Percutaneous vertebral surgery. Technics and indications]. *J Neuroradiol* 1997;24:45–59.
13. Jensen ME, Evans AJ, Mathis JM, et al. Percutaneous polymethylmethacrylate vertebroplasty in the treatment of osteoporotic vertebral body compression fractures: technical aspects. *Am J Neuroradiol* 1997;18:1897–1904.
14. Cotten A, Boutry N, Cortet B, et al. Percutaneous vertebroplasty: state of the art. *Radiographics* 1998;18:311–320.
15. Deramond H, Wright NT, Belkoff SM. Temperature elevation caused by bone cement polymerization during vertebroplasty. *Bone* 1999;25(2 Suppl):17S–21S.
16. Lieberman IH, Dudeney S, Reinhardt M-K, et al. Initial outcome and efficacy of "kyphoplasty" in the treatment of painful osteoporotic vertebral compression fractures. *Spine* 2001;26:1631–1638.
17. Galibert P, Deramond H, Rosat P, et al. [Preliminary note on the treatment of vertebral angioma by percutaneous acrylic vertebroplasty.] *Neurochirurgie* 1987;33:166–168.
18. Bai B, Jazrawi LM, Kummer FJ, et al. The use of an injectable, biodegradable calcium phosphate bone substitute for the prophylactic augmentation of osteoporotic vertebrae and the management of vertebral compression fractures. *Spine* 1999;24:1521–1526.
19. Barr JD, Barr MS, Lemley TJ, et al. Percutaneous vertebroplasty for pain relief and spinal stabilization. *Spine* 2000;25:923–928.
20. Mathis JM, Petri M, Naff N. Percutaneous vertebroplasty treatment of steroid-induced osteoporotic compression fractures. *Arthritis Rheum* 1998;41:171–175.
21. Cotten A, Dewatre F, Cortet B, et al. Percutaneous vertebroplasty for osteolytic metastases and myeloma: effects of the percentage of lesion filling and the leakage of methyl methacrylate at clinical follow-up. *Radiology* 1996; 200:525–530.
22. Dean JR, Ison KT, Gishen P. The strengthening effect of percutaneous vertebroplasty. *Clin Radiol* 2000;55: 471–476.
23. O'Brien JP, Sims JT, Evans AJ. Vertebroplasty in patients with severe vertebral compression fractures: a technical report. *Am J Neuroradiol* 2000;21:1555–1558.
24. Cortet B, Cotten A, Boutry N, et al. Percutaneous vertebroplasty in the treatment of osteoporotic vertebral compression fractures: an open prospective study. *J Rheumatol* 1999;26:2222–2228.
25. Martin JB, Jean B, Sugiu K, et al. Vertebroplasty: clinical experience and follow-up results. *Bone* 1999;25 (2 Suppl):11S–15S.
26. Padovani B, Kasriel O, Brunner P, et al. Pulmonary embolism caused by acrylic cement: a rare complication of percutaneous vertebroplasty. *Am J Neuroradiol* 1999;20:375–377.
27. Cunin G, Boissonnet H, Petite H, et al. Experimental vertebroplasty using osteoconductive granular material. *Spine* 2000;25:1070–1076.
28. Leeson MC, Lippitt SB. Thermal aspects of the use of polymethylmethacrylate in large metaphyseal defects in bone: a clinical review and laboratory study. *Clin Orthop* 1993;(295):239–245.
29. Phillips H, Cole PV, Lettin AW. Cardiovascular effects of implanted acrylic bone cement. *BMJ* 1971;3:460–461.
30. Ware JE Jr, Gandek B, for the IQOLA Project. Overview of the SF-36 Health Survey and the International Quality of Life Assessment (IQOLA) Project. *J Clin Epidemiol* 1998;51:903–912.

21

Vertebroplasty and Use of Methylmethacrylate

Norbert Passuti and Joel Delécrin

Clinique Orthopédique, Hôtel Dieu, Nantes cedex 1, France

The most common consequences of spinal osteoporosis are the vertebral compression fractures. With the aging of the population, osteoporosis and its complications will have staggering implications for all physicians involved in spine care. Vertebral compression fracture care includes bed rest, bracing, narcotic analgesics, and nasal calcitonin. Most patients experience improvement with this approach, but inactivity contributes to a further bone loss, subsequent fracture, and functional decline. Moreover, multiple vertebral compression fractures can lead to decreased pulmonary function; thus, there is a question of whether there is any surgical possibility of stabilizing these lesions without medical morbidity in old patients.

Vertebroplasty was developed in the mid-1980s by Galibert and Deramond to address the limitations of more invasive surgical techniques, particularly for hemangiomas and metastatic tumors. Cement is injected through a transpedicle approach under fluoroscopic control. The polymethylmethacrylate (PMMA) may increase vertebral stiffness and provide pain relief, but the exact effect of cement is unknown. It has been hypothesized that this exothermic reaction of the PMMA, in combination with the neurotoxic effect, contribute to the marked pain relief of patients, but there remain several questions concerning complications, indications, and the volume of injected cement that is needed for good results.

BIOMECHANICS OF VERTEBROPLASTY

The first problem is the volume of cement that must be injected to restore the strength and stiffness of the vertebral body. Belkoff (1) experimentally created compression fractures in 144 vertebral bodies (T-6 to -L-5) obtained from 12 cadaver porotic spines. Two investigational cements were studied: Orthocomp and Simplex 20 with barium sulfate content.

Results suggested that strength could be restored with the injection of 2 mL of cement (Simplex 20 or Orthocomp). In general, stiffness was restored with 4 mL of either cement, except that the lumbar region treated with Orthocomp required 6 mL) and the thoracolumbar region treated with Simplex 20 (required 8 mL). Preliminary clinical data suggest that pain relief may be experienced with the injection of smaller volumes of cement (as little as 2.1 mL). Smaller amounts of injected cement would have the additional benefit of decreased risk of extravasation. In this study, leakage was noted in eight of the vertebrae, but it amounted to 1 mL or less, and in all cases, extravasation occurred with injection volume of 6 mL or more; thus, strength was restored with 2 mL of either of the two cements studied. Also, Heini et al. (2) observed a significant effect even with cement volumes of 6 to 7 mL, which represented filling of about one quarter of the vertebral body volume. In fact, only a small amount of bone cement (15% volume fraction) is needed to restore stiffness to predamage levels. Large filling volumes may not be the most biomechanically optimal configuration.

Little information is available on the biomechanical efficacy of unipedicular versus bipedicular vertebroplasty. Tohmeh et al. (3) performed a cadaveric study on the biomechanics of osteoporotic fractured vertebral bodies treated with unipedicle vertebroplasty (6 cm^3 of bone cement) or bipedicle vertebroplasty (5 cm^3 of bone cement through each pedicle). Their results demonstrated that unipedicle and bipedicle vertebroplasty increased strength and restored stiffness of vertebral bodies with compression fractures. Therefore, the authors believed that a unipedicle cement injection is adequate and may be considered an alternative when a bipedicle injection is obviated; they also believed that unipedicle injection into high thoracic vertebrae theoretically reduces the technical risks by reducing the total number of injected pedicles, thereby reducing the potential for cement extravasation and potential complications.

The different data suggest that only a small amount of bone cement is needed to restore stiffness to predamage levels and that greater filling can result in substantial increases in stiffness and presents problems to the adjacent vertebrae.

COMPARISON OF BONE CEMENT AND HYDROXYAPATITE CEMENTS

Belkoff et al. (1) performed a biomechanical evaluation on vertebral bodies of 10 fresh cadaver spines and compared PMM1 (Simplex P) with or without barium sulfate and bone source (hydroxyapatite cement). The authors injected 6 mL of Simplex 20 cement into L-2, bone source into L-3, and Simplex into L-4. They observed that all three materials restored or increased vertebral body strength. Posttreatment stiffness values for both cements were similar; both cements exhibited injectability similar to that of regular Simplex and may be candidates for use clinically with percutaneous transpedicle vertebroplasty.

Heini at al. (2) compared different bone cements, such as PMMA and calcium phosphate (CaP) cement. The study was performed on 39 porotic cadaver vertebrae; vertebral filling of 20% to 50% was achieved, with PMMA stiffness increases at 174% and 120% with CaP cement and with 6 to 7 mL of volume, respectively. Filling of about one quarter was achieved, but the degree of local stiffness and force augmentation that is desirable remains unclear. A large difference in stiffness between two adjacent vertebrae results in damage to the weaker vertebra with time; furthermore, leakage, which was observed in 12% of cases, may lead to neurological compromise, and continuous fluoroscopic control *in vivo* is recommended.

CLINICAL STUDIES

The clinical studies are only retrospective or prospective without randomization. Nine publications, which represent 115 patients with 195 vertebral procedures, reported 78% to 100% of pain relief, but with only on average of 14 months of follow-up. Jensen et al. (4) reported results from managing 47 osteopenic or steroid-induced compression fractures with vertebroplasty in 29 patients. They reported reduction in pain in 90% within

24 hours, but they did not precisely describe the evolution of the pain at the time of vertebroplasty, and follow-up was only short term.

Heini et al. (5) described the results of a study of 17 patients undergoing procedures in a total of 45 vertebral bodies with injection of a mean volume of 5.9 mL of PMMA. Leakage was noted in 20% with no complications. All patients reported a considerable pain benefit, but 1 year later in two patients, additional new compression fractures were noted with secondary osteoporosis.

Cortet et al. (6), in a prospective study, used as inclusion criteria a rate superior to 50 mm (severe pain) on a visual analogue scale. The results were good after 3 and 6 months, but only 44% of patients described a decrease of pain of approximately 50%; 75% of patients described a decrease of pain of at least 33%.

Barr et al. (7) published a retrospective review of 38 consecutive patients treated for osteoporotic fractures; 24 (63%) had marked to complete pain relief, 12 (32%) had moderate relief, and two (5%) experienced no significant change. The follow-up period ranged from 2 to 42 months, with a mean of 18 months, and five patients had recurrent painful episodes during this time.

The first question to be discussed is whether the reinforcement of the affected and already fractured vertebra alone is sufficient or whether a more extensive treatment that includes the adjacent vertebrae should be performed. With a much larger sample, the importance of other factors such as the degree of vertebral compression and associated kyphosis, fracture location, fracture age, and patient gender should be determined. Furthermore, markedly increased stiffness of a treated vertebra places increased stress on the inferior and possibly even the superior vertebrae. But if the patient's pain seems more related to an advanced kyphotic deformation and loss of spinal balance, more aggressive measures, such a multisegment correction and stabilization, may be indicated.

COMPLICATIONS AND DISADVANTAGES

Root compression is possible, as described by Ratliff et al. (8) or Grados et al. (9) (2 root pain). Cortet et al. revealed that in two of 37 patients, symptomatic foraminal cement extravasation necessitated surgical intervention; cement leakage and pulmonary embolism were noted in 4 (3%) by Jensen et al., but fracture risk at adjacent levels is higher around a vertebroplasty, as reported, for example, by Grados et al. (9) after 4 years' follow-up. . The relative risk of fracture was 1.44 around a nontreated fractured vertebra and 2.27 for the vertebrae around a vertebra treated with PMMA. Cyteval et al. (10) demonstrated a new vertebral fracture in 25% of cases after 6 months' follow-up.

Other questions concern whether it is necessary to perform an hyperextension in an attempt to restore vertebral height; whether prophylactic treatment is indicated for noncompressed vertebrae in patients with severe osteoporosis; and whether, for patients with severe and multiple levels of vertebral compression, it is mandatory to inject cement at all the levels or only one level andhow to determine the painful localization. In addition, if a patient presents a loss of sagittal balance, the pain seems more related to an advanced kyphotic deformation and, therefore, multisegmental correction and stabilization may be indicated; however, it must be remembered that cement injection does not restore vertebral height and is only a palliative treatment.

In conclusion, vertebroplasty is being increasingly used to treat osteoporotic vertebral compression fractures, although no controlled studies supporting this trend have been published. Vertebroplasty remains controversial as a treatment for osteoporotic fractures because it is a local response to a systemic disease and because the pain caused by porotic fractures usually subsides within a few days or weeks. Current data suggest that pain severity may decrease by half, on average, in 90% to 100% of patients. Although vertebroplasty is usually well tolerated, some neurological complications have been reported in a few patients. The most common is root pain, caused by leakage of cement into the foramen. Whether vertebroplasty is followed by an increased risk of porotic fractures in the adjacent vertebras remains unclear. Also, indications must be defined in cases of severe sagittal imbalance, perhaps in combination with correction of the kyphosis by instrumentation and precise indications for prevention of compression in patients at risk.

At present, acrylic cement vertebroplasty to treat porotic fractures is appropriate in only a minority of patients selected carefully by a multidisciplinary team and with prospective and controlled studies.

REFERENCES

1. Belkoff SM, Mathis JM, Jasper LE, et al. The biomechanics of vertebroplasty. The effect of cement volume on mechanical behaviors. *Spine* 2001;26:1537–1542.
2. Heini PF, Berlemann V, Kaufmann M, et al. Augmentation of mechanical properties in investigation of vertebroplasty efficacy with different bone cements. *Eur Spine J* 2001;10:164–171.
3. Tohmeh AG, Mathis JM, Fenton DC, et al. Biomechanical efficacy of unipedicular versus bipedicular vertebroplasty for the management of osteoporotic compression fractures. *Spine* 1999;24:1772–1776.
4. Jensen ME, Evans AJ, Mathis JM, et al. Percutaneous PMMA vertebroplasty in the treatment of osteoporotic vertebral body compression fractures: technical aspects. *AJNR Am J Neuroradiol* 1997;18:1897–1904.
5. Heini PF, Wälchli B, Berlemann U. Percutaneous transpedicular vertebroplasty with PMMA, operative technique and early results. *Eur Spine J* 2000;9:445–450.
6. Cortet B, Cotten A, Boutry N, et al. Percutaneous vertebroplasty in the treatment of osteoporotic fracture: on open prospective study. *J Rheumatol* 1999;26:2222–2228.
7. Barr JD, Barr MS, Lemley JJ, et al. Percutaneous vertebroplasty for pain relief and spinal stabilization. *Spine* 2000;25:923–928.
8. Ratliff J, Nguyen T, Heiss J. Root and spinal cord compression from methylmethacrylate vertebroplasty. *Spine* 2001;26(13):E300–E302.
9. Grados F, Depriester C, Fardellone P. Long term observations of vertebral osteoporotic fractures treated by percutaneous vertebroplasty *Rheumatology* 2000;39:1410–1414.
10. Cyteval C, Baron-Sarrebere MP, Pous JO, et al. Acute osteoporotic vertebral collapse: open study on percutaneous injection of acrylic surgical cement in 20 patients. *AJR Am J Roentgenol* 1999;173:1685–1690.

22

Percutaneous Injection of Cortoss Synthetic Bone Void Filler in the Repair of Fractures in the Vertebral Body

[*]Marek Szpalski, †Robert Gunzburg, and ‡Hervé Deramond

[*]Hôpitaux Iris Sud-Molière Longchamp, Université Libre de Bruxelles, Bruxelles, Belgium;
†Department of Orthopaedics, Eeuwfeestkliniek, Antwerpen, Belgium;
‡Service de Radiologie A, CHU Amiens-Hôpital Nord, Amiens, France

Vertebral compression fractures are common causes of pain and disability. Each year more than 270,000 painful vertebral compression fractures are clinically diagnosed in the United States alone, and this number is increasing (1). According to the U.S. National Osteoporosis Foundation, 700,000 vertebral fractures occur annually (2). The most common etiologies of vertebral compression fractures are osteopenia associated with aging or chronic steroid use and metastatic disease. All patients experience pain, the intensity and duration of which varies. The pain can last from weeks to months (3). Most patients with osteoporotic fractures are treated conservatively with external bracing, analgesics, and bed rest, but a small percentage is left with persistent pain and limited mobility (4). Standard medical therapy for vertebral compression fractures may compound the problem of bone mineral loss due to the lack of mobility, thereby increasing the risk of subsequent fractures (5–7). These fractures may impact health and daily living and may increase medical costs through loss of lung capacity, decreased appetite, impaired mobility, chronic pain, or psychiatric effects (3,8–10).

Vertebroplasty with injection of polymethylmethacrylate (PMMA) has previously been reported (11–14). Since the early 1990s, PMMA has been injected in vertebral bodies for the treatment of pain related to osteoporotic compression fractures or tumor invasion, with good results (15,16). There remain, however, significant concerns about the filler material that is used for fixation. PMMA cement has been used mostly in vertebroplasty. However, it does have some important drawbacks. The curing temperature is very high, sometimes over 100°C; the visualization is suboptimal; and repeated delivery often requires mixing a new PMMA unit. Moreover, in order to obtain good injection characteristics, surgeons have increased the monomer-to-powder ratio from the standard recommended composition, which increases the concentration of toxic components (17).

As a result, many new devices have been developed to make the procedure of filling the vertebral bodies with PMMA easier and more reliable. So far, only one new material that, according to its chemical mechanical and biological characteristics, in theory is superior to PMMA for this indication has been developed.

MATERIALS AND TECHNIQUES

Cortoss cement is a new synthetic cortical bone void filler that contains bis-glycidyl-methylmethacrylate (bis-GMA), bisphenol A polyethylene glycol diether dimethylacrylate (bis-EMA), and triethyleneglycol dimethylacrylate (TEGDMA) monomers, as well as radiopaque glass and bioactive glass-ceramic fillers. It is provided in a double-lumen cartridge with specially designed tips for mixing. After the composite is expressed through these tips, polymerization begins, and the material is ready for use. The delivery system with changeable mix tips allows the physician to prepare fresh material any time it is needed during the procedure. The difunctional monomers described are not volatile, and because of the two double bonds, they polymerize in a three-dimensional network, which minimizes the chances of leaking. After mixing, the material has a consistency that is similar to that of toothpaste and stays that way until it polymerizes quickly in a matter of seconds. This characteristic provides a consistent tactile feedback and allows for an even injection.

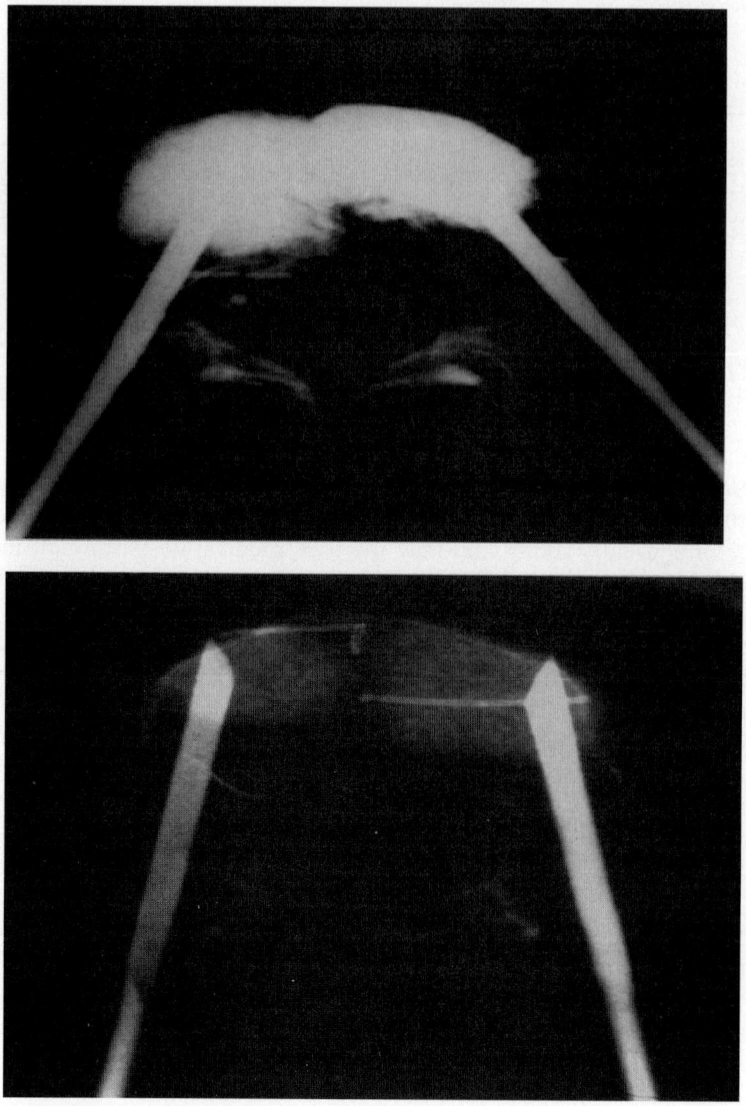

FIG. 22.1. The difference in radiodensity between Cortoss cement (top) and Simplex P (bottom) in an osteoporotic vertebral body.

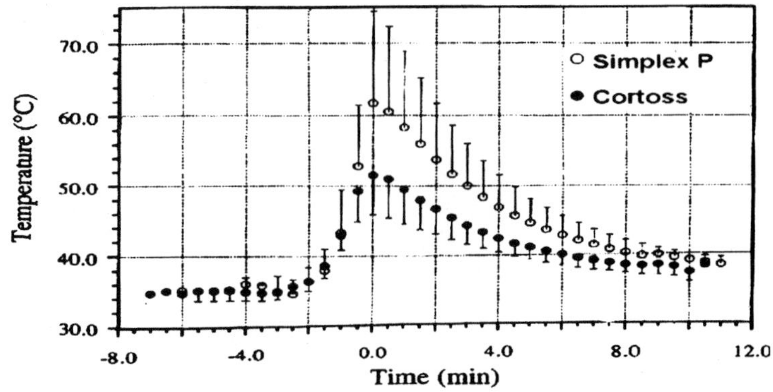

FIG. 22.2. Temperature elevation during curing of Cortoss cement and Simplex P, measured in the vertebral body.

The polymerization itself has a much lower exotherm than PMMA (63°C vs 84°C to 105°C), which reduces the risk of thermal necrosis. Because of the fillers, Cortoss cement is inherently radiopaque, making for excellent visualization of its placement under fluoroscopic guidance (Fig. 22.1), or on postoperative imaging studies. Biomechanically, the composite material is stronger than PMMA under static and dynamic loading in tension and compression. Its modulus of elasticity is close to that of bone and three times higher than that of PMMA (18–21) (Fig. 22.2).

This composite has bioactive properties as a result of combeite bioactive glass particles. In animal studies, the Cortoss cement–bone interface continues to be strengthened over time, with bone apposition occurring at the interface without any fibrous interposition (Fig. 22.3),

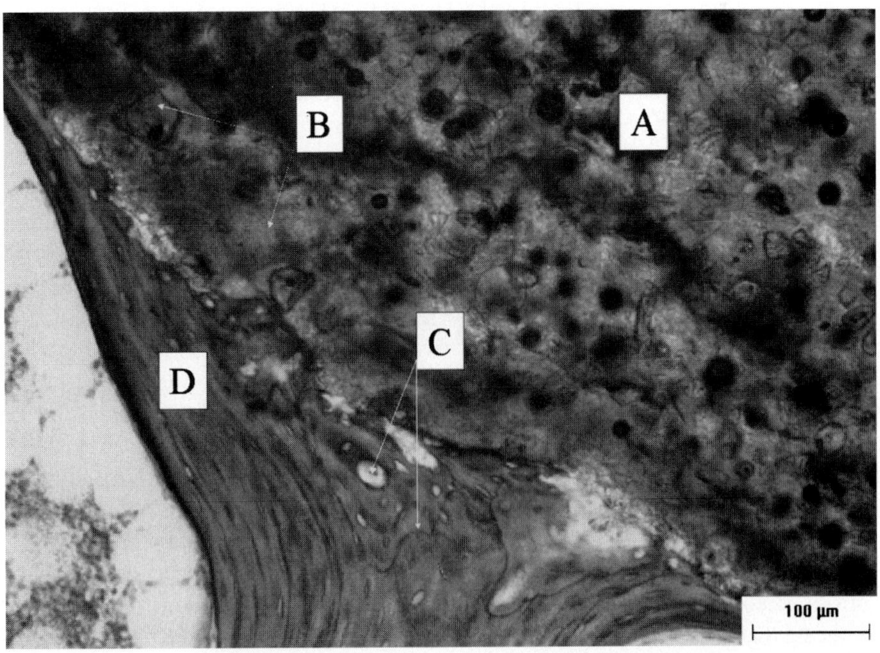

FIG. 22.3. Images captured after 52 weeks of implantation in a rabbit diaphysis. These are nondecalcified histological sections stained with hematoxylin and eosin. **A:** Cortoss cement. **B:** Bioactive filler. **C:** Osteon with cement lines. **D:** Mature bone with osteocytes.

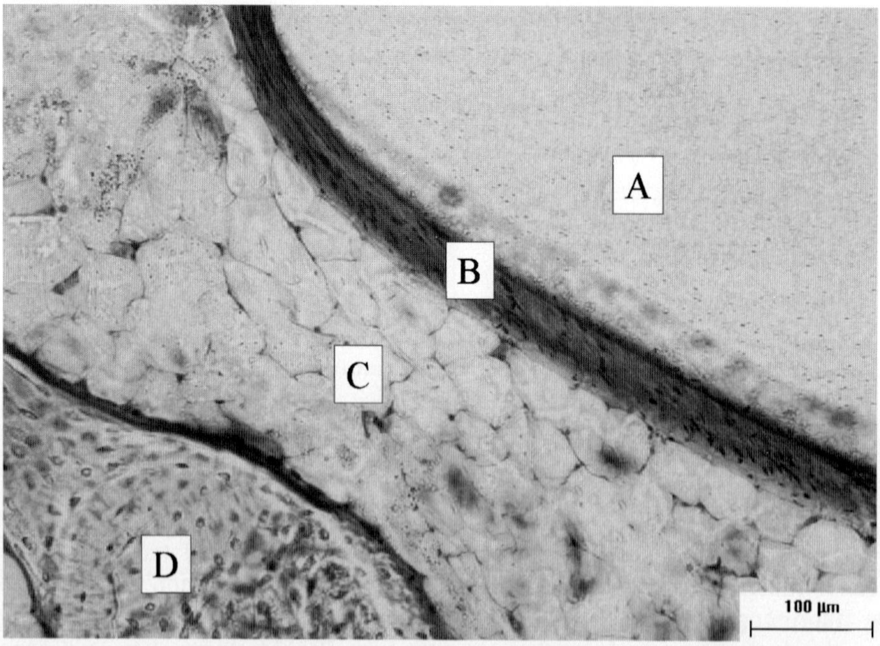

FIG. 22.4. This 78-week polymethylmethacrylate (PMMA) histologic specimen (from a sheep) illustrates the soft tissue encapsulation of PMMA. **A:** PMMA. **B:** 50 μm fibrous tissue encapsulation. **C:** 200 μm adipose tissue layer. **D:** Bone.

whereas in the same studies, the PMMA–bone interface develops into a fibrous layer (Fig. 22.4) (2).

IN VITRO EVALUATIONS

An *in vitro* evaluation was conducted to assess the benefits of Cortoss cement as an injectable material for use in percutaneous vertebroplasty procedures. In addition, a unique delivery system for Cortoss cement, the Aliquot™ system, was tested in a clinical percutaneous vertebroplasty case.

Cortoss cement was obtained by Orthovita, Inc. (Malvern, PA), whereas Simplex was obtained from Stryker-Howmedica-Osteonics (East Rutherford, NJ). *In vitro* evaluations were performed at the Orthopaedics Biomechanics Laboratory at the University of Maryland (College Park). Radiographic and temperature evaluations were performed after 5-mL bipedicular injections into cadaver vertebral bodies T-11 to L-2 with dual x-ray absorptiometry (DEXA) T-scores of −7.8 to −0.1. Mechanical testing was performed before and after 4-mL bipedicle injections into cadaver vertebral bodies L-1 to L-5 with DEXA T-scores of −3.4 to −6.4. An anteriorly offset compression test was performed at a rate of 5 mm per minute.

The radiographic evaluation displayed in Fig. 22.1 illustrates the difference in radiodensity between Cortoss and Simplex P in an osteoporotic vertebral body (20). Cortoss is readily visualized during and after injection. The temperature elevation during cure in the vertebral bodies is shown in Fig. 22.2. The peak temperature measured during curing was 51°C for Cortoss, in comparison with 61°C for Simplex P (20). Mechanical testing results in Fig. 22.5 indicate that Cortoss injected vertebral bodies rupture at a load of 6700 N, whereas the Simplex P–treated vertebral bodies succumbed to a failure load of only 3600 N (19). In addition, Fig. 22.6 shows that Cortoss restores the vertebral bodies to normal stiffness, whereas

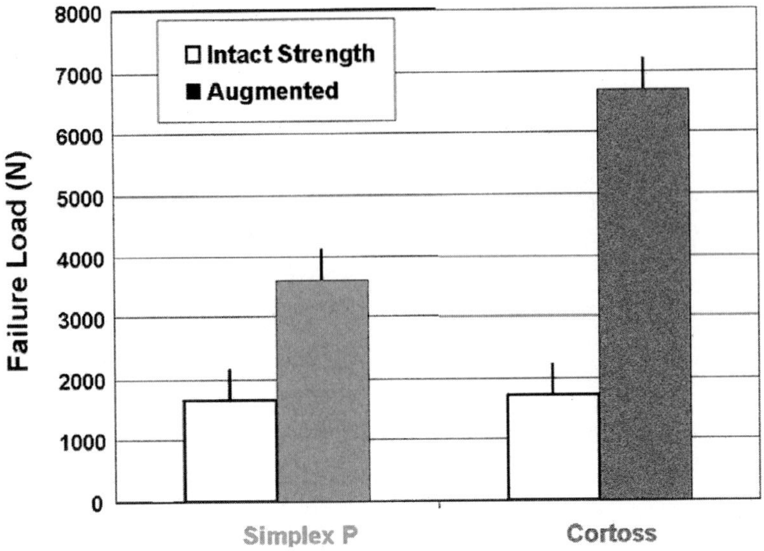

FIG. 22.5. The intact and augmented (Cortoss cement, Simplex P) strength.

Simplex P does not (19). This is important in considering not only the immediate biomechanical stability of the augmented vertebral body but also the effect of transmitting load to the adjacent vertebral segments. Clearly, if the Cortoss cement—augmented vertebral body is similar in stiffness to the original intact vertebral body, there is less chance of creating a stress riser or stiffness zone that could lead to the failure of adjacent vertebral bodies.

A specific delivery system was developed. The Aliquot™ delivery system and instruments designed by Orthovita, Inc.

Clinically, use of the new Aliquot delivery system gives the surgeon greater control of the material during injection. Figure 22.7 represents the injection phase of the

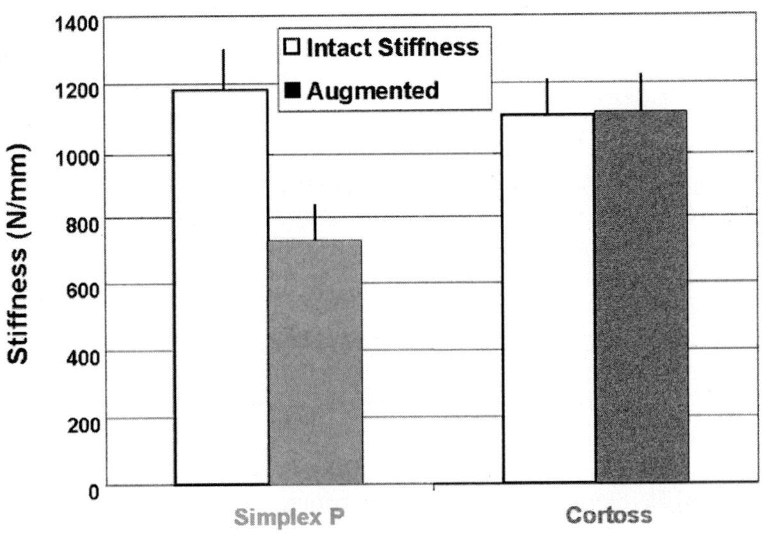

FIG. 22.6. The intact and augmented (Cortoss cement, Simplex P) stiffness.

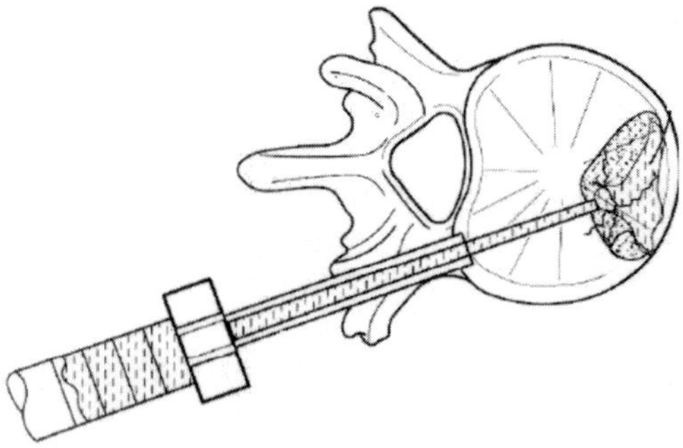

FIG. 22.7. Schematic representation of the injection phase of the Aliquot™ delivery system.

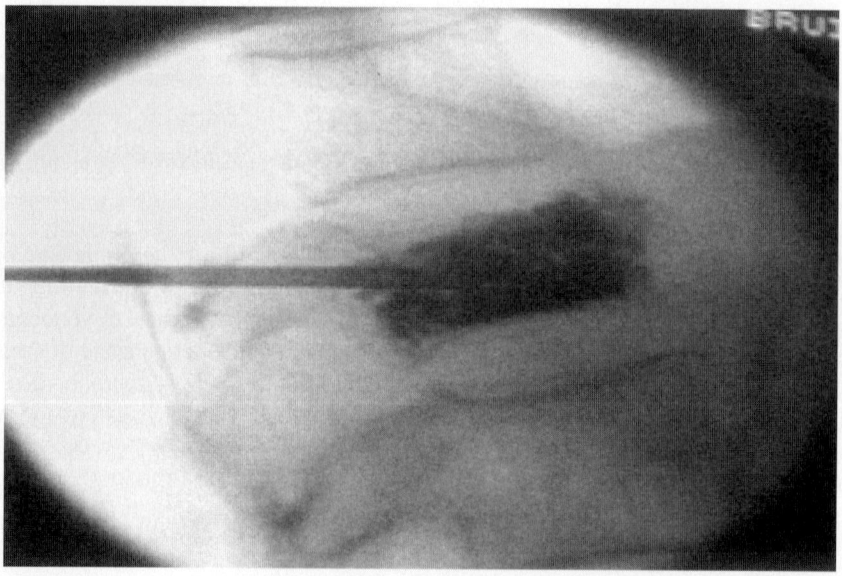

FIG. 22.8. Fluoroscopic image illustrating a vertebral body augmented with Cortoss cement with the Aliquot™ delivery system.

Aliquot delivery system. The material is injected through an internal catheter, with the access cannula kept open for multiple catheter injections. In view of the injection and observed nature of the vertebral augmentation procedure, this flexibility is a required feature. As illustrated in Fig. 22.8, visualization of the material being injected into the vertebral body is critical.

DISCUSSION

This chapter has described the characteristics of a new bioactive material, specially designed to replace and reinforce load-bearing bone, in vertebroplasty.

In comparison with PMMA, Cortoss cement shows better mechanical properties and a reduced potential for thermal injuries. Its radiopaque properties make the monitoring of delivery safe and easy.

The bioactivity of the composite induces close integration with surrounding bone; this property may be interesting for the long-term evolution of the construct.

Cortoss cement appears well suited for use in the treatment of vertebral compression fractures. Results indicate that Cortoss cement addresses the shortcomings of using a PMMA material for vertebral augmentation, being stronger than PMMA when injected into the spine, which results in easier radiographic visualization, and yielding a lower peak curing temperature. The Aliquot delivery system allows for accurate amounts of Cortoss cement to be injected directly to the region of interest.

ACKNOWLEDGMENTS

I would like to thank Steve Belkoff, PhD, University of Maryland, College Park, Maryland for help in realizing this study.

REFERENCES

1. Cooper C, Atkinson EJ, O'Fallon WM, et al. Incidence of clinically diagnosed vertebral fractures: a population-based study in Rochester, Minnesota, 1985–1989. *J Bone Miner Res* 1992;7:221–227.
2. National Osteoporosis Foundation. Fast facts on osteoporosis. http://www.nof.org/osteoporosis/stats.htm.
3. Silverman SL. The clinical consequences of vertebral compression fractures. *Bone* 1992;13(Suppl 2):S27–S31.
4. Karjalainen M, Aho AJ, Katevuo K. Painful spine after stable fractures of the thoracic and lumbar spine: what benefit from the use of extension brace? *Ann Chir Gynaecol* 1991;80:45–48.
5. Genant HK, Li J, Wu CY, et al. Vertebral fractures in osteoporosis: a new method for clinical assessment. *J Clin Densitom* 2000;3(3):281–290.
6. Heany RA. The natural history of vertebral compression fractures. *Bone* 1992;13:S23–S26.
7. Huopio J, Kroger H, Honkanen R. Risk factors for perimenopausal fractures: a prospective study. *Osteoporos Int* 2000;11(3):219–227.
8. Cook DJ, Guyatt GH, Ryan G, et al. Quality of life issues in women with vertebral fractures due to osteoporosis. *Arthritis Rheum* 1993;36:750–756.
9. Gold DT. The clinical impact of vertebral fractures: quality of life in women with osteoporosis. *Bone* 1996;18(3 Suppl):185S–189S.
10. Lyles KW, Gold DT, Shipp KM, et al. Association of osteoporotic vertebral compression fractures with impaired functional status. *Am J Med* 1993;94:595–601.
11. Cortet B, Cotten A, Deprez X, et al. [Value of vertebroplasty combined with surgical decompression in the treatment of aggressive spinal angioma. Apropos of 3 cases]. [In French.] *Rev Rhum Ed Fr* 1994;61(1):16—22.
12. Cybulski GR. Methods of surgical stabilization for metastatic disease of the spine. *Neurosurgery* 1989;25:240-252.
13. Harrington KD. Anterior decompression and stabilization of the spine as a treatment for vertebral collapse and spinal cord compression from malignancy." *Clin Orthop* 1988;233:177–197.
14. Nicola N, Lins E. Vertebral hemangioma: retrograde embolization-stabilization with methyl methacrylate. *Surg Neurol* 1987;27:481–486.
15. Deramond H, Depriester C, Galibert P, et al. Percutaneous vertebroplasty with polymethylmethacrylate. Technique, indications, and results. *Radiol Clin North Am* 1998;36(3):533–546.
16. Gangi A, Dietemann JL, Guth S, et al. CT & Fluoroscopic VP: Results & complications in 187 pts. *Sem Interven Radiol* 1999;16:137–142.
17. Jasper LE, Deramond H, Mathis JM, et al. Effect of monomer-to-powder ratio on the material properties of cranioplastic. *Bone* 1999;25(2 Suppl):27S–29S.
18. Belkoff SM, Maroney M, Fenton DC, et al. An *in vitro* biomechanical evaluation of bone cements used in percutaneous vertebroplasty. *Bone* 1999;25(2 Suppl):23S–26S.
19. Belkoff SM, Mathis JM, Erbe EM, et al. Biomechanical evaluation of a new bone cement for use in vertebroplasty. *Spine* 2000;25:1061–1064.
20. Deramond H, Wright NT, Belkoff SM. Temperature elevation caused by bone cement polymerization during vertebroplasty. *Bone* 1999;25(2 Suppl):17S–21S.
21. Erbe E, Pomrink GJ, Murphy CA. The static and dynamic mechanical properties of Cortoss synthetic cortical bone void filler. Presented at WorldSpine 1, Berlin, Germany, 2000.

23

Treatment of Severe Osteoporotic Fractures through a Microsurgical Interlaminary Approach

Bronek M. Boszczyk, Michael Bierschneider, Björn Robert, and Hans Jaksche

Neurochirurgie, Berufsgenossenschaftliche Unfallklinik Murnau, Murnau, Germany

Percutaneous vertebroplasty and kyphoplasty have been shown to provide rapid clinical improvement in the management of osteoporotic vertebral collapse. In patients with isolated back pain, these percutaneous procedures are minimally invasive and lead to immediate stabilization of the affected vertebral body.

There are, however, several limitations to the percutaneous approach: In cases with severe loss of vertebral body height, the angle of the transpedicle approach may be too steep to effectively enter the anterior or middle portion of the vertebral body (Fig. 23.1A). When the spinal canal is compromised as a result of fragmentation of the posterior vertebral wall, causing neurological symptoms, decompression of the neural structures cannot be undertaken (Fig. 23.2). Mechanical or thermal neural damage is rare in the frequently occurring minor cement extrusions (1,2); the risk of neural damage from extruded cement (3,4), however, is increased and difficult to control percutaneously, in cases of severe disruption of the posterior wall.

For safe treatment of these severe cases of collapse, Wenger and Markwalder (5) developed the technique of open surgical vertebroplasty, which allows bilateral decompression of the spinal canal and affords control over the neural structures during bipedicle augmentation.

In the application of a microsurgical interlaminary approach to the principle of open surgical augmentation, soft tissue trauma is limited by minimal unilateral muscle dissection. Neural decompression is accomplished, and access is provided to both adjacent vertebrae without extension of the approach. Safety during augmentation is increased through control of the spinal canal.

SURGICAL TECHNIQUE

The microsurgical interlaminary augmentation procedure is performed with the patient under general anesthesia. The patient is positioned prone on a spine frame or on cushions with legs extended, to avoid abdominal compression. An image intensifier is mounted in the lateral fluoroscopy position, and the affected vertebral bodies are identified. When a single vertebra is to be treated, the cranial interlaminary space should be targeted, because

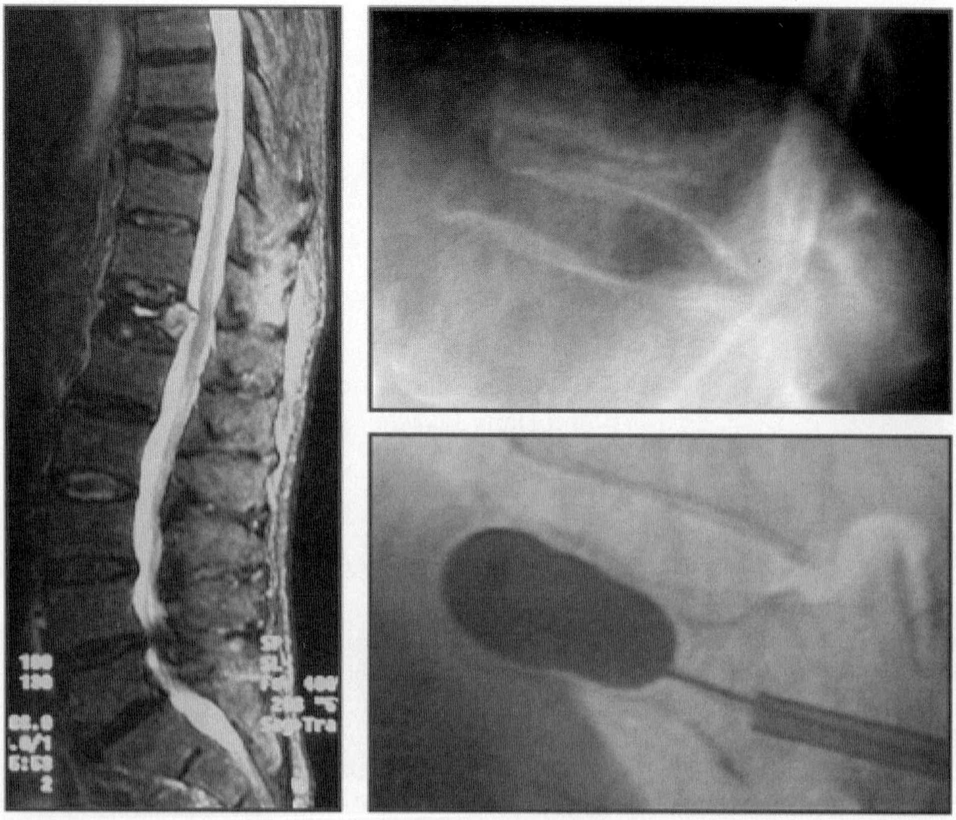

A

FIG. 23.1. A: Case illustration of an 81-year-old man with an osteoporotic fracture of T-12, severe loss of height, and fragmentation of the posterior wall (*left,* magnetic resonance image; *right,* lateral radiograph). The very steep angle of the pedicle precludes anterior placement of the kyphoplasty balloon by the percutaneous route. Through an open interlaminary approach, ideal placement of the balloon is achieved (*lower right,* fluoroscopy image).

this will be in projection to the superior aspect of the affected vertebral body. Should adjacent vertebral bodies need to be treated, the common intervertebral space is approached. The approach should be performed on the side with the predominant radicular symptoms.

A longitudinal midline incision approximately 5 cm long is centered above the interlaminary space as for microdiscectomy. Minimal unilateral muscle dissection is performed, exposing the ligamentum flavum between the vertebral arches. Conventional retractors are introduced. With the use of a surgical microscope or loupes, an interlaminar fenestration and unilateral flavectomy are accomplished, exposing the thecal sac and the segmental nerve root (Fig. 23.3). At this stage, decompression of the neural structures is undertaken as necessary. The fenestration is extended laterally, avoiding excessive destruction of the facet joint, until the lateral border of posterior wall of the affected vertebral body is exposed by gentle medial retraction of the thecal sac. With advanced degeneration of the facet joints, it may be necessary to resect the medial joint portion.

In treatment of the thoracolumbar to midthoracic levels, partial resection of the facet joint and medial pedicle wall may be necessary in order to gain access to the posterior wall without exerting pressure on the spinal cord.

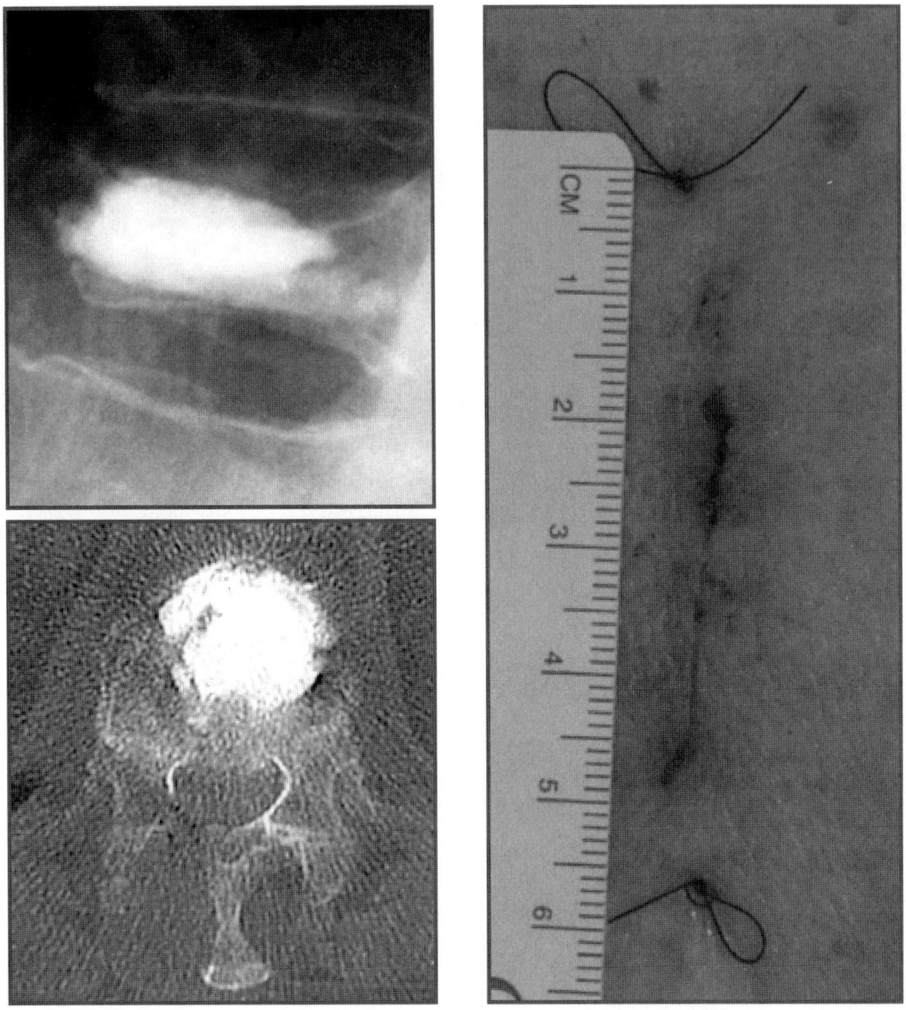

B

FIG. 23.1. *Continued.* **B:** The postoperative lateral view (*upper left*) shows good filling of the anterior and middle portions of the vertebral body. The postoperative computed tomographic scan confirms central placement of the augmentation (*lower left*). The required skin incision is less than 6 cm in length (*right*).

Under fluoroscopic control, a vertebroplasty cannula or kyphoplasty trochar is then introduced into the vertebral body directly through the posterior wall (Fig. 23.4). Slight convergence leads to central positioning of the tip of the instrument in the vertebral body. A biopsy sample is routinely taken at this point. Because the approach is not dependant on the angle of the pedicle, the cannula or trochar may be introduced at the ideal angle, with regard to the endplates, that allows it to be advanced to the anterior third of the vertebral body (see Fig. 23.1A). Through the same interlaminary approach, both the superior and the inferior vertebral bodies of a motion segment may be reached, if necessary, without additional soft tissue trauma (see Fig. 23.3).

When vertebroplasty is to be performed, contrast medium is injected to assess the vertebral venous blood flow (Fig. 23.5). When epidural drainage is rapid, slight

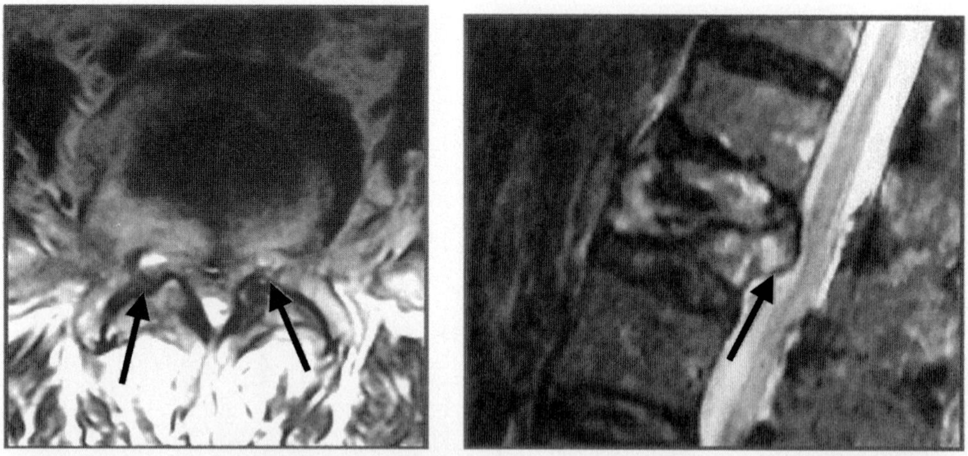

FIG. 23.2. Osteoporotic fractures may result in compromise of the neural structures through narrowing of the lateral recess (*left*) or through fragmentation of the posterior wall (*right*), which, in addition, increases the risk of epidural cement leakage.

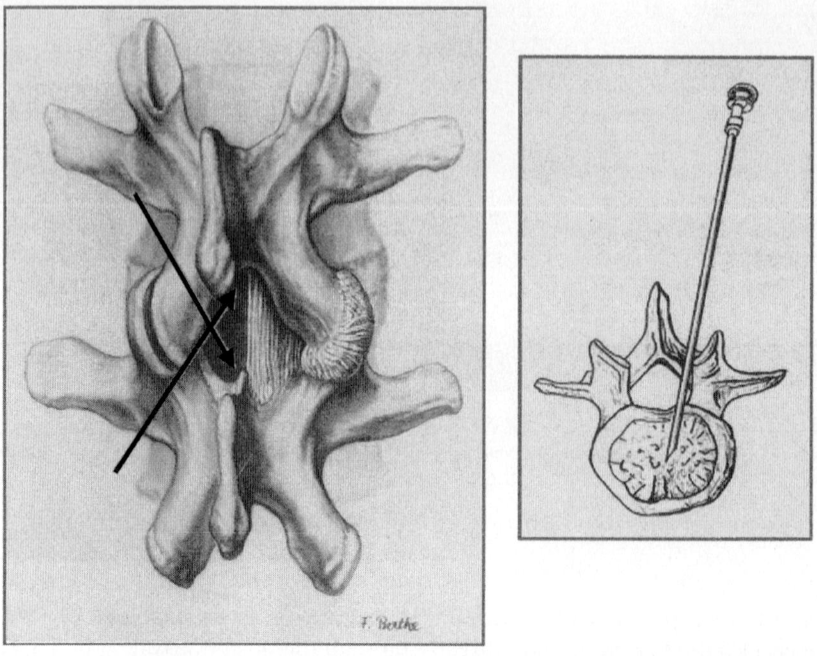

FIG. 23.3. The interlaminary approach requires a unilateral fenestration of the spinal canal (*left*). After lateral flavectomy, the thecal sac is gently retracted medially, which exposes the posterior vertebral wall, through which a tool may be introduced into the vertebral body (*right*). Both adjacent vertebrae may be reached through the same approach. (*Left:* from Putz R. Funktionelle Anatomie der Wirbelgelenke. Thieme, 1981.)

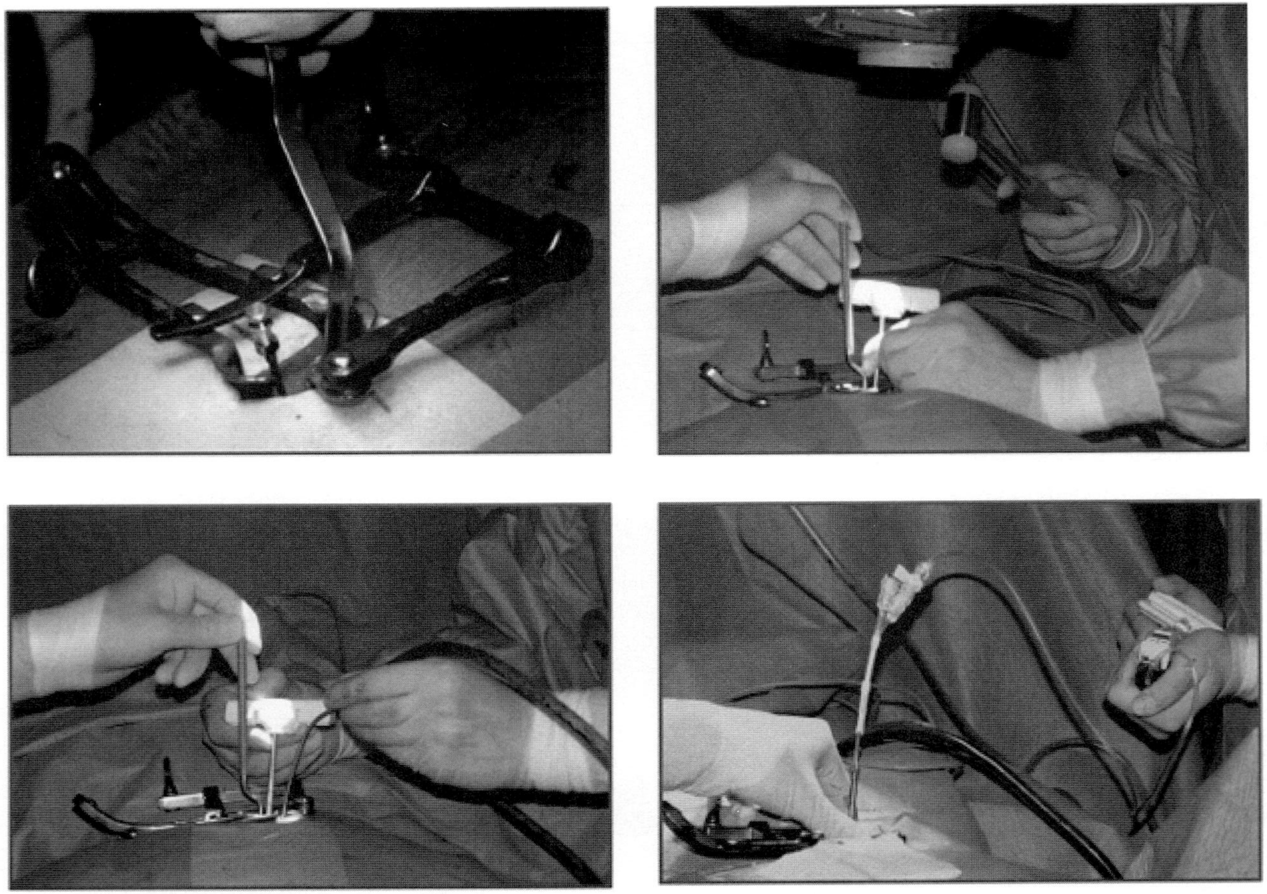

FIG. 23.4. Conventional retractors are used for the microsurgical interlaminary approach. The thecal sac is gently retracted medially, which allows a vertebroplasty trochar to be placed (**A**). Alternatively, a kyphoplasty cannula may be tapped into the vertebral body through the posterior wall (**B,C**), which allows introduction of a kyphoplasty balloon (**D**).

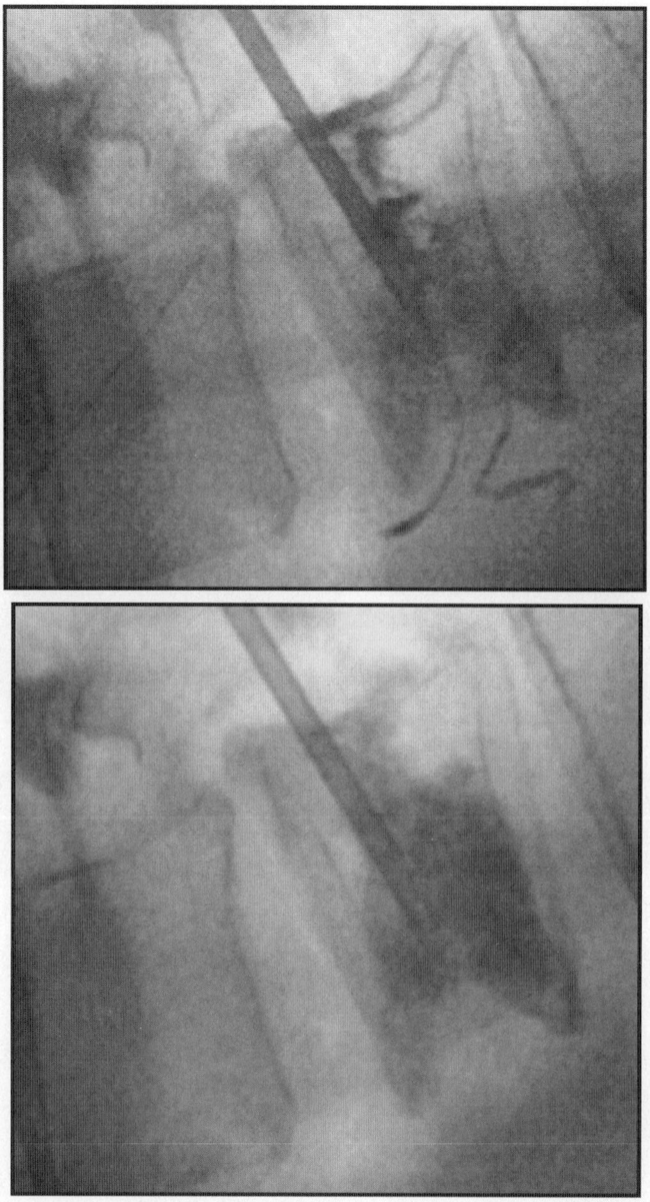

A

B

FIG. 23.5. In interlaminary vertebroplasty, contrast medium is injected before augmentation in order to assess vertebral venous blood flow. When rapid epidural filling is present (**A**), slight advancement of the trochar usually improves trabecular filling. Injection of low-viscosity acrylic cement is performed under live fluoroscopic guidance (**B**).

advancement of the cannula toward the anterior third of the vertebral body usually increases vertebral body filling. Care must be taken not to create additional perforations of the cortex, because the injected acrylic cement will leak through them easily. A low-viscosity acrylic cement (e.g., Osteopal, manufactured by Biomet Merck) is mixed with contrast medium (e.g., tantalum powder, manufactured by Cook) or a radiopaque cement (e.g., Vertebroplastic, manufactured by DePuy AcroMed) is prepared and injected under live fluoroscopy at low viscosity to achieve trabecular filling (see Fig. 23.5).

In kyphoplasty, injection of contrast medium is not mandatory. A kyphoplasty balloon is introduced through the cannula and inflated as usual. A 20-mm balloon, used for the lumbar levels and lower thoracic levels, creates a cavity with a maximum capacity of 6 mL. In the midthoracic levels, a 15-mm balloon may be used for a cavity with a maximum capacity of 4 mL. The created cavity is filled with the prepared acrylic cement at a higher viscosity than for vertebroplasty. As for vertebroplasty, the augmentation is monitored under live fluoroscopy.

If epidural leakage is detected with either technique during augmentation, the spinal canal may be inspected with the surgical microscope. Extruded cement is usually removed easily as long as it has a pasty consistency.

CLINICAL EXPERIENCE

Using the microsurgical interlaminary augmentation techniques, the authors have treated 21 patients suffering from severe osteoporotic vertebral collapse and neurological symptoms or from posterior wall fragmentation and pain that is unresponsive to conservative therapy (Figs. 23.6, and 23.7; see Fig. 23.1). Affected vertebrae ranged from T-10 to L-5. In patients with neoplastic disease, the authors have approached the midthoracic spine up to T-8. A single vertebra was treated in 15 patients, and adjacent vertebrae were treated in four patients. Three and four vertebrae were treated in two patients, respectively, through two separate interlaminary approaches each.

The average amount of blood loss, less than 100 mL, is not significantly more than for a conventional fenestration or decompression. The actual augmentation procedure adds 15 to 40 minutes to the operation per treated vertebra.

Homogenous filling of the vertebral body with acrylic cement may be achieved in both vertebroplasty and kyphoplasty, whereby augmentation volumes range from 2 to 6 mL, depending on the severity of collapse and the size of the vertebra (Fig. 23.8). Minor subligamentary cement leakage, which did not need to be removed, occurred in a third of patients. In the authors' experience, leakage is more frequent in patients undergoing vertebroplasty. Larger amounts of epidural leakage occurred in two such patients and in one patient undergoing kyphoplasty who had pronounced posterior wall fragmentation. The epidural cement was easily removed, but an additional depot of subligamentary cement was not removable in one of the patients undergoing vertebroplasty. There were no neurological complications and no new radicular symptoms among the patients.

DISCUSSION

The conventional percutaneous approach for vertebroplasty and kyphoplasty limits the application to patients without symptomatic encroachment of neural structures that mandates operative decompression. Moreover, the transpedicle approach becomes increasingly difficult with the degree of collapse, because the angle of the instruments entering the vertebral body from the pedicle increases in steepness, ultimately precluding placement in the middle or anterior third of the vertebral body. Finally, with fragmentation of the posterior wall, the risk of neural damage from epidural cement leakage is increased, because it cannot be removed percutaneously. The alternative, conventional operative treatment for patients with such vertebral collapse is posterior internal fixation, potentially combined with anterior reconstruction.

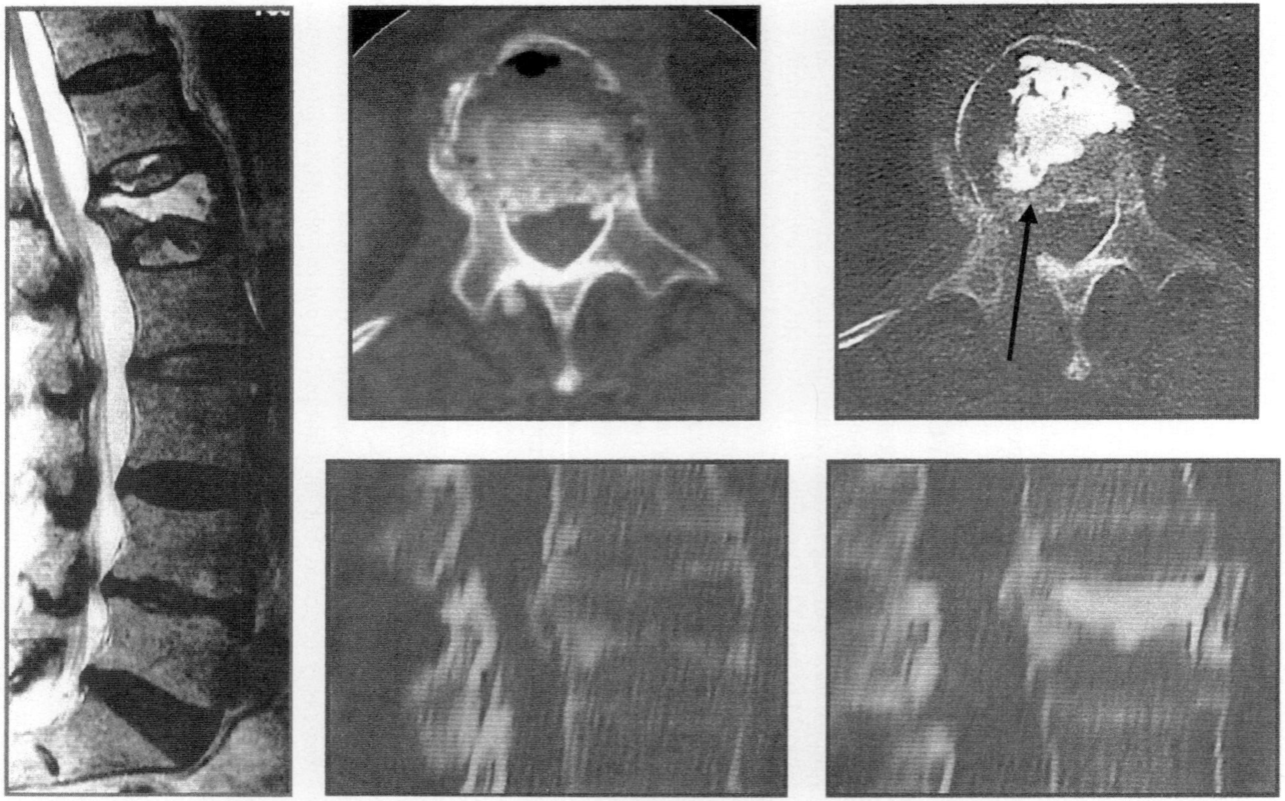

FIG. 23.6. Case illustration of a 91-year-old woman with an osteoporotic fracture of L-1. Open interlaminary vertebroplasty was performed because of the fragmentation of the posterior wall (*left:* magnetic resonance image; *middle:* computed tomographic scans). The postoperative computed tomographic scans (*right*) confirm adequate filling of the vertebral body. The *arrow* indicates the track of the vertebroplasty trochar.

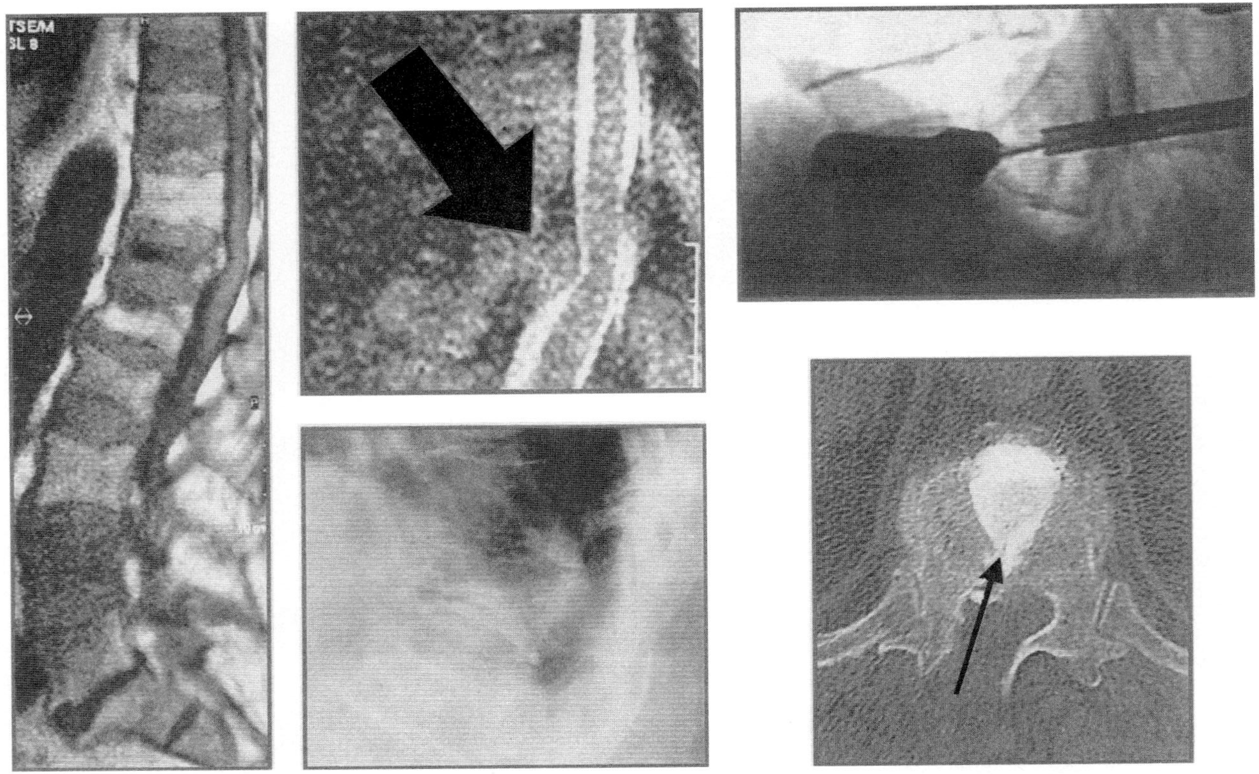

FIG. 23.7. Case illustration of a 64-year-old man with multiple osteoporotic fractures (*left:* magnetic resonance image). Upon weight bearing, neurogenic claudication developed as a result of the posterior wall fragment of T-12 (*arrow* on *upper middle* magnetic resonance image). Because of this fragment and the severe loss of height (lateral radiograph, *lower middle*), an interlaminary approach was chosen. The kyphoplasty balloon was advanced into the anterior third of the vertebral body (fluoroscopy image, *upper right*), and adequate central augmentation was achieved with minor subligamentary leakage (postoperative computed tomographic scan, *lower right*). The slender *arrow* indicates the track of the kyphoplasty cannula.

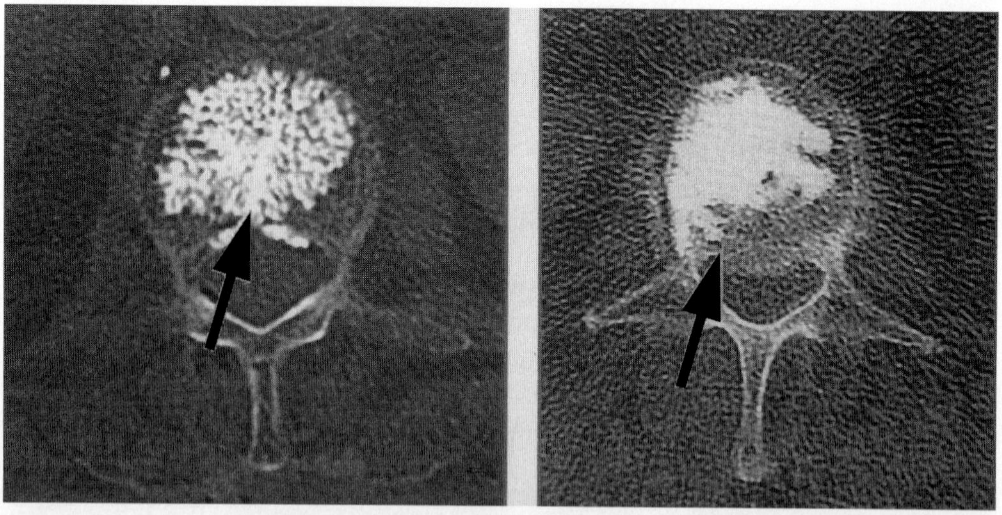

FIG. 23.8. Both interlaminary vertebroplasty (postoperative computed tomographic scan, *left*) and kyphoplasty (postoperative computed tomographic scan, *right*) enable central augmentation with acrylic cement. The trabecular filling pattern in vertebroplasty is a result of the injection of acrylic cement at low viscosity. The cavity produced through kyphoplasty is filled with acrylic cement at a higher viscosity. Minor subligamentary cement leakage, as seen on the vertebroplasty image, has not been shown to be of clinical significance in the authors' experience and is therefore not usually removed.

Microsurgical interlaminary augmentation provides a less invasive approach for this group of patients, who are generally poor candidates for extensive surgery but cannot be adequately treated percutaneously. Soft tissue trauma is kept to a minimum because the approach is unilateral and the pedicle entry zone does not need to be exposed. Both adjacent vertebrae may be treated through the same interlaminary approach, when required, without significant extension of the approach. Neural structures are decompressed, and epidural cement leakage is controllable. The interlaminary approach is easily converted to include laminectomy and instrumentation as needed, so that no options are lost through initiating this procedure.

As with the percutaneous techniques, patients are rapidly mobilized, which reduces comorbidity.

Because no additional specialized instruments are needed for the approach, spine surgeons accustomed to microsurgical procedures are able to apply this method easily, expanding the indications for these procedures in vertebroplasty and kyphoplasty.

REFERENCES

1. Bostrom MP, Lane JM. Augmentation of osteoporotic vertebral bodies. *Spine* 1997;22(24S):38S–42S.
2. Martin JB, Jean B, Sugiu K, et al. Vertebroplasty: Clinical experience and follow-up results. *Bone* 1999;25S: 11S–15S.
3. Deramond H, Wright NT, Belkoff SM. Temperature elevation caused by bone cement polymerization during vertebroplasty. *Bone* 1999;25S:17S–21S.
4. Ratliff J, Nguyen T, Heiss J. Root and spinal cord compression from methylmethacrylate vertebroplasty. *Spine* 2001;26:E300–E302.
5. Wenger W, Markwalder TM. Surgically controlled, transpedicular methyl methacrylate vertebroplasty with fluoroscopic guidance. Acta Neurochir 1999;141:625–631.

24

Percutaneous Vertebroplasty in the Treatment of Osteoporotic Vertebral Compression Fractures

What Can We Learn from the Bad Results?

G. Michael Hess and H. Michael Mayer

Spine Center, Orthopädische Klinik München-Harlaching, 81547 München, Germany

Percutaneous vertebroplasty was developed in France in the mid-1980s for the treatment of vertebral hemangioma (1). The indication was later extended to include the treatment of other osteolytic lesions and painful affections of the spine (2), as well as the treatment of osteoporotic vertebral compression fractures (VCFs). The first series in the United States was reported in 1997 (3). In the late 1990s, vertebroplasty was re-imported to Europe and became increasingly popular.

Reasons for the popularity of percutaneous vertebroplasty are (a) the limited therapeutic alternatives for this group of patients, in whom severe pain is refractory to conservative treatment, including analgesics, and (b) the excellent early results.

The polymethylmethacrylate (PMMA) cement augmentation of the vertebral body reportedly results in early postoperative pain relief in the majority of patients. One study reported vertebroplasty in 104 patients treated over a period of 5 years. Of the patients with preoperative edema evident on magnetic resonance images (MRIs), 90% experienced excellent results, and of the patients in whom the compression fracture affected less than 50% of the original vertebral height, 87% experienced excellent results (4). Another study, of 38 patients with 70 osteoporotic fractures, showed marked or complete pain relief in 63% and moderate pain relief in 32% of the patients (5).

The reported complication rate is low. Extravertebral leakage of the PMMA to the epidural space and the paravertebral tissue occurs in up to 74% of the patients (4). Fortunately, these leakages remain clinically insignificant in most cases. But a finding that is clinically insignificant in one patient may be a severe complication in another: Fig. 24.1 shows the MRI of a patient with a VCF of L-2 and an asymptomatic spinal stenosis at the same level. It is obvious that a small amount of PMMA leaking into the epidural space would cause severe neurological complications. In this patient, percutaneous vertebroplasty was performed without any complications and yielded an excellent result.

Serious complications have also been reported; these include transient or persistent radicular neuritis (5) and nerve root and spinal cord compromise, as well as pulmonary embolism (6).

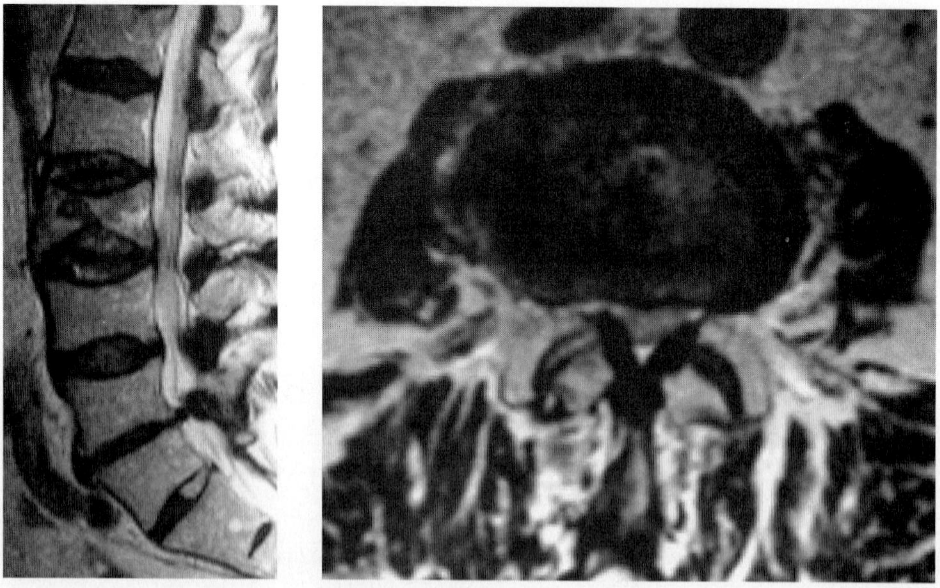

FIG. 24.1. Sagittal **(A)** and axial **(B)** T-2 magnetic resonance images of a vertebral compression fracture of L-2 and an asymptomatic absolute spinal stenosis at the same level in a 71-year-old man.

As with other relatively new therapeutic options, long-term follow-up results of prospective controlled randomized clinical trials are lacking. This explains why, despite a multitude of published articles on percutaneous vertebroplasty, many questions have been left unanswered and why several articles concluded that this procedure is still in the investigational stage (7,8).

This chapter is based on a review of the authors' first 40 patients, in whom percutaneous vertebroplasty with PMMA (low-viscosity Osteopal™ mixed with 10 mL of Solutrast™ as opacifier) has been performed in order to alleviate pain resulting from an osteoporotic VCF. The fractured vertebrae ranged from T-4 to L-5 and were located predominantly around the thoracolumbar junction. All operations have been performed by an orthopedic surgeon (G. Michael Hess) or a neurosurgeon, trained in percutaneous and minimal invasive procedures.

The following cases represent an analysis of the authors' experience with percutaneous vertebroplasty, focusing on the topics *indication*, *biomechanical considerations,* and *complications,* as well as an attempt to elaborate more detailed guidelines for a safe performance of vertebroplasty.

INDICATION: CASE 1

A 71-year-old man with a history of prostate cancer for 2 years had chronic low back pain for 1 year [Visual Analogue Scale (VAS) score, 7]. No diagnostic or therapeutic efforts had yet been undertaken. The pain was located around the thoracolumbar junction, and radiographs of the lumbar spine revealed VCFs of L-1 and L-2 with a vacuum phenomenon at L-1 (Fig. 24.2A–C). An MRI and a bone scan were obtained but did not pro-

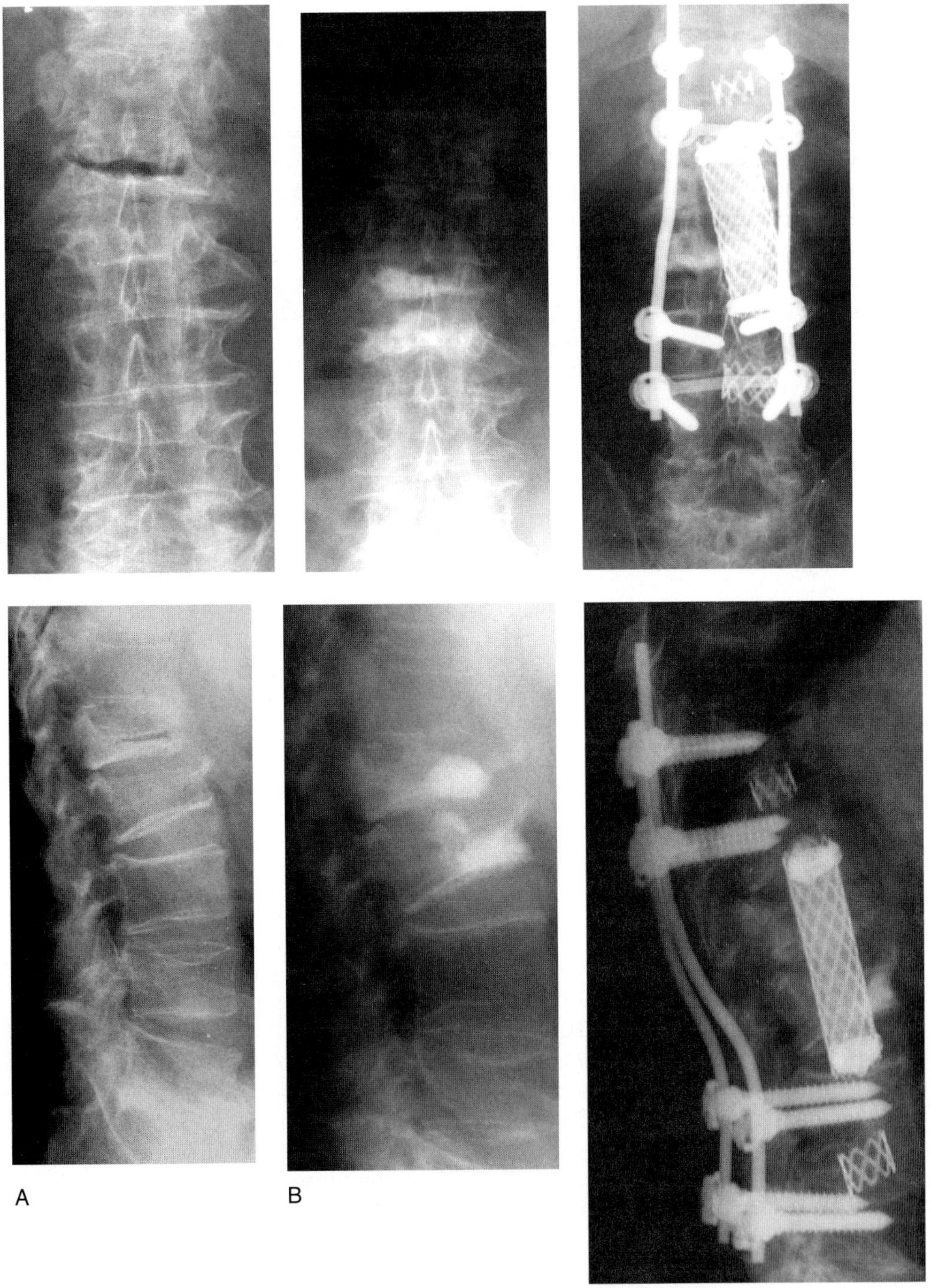

FIG. 24.2. Case 1: Anteroposterior and lateral radiographs of L-1 and L-2 vertebral compression fractures **(A)** in a 71-year-old man, which were treated with vertebroplasty **(B).** Anterior-posterior decompression and instrumentation was necessary because of a progressive compression of L-1 with retropulsion of a fragment of the posterior cortical wall and neurological compromise **(C).**

vide any further information in determining whether the fracture was osteoporotic or metastatic in origin. Percutaneous needle biopsy specimens of L-1 and L-2 revealed no material indicative of a metastasis.

The authors performed percutaneous vertebroplasty on L-1 and L-2. Correct needle placement in the severely collapsed vertebral body of L-1 was nearly impossible, and the injection of PMMA had to be stopped after a small amount because of a leakage to the upper disc space. However, the patient experienced alleviation of pain (VAS 4), could be well mobilized with a brace, and transferred to an inpatient rehabilitation center.

Four weeks after surgery, he experienced acute nontraumatic back pain and developed a progressive paraplegia of the lower limbs. A computed tomographic scan highlighted a retropulsed fragment at the posterior cortical wall of L-1, which caused dural compromise. The authors performed immediate anterior and posterior decompression with corporectomy of L-1 and L-2 and stabilization with an anterior titanium mesh cage and a posterior pedicle screw system, and a high-dose intravenous corticosteroid medication according to the National Acute Spinal Cord Injury Study (NASCIS) scheme was administered.

At the last follow-up visit 6 months later, the patient had moderate back pain (VAS 4), and the neurological deficits had improved to Frankel grade D.

BIOMECHANICAL CONSIDERATIONS: CASE 2

A 74-year-old woman had acute nontraumatic back pain (VAS 8). An acute VCF of T-12 with a marked kyphotic deformity (vertebral kyphosis angle of 30 degrees) was radiologically visible (Fig. 24.3A–E). Because of this kyphotic deformity at the thoracolumbar junction, an anterior corrective procedure with a titanium mesh cage and an anterolateral constrained screw/plate device from T-11 to L-1 was performed. However, the poor quality of bone led to an early implant migration with a loss of correction. Therefore, a posterior corrective procedure with a pedicle screw system from T-9 to L-3 was performed. The patient was discharged with a moderate pain relief (VAS 5). Two months later, she again had a sudden increase of low back pain without any prior trauma. Radiographs of the lumbar spine demonstrated a compression fracture of the upper endplate of L-4, which was treated successfully with a unipedicle percutaneous vertebroplasty: The patient's low back pain improved within a few days (VAS 3). Six months later, a fall onto her back caused immediate debilitating lower back pain (VAS score, 10) and the patient became bedridden. Radiographs of the lumbar spine revealed a coronary split fracture of L-4 at the bone-PMMA interface.

One treatment option was a corporectomy of L-4 and a prolongation of the anterior-posterior fusion to the sacrum; the authors decided instead to treat the patient conservatively with analgesics and antiinflammatory medication and mobilized her with a brace. At the last follow-up visit 6 months later, she complained of moderate chronic low back pain (VAS score, 5) but was more or less satisfied with the result and reported no major restrictions in her activities of daily living.

COMPLICATIONS: CASE 3

A 65-year-old woman had acute back pain after a fall on her back (VAS 7). Radiographs of the lumbar spine and an MRI 3 weeks later showed acute VCFs of T-12 and L-2 (Fig. 24.4A–E), which were treated with a percutaneous vertebroplasty over a unipedicle approach at both levels. Several repositioning maneuvers of the Jamshidi needle were nec-

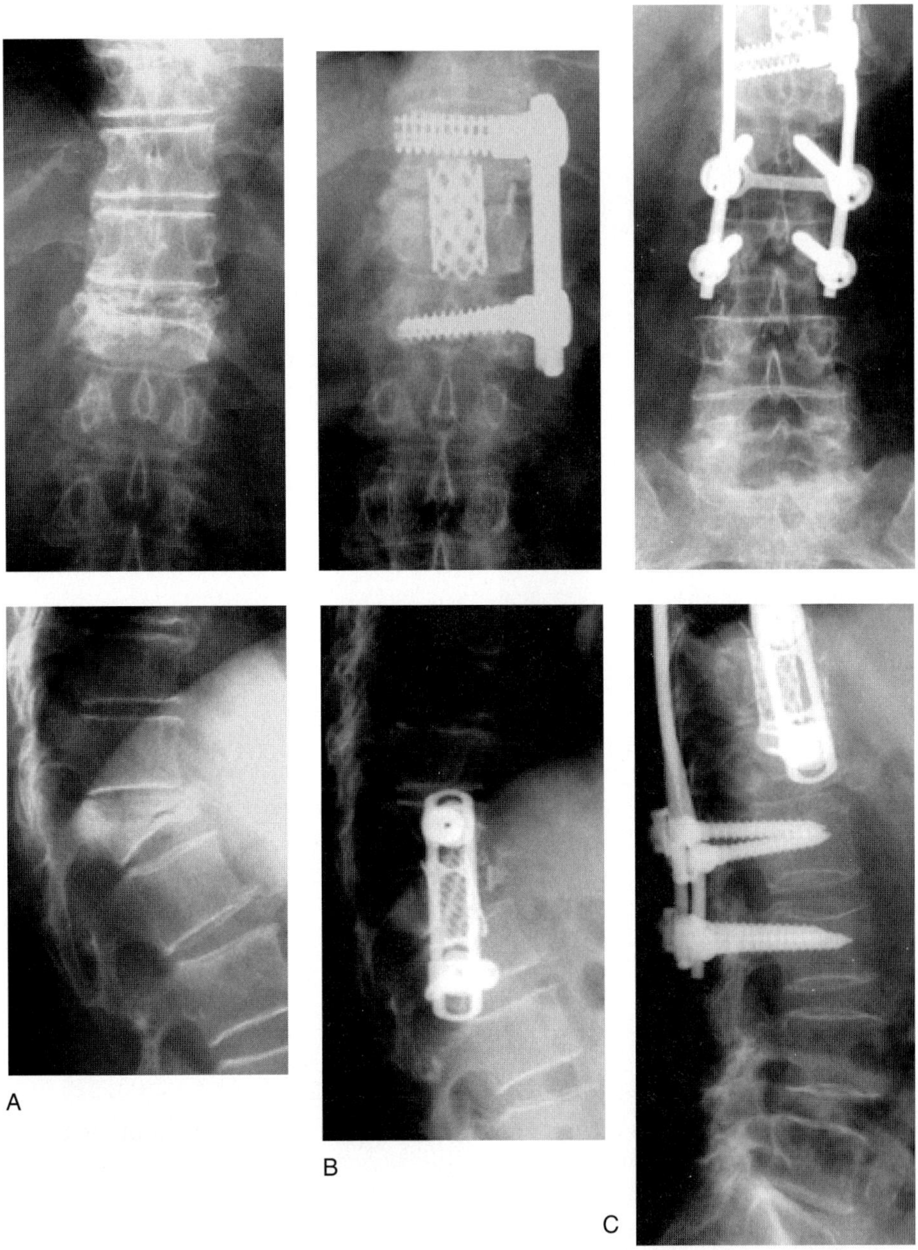

A B C

FIG. 24.3. Case 2: Anteroposterior and lateral radiographs of with a T-12 vertebral compression fracture in a 74-year-old woman **(A),** an anterior corrective procedure in T-11 to L-1 with implant migration **(B),** a posterior procedure in T-9 to L-3 **(C).**

(continued on next page)

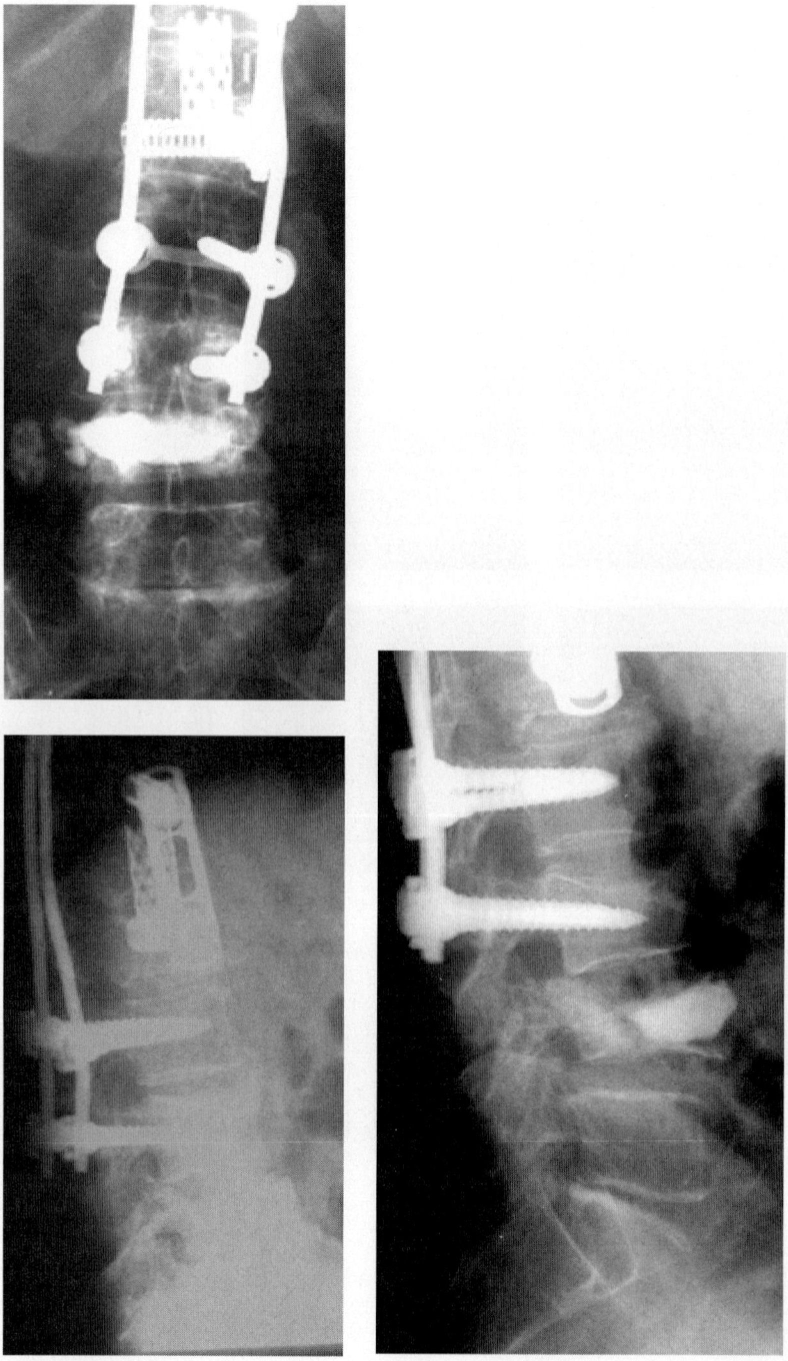

D E

FIG. 24.3. *Continued.* Case 2: A consecutive vertebral compression fracture of L-4 that was treated with vertebroplasty **(D).** Posttraumatic split fracture of L-4 at the bone-polymethylmethacrylate interface **(E).**

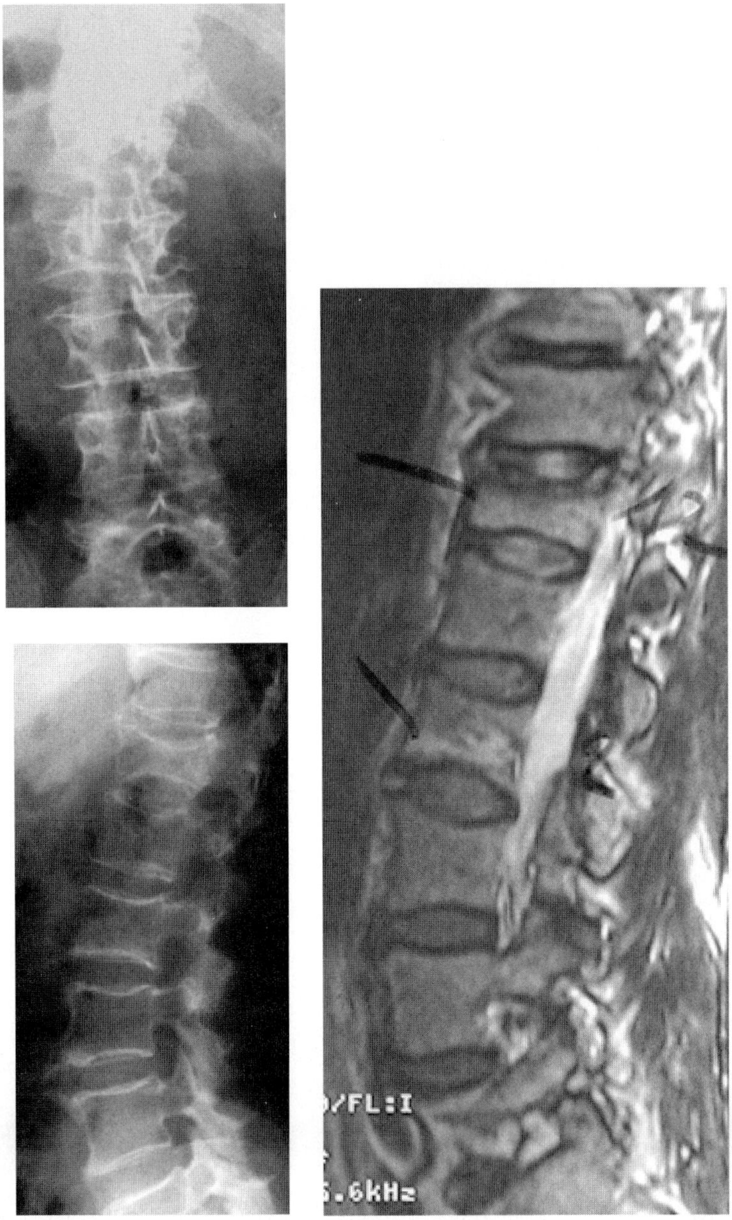

A B

FIG. 24.4. Case 3: **A,B:** Anteroposterior and lateral radiographs and a sagittal T-2 magnetic resonance image of acute vertebral compression fractures of T-12 and L-2 in a 65-year-old woman.

(continued on next page)

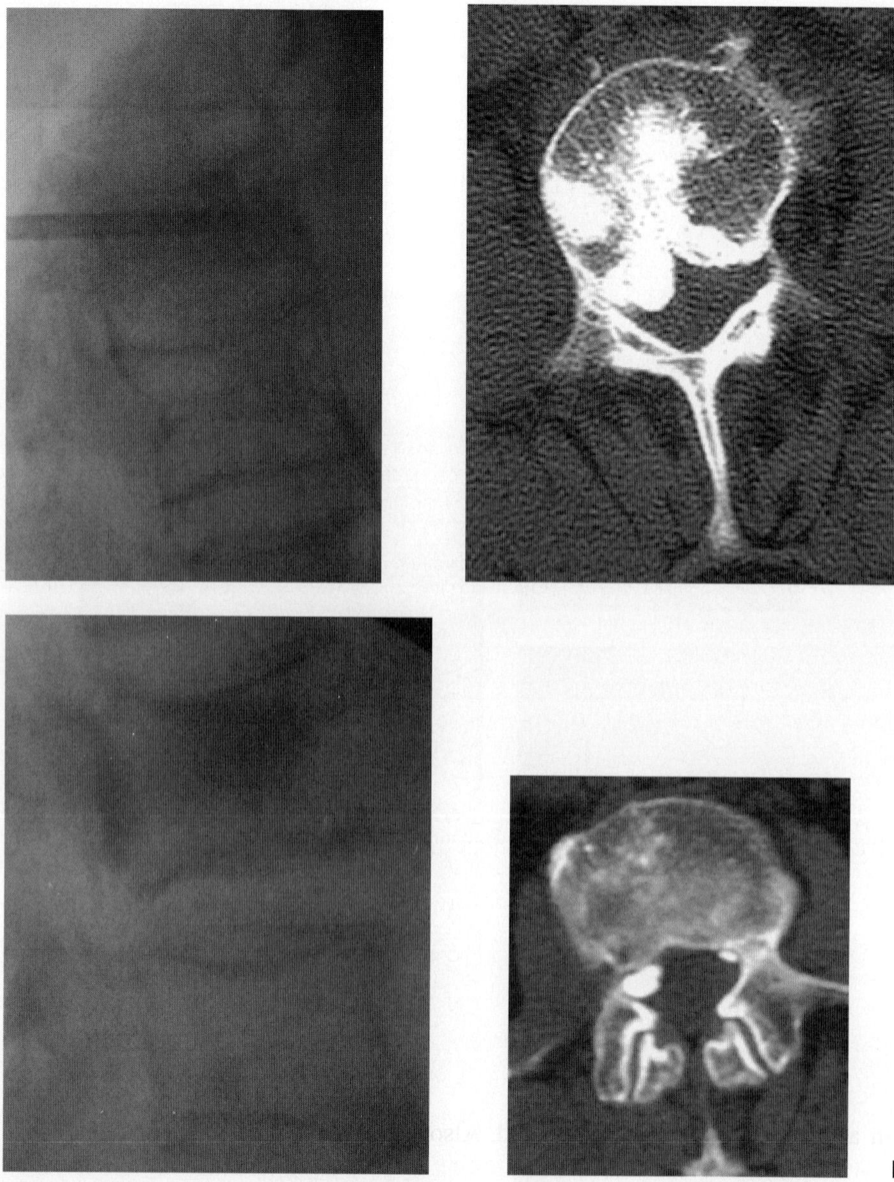

C

D

E

FIG. 24.4. *Continued.* Case 3: **C:** Intraoperative placement of the Jamshidi needle in L-2. **D:** Postoperative lateral fluoroscopic printout, revealing the epidural polymethylmethacrylate (PMMA) leakage at L-2 **E:** Postoperative computed tomographic scan, highlighting the PMMA in the spinal canal and the right recess of L-2 to L-3.

essary in order to obtain a more convergent needle position in L-2. The intraoperative fluoroscopic printouts showed obvious PMMA leakage to the epidural space. A computed tomographic scan gave definite evidence of a compromise of the L-2- and L-3 nerve roots on the right side. The clinical picture with pain radiating into the anterior right thigh and a grade 2 paresis of the hip flexion on the right side corresponded to that finding.

The patient was treated with a microsurgical hemilaminectomy on the right side and decompression of the roots L-2 and L-3. At the last follow-up visit 6 months later, she still had a neuropathic pain radiation; the hip flexion paresis had slightly improved one grade.

CONCLUSIONS

The three cases just reported represent the authors' negative experiences with percutaneous vertebroplasty in the treatment of osteoporotic VCFs. One other patient had a transient intercostal neuritis. All the other 36 patients (90%) of this initial series had excellent or good outcomes. This overall result compares favorably with the results reported in the literature (3–5).

The root causes for the suboptimal results are two learning curves: one concerning the indication and one concerning technical and surgical aspects. Whereas the first case was not an indication for vertebroplasty, the very complex second case was worth the attempt. To the authors' best knowledge, no precedent case has been reported in the literature.

In conclusion, the authors see an indication for percutaneous vertebroplasty in patients with (a) severe debilitating pain corresponding to the level of the fracture, (b) a fracture affecting 50% or less of the original vertebral body height, and (c) edema visible on MRI, which highlights an acute or nonhealed fracture.

The technical aspects of percutaneous vertebroplasty have been reported and discussed in detail (3,9,10). Our third case points out the necessity of an initial correct needle placement. At the lumbar spine, the authors prefer a bilateral approach, which has the advantage of a less convergent needle placement (destruction of medial cortex of the pedicle) as well as a lower injection pressure and a shorter way for the distribution of the PMMA within the vertebral body.

A PMMA cement with adequate radiopacity and a prolonged working time would be very helpful and would make the procedure safer.

We support the demand of most authors reporting on percutaneous vertebroplasty that the procedure must be standardized (7,8,11). First, a randomized clinical multicenter trial with a long-term follow-up is needed. Also needed is more knowledge about possible long-term complications and the biomechanical properties *in vivo,* such as the fracture risk of adjacent vertebrae (12).

OUTLOOK TO THE FUTURE

The correct placement of the Jamshidi needle is the key procedure in order to obtain good results and to avoid complications, as mentioned earlier. A prospective clinical trial performed by the authors examines the technical feasibility and accuracy of fluoroscopy-based computer-assisted percutaneous vertebroplasty (13).

In the future, the injection of PMMA cement may be replaced by the percutaneous instillation of osteoconductive and osteoinductive material or osteogenic growth factors, which would be a revolutionary step in the treatment not only of osteoporotic VCFs.

REFERENCES

1. Galibert P, Deramond H, Rosat P, et al. Note préliminaire sur le traitement des angiomes vertébraux par vertébroplastie percutanée. *Neurochirurgie* 1987;33:166–168.
2. Galibert P, Deramond H. La vertébroplastie acrylique percutanée comme traitement des angiomes vertébraux et des affections dolorigènes et fragilisantes du rachis. *Chirurgie* 1990;116:326–335.
3. Jensen ME, Evans AJ, Mathis JM, et al. Percutaneous polymethylmethacrylate vertebroplasty in the treatment of osteoporotic vertebral body compression fractures: technical aspects. *AJNR Am J Neuroradiol* 1997;18: 1897–1904.
4. Alvarez L, Perez-Higueras A, Rossi RE, et al. Vertebroplasty in osteoporotic fractures: Clinical and radiological results after 5 years. *Eur Spine J* 2001;10:S8.
5. Barr JD, Barr MS, Lemley TJ, et al. Percutaneous vertebroplasty for pain relief and spinal stabilization. *Spine* 2000;25:923–928.
6. Padovani B, Kasriel O, Brunner P, et al. Pulmonary embolism caused by acrylic cement: a rare complication of percutaneous vertebroplasty. *AJNR Am J Neuroradiol* 1999;20(3):375–377.
7. Einhorn TA. Vertebroplasty: an opportunity to do something really good for patients. *Spine* 2000;25:1051–1052.
8. Levine SA, Perin LA, Hayes D, et al. An evidence-based evaluation of percutaneous vertebroplasty [Abstract]. *Manag Care* 2000;9:56–60,63.
9. Deramond H, Depriester C, Galibert P, et al. Percutaneous vertebroplasty with polymethylmethacrylate. Technique, indications and results. *Radiol Clin North Am* 1998;36:533–546.
10. Heini PF, Wälchli B, Berlemann U. Percutaneous transpedicular vertebroplasty with PMMA: operative technique and early results. A prospective study for the treatment of osteoporotic compression fractures. *Eur Spine J* 2000; 9(5):445–450.
11. Cortet B, Cotten A, Boutry N, et al. Percutaneous vertebroplasty in the treatment of osteoporotic vertebral compression fractures: an open prospective study. *J Rheumatol* 1999;26:2222–2228.
12. Ferguson S, Berlemann U, Polikeit A, et al. Are adjacent vertebrae at risk following vertebroplasty? *Eur Spine J* 2001;10:S7.
13. Hess GM, Mayer HM. Computer-assisted percutaneous vertebroplasty in the treatment of vertebral body compression fractures. Unpublished data.

25

Toward a Safer Method of Vertebroplasty: Elevation and Stabilization of Vertebral Compression Fractures with a Novel, Inflatable, Implantable, Minimally Porous Mesh Container

Stephen D. Kuslich

The Spineology Research Group, Stillwater, Minnesota

The orthopedic and radiological literature has been flooded with articles describing the benefits of vertebroplasty, a procedure in which osteoporotic vertebral compression fractures are treated by injection with bone cement. The clinical results are good, and the effect is long lasting. Most patients obtain significant relief of pain, and their ability to perform the activities of daily living dramatically improves (1–17). Other reports are less enthusiastic about the procedure (18–20). Several biomechanical studies have concluded that cement-filled osteoporotic vertebral bodies are stronger and somewhat stiffer than unfilled specimens (21–26). The procedure seems to work best when the following guidelines are observed:

1. When only one or two levels are treated.
2. When the fractures are treated early.
3. When the fracture is not the result of tumor.
4. When the cement is injected with low pressure.
5. When the injection step is monitored radiographically.
6. When the patient is otherwise healthy.

Complications appear to be few and occur at low incidence. Unfortunately, a small number of patients suffer serious complications, the most significant of which involve the migration of cement into unintended areas. Cement leakage into adjacent neurological structures has caused paralysis (27,28). Embolization into the pulmonary vasculature has resulted in death (27–31). Any technology that could reduce or eliminate cement leakage would be a worthwhile addition to the vertebroplasty procedure.

DEVELOPMENT OF A NEW METHOD OF VERTEBROPLASTY

The author's colleagues at the Spineology Research Group have been developing a new technology for interbody fusion with the use of novel methods and devices. That technology consists of techniques, tools, and devices that allow the surgeon to prepare and fill body cavities through very small portals. First, this group developed expandable reamers that can create spherical or elliptical cavities up to 25 mm in diameter in bone or joint tissue, by use of reamers that are only 8 to 10 mm in cross-sectional diameter. Second, this group devised tools and methods by which to process and inject bone graft and bone graft substitutes through tubes with very small diameters. Finally, this group designed, patented, fabricated, and tested a variety of porous mesh containers and annular rings that, when filled appropriately, cause the cavity to be tightly and intimately filled with a bolus of compressed material. This compressed material is capable of withstanding physiologic loads without collapse. The fabric material has been named *OptiMesh*™.

The mesh containers simply provide a means for containing and retaining bone graft or bone graft substitute materials. Common dictionary definition (33) for “contain.”

con-tain (verb, transitive) 1. To have something inside, or to hold something. 2. To be capable of holding something within, especially a particular amount.

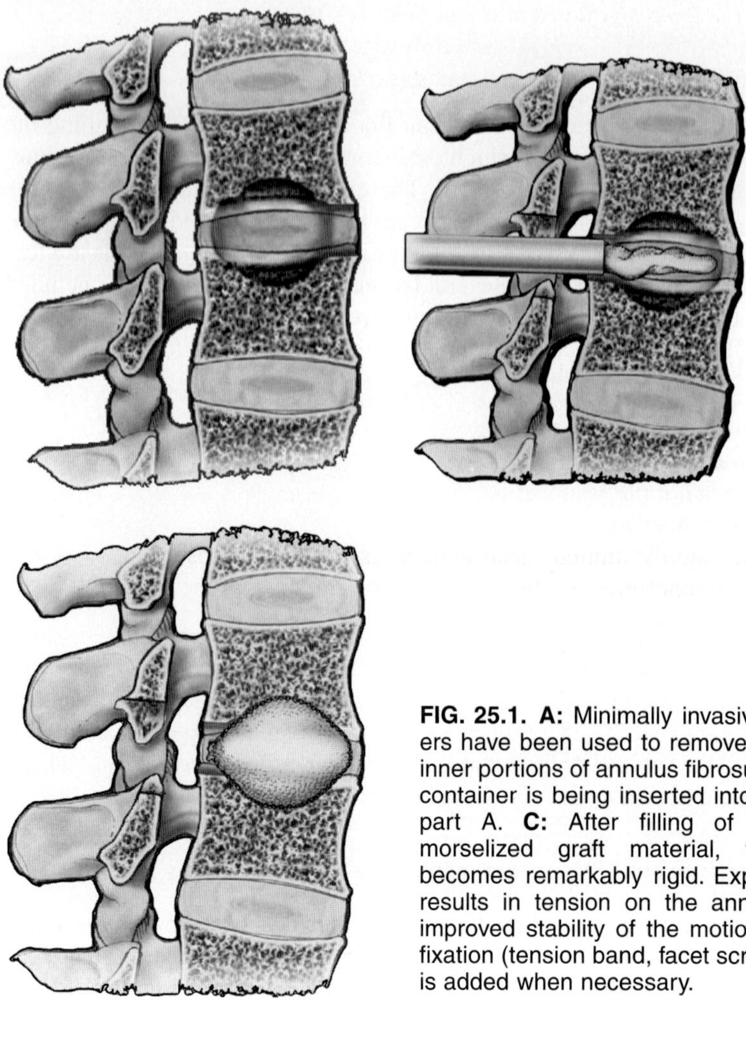

FIG. 25.1. A: Minimally invasive expandable reamers have been used to remove the nucleus and the inner portions of annulus fibrosus. **B:** A porous mesh container is being inserted into the cavity shown in part A. **C:** After filling of the container with morselized graft material, the resultant pack becomes remarkably rigid. Expansion of the cavity results in tension on the annulus and, therefore, improved stability of the motion segment. Ancillary fixation (tension band, facet screws, pedicle fixation) is added when necessary.

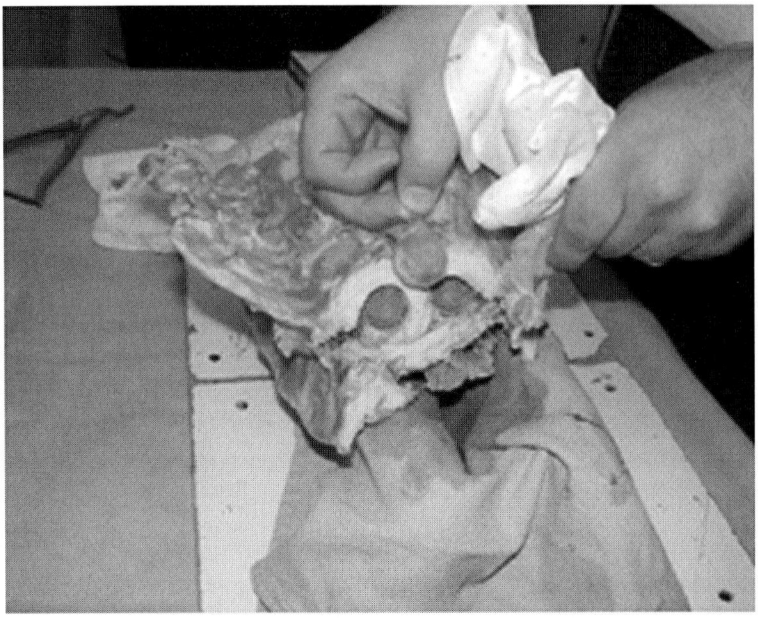

FIG. 25.2. This calf spine disc was enucleated by the expandable reamer. The OptiMesh container was then filled with morselized graft. The disc has been split transversely to show the nature of the cavity and the rigidity and porosity of the OptiMesh graft construct.

These balloons are not intended to be fixation or stabilization devices. Rather, the fixation or stabilization function is performed by the grafted material itself, sometimes by the addition of traditional fixation devices.

Figures 25.1 and 25.2 illustrate the use of the OptiMesh system in the case of interbody fusion with morselized bone graft. The Spineology Research Group tested these and other techniques, tools, and devices in a variety of *in vitro* and *in vivo* models. The technology appears to be a valuable contribution to the science of interbody fusion, joint arthrodesis, tendon reattachment, and, perhaps, other situations (33).

The Spineology Research Group realized that the system might also be useful for the containment of bone cement during vertebroplasty. The group therefore developed and tested small-diameter, tightly knitted mesh containers that were subsequently used to reduce and stabilize osteoporotic vertebral compression fractures in the pathology laboratory. This chapter reports the methods and results.

METHODS

OptiMesh Vertebroplasty

OptiMesh is used to contain and reinforce graft or bone cement when they are used to elevate and stabilize compression fractures of vertebral bodies.

The OptiMesh System consists of novel techniques, tools, and devices for creating cavities within skeletal structures and for filling these cavities with the use of porous balloons or annular rings. The entire technology was developed with the intention of producing a new, minimally invasive system that would allow the surgeon to remove and correct pathological processes by the least traumatic means.

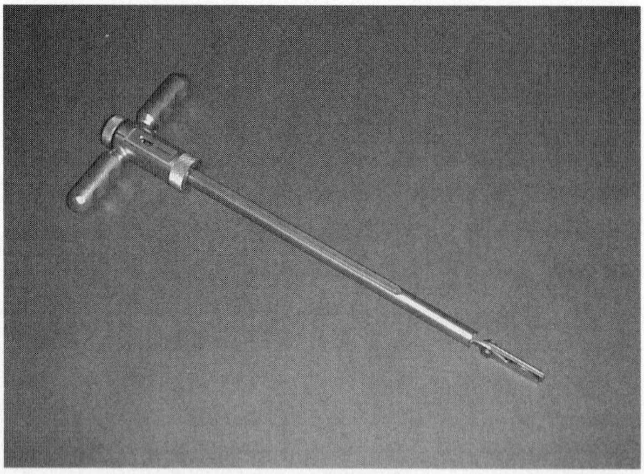

FIG. 25.3. One version of the expandable reamer, with the cutting blades in the retractable position.

Tools

The first tool developed was the **expandable, rotating reamer** (Figs. 25.3, 25.4). The tool is available in 5-, 8-, and 10-mm—diameter models. The surgeon is able to pass the instrument through a very small entrance portal and then gradually increase the diameter of the cutting blade extension by turning a knob at the proximal end of the instrument. Rotating the entire instrument cuts out an elliptical, spherical, or cylindrical cavity, depending on the geometric shape of the cutting blades. The 5-, 8-, and 10-mm models cut cavities that can be as large as 14, 22 or 25 mm in diameter, respectively.

The second tool is the **circumferential, peripheral resecting reamer** (Figs. 25.5, 25.6). This tool allows the surgeon to create a toroid-shaped cavity. A toroid is a dough-nut-shaped geometric surface generated by rotating a circle about a line in the same plane as the circle but not intersecting it.

Devices

The Spineology Research Group has been experimenting with various soft, pliable, porous containers that might be used to contain and retain bone graft and bone graft substitutes (Figs. 25.7, 25.8).

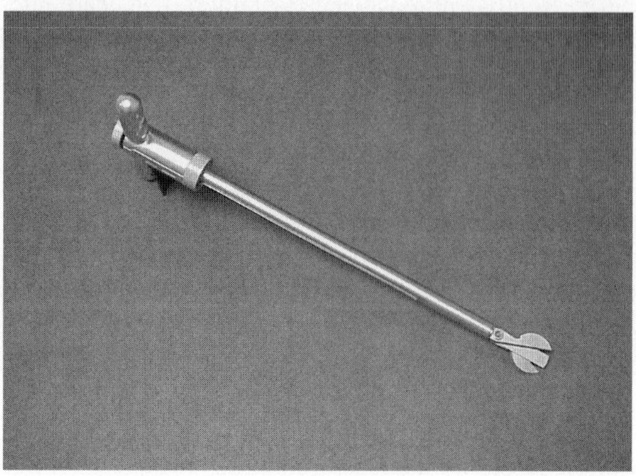

FIG. 25.4. The reamer of shown in Fig. 25.3, with the cutting blades fully extended.

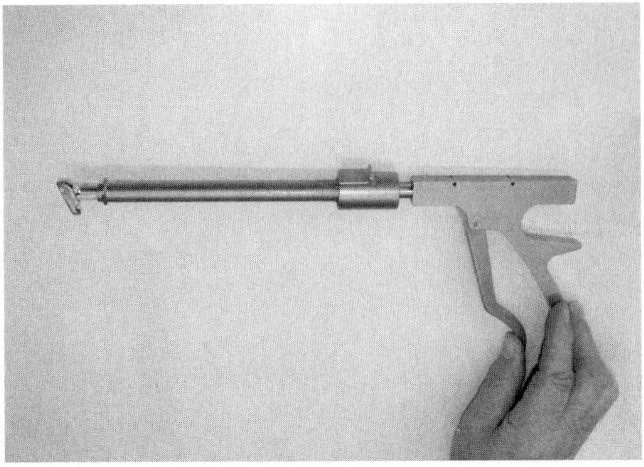

FIG. 25.5. This reamer removes the inner annulus, producing the toroid portion of the cavity seen in Fig. 25.6.

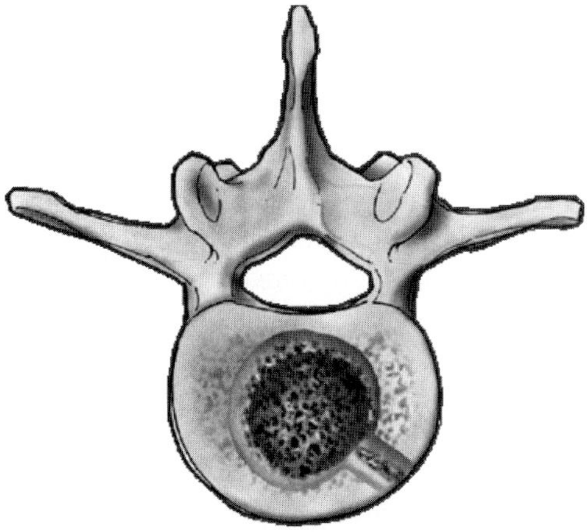

FIG. 25.6. The flattened, Saturn-shaped cavity that results from the use of both reamers.

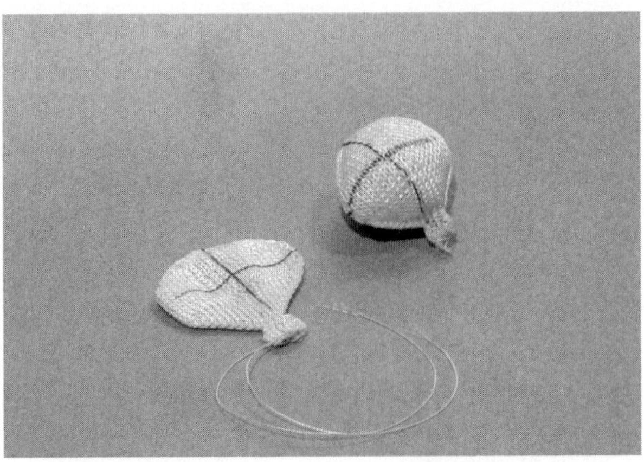

FIG. 25.7. OptiMesh containers made from polyester.

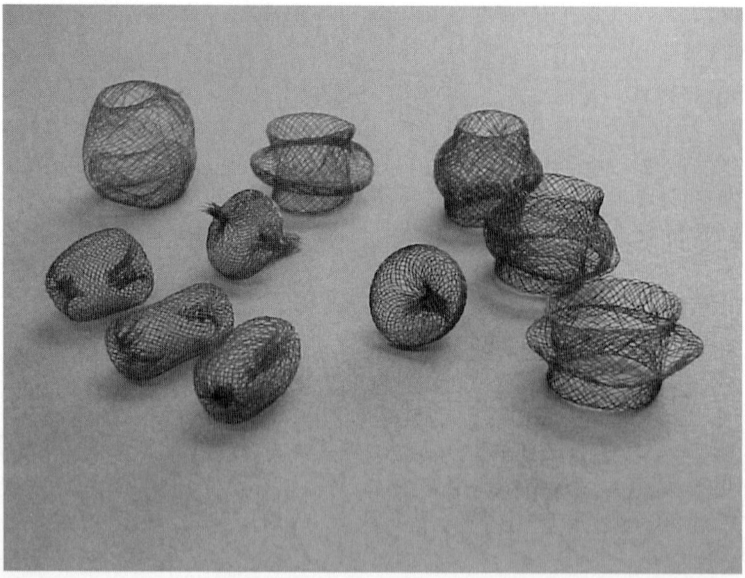

FIG. 25.8. OptiMesh containers made from metal filaments—in this case, nitinol.

After a great deal of trial and error, the group succeeded in manufacturing fabric and other forms of porous balloons and annular rings that completely contain morselized bone graft material but allow fluids, electrolytes, and cellular elements to penetrate the surfaces of the balloons and rings. These devices are capable of containing and retaining granular materials in such a way that they allow the injected filler materials to change phase from liquid to solid by the application of the appropriate injection pressure. Furthermore, because the devices do not impair the ingrowth and throughgrowth of cellular elements, they are capable of inducing arthrodesis (such as interbody fusion) when properly placed within certain skeletal locations.

Of specific relevance to the topic of this chapter, the Spineology Research Group discovered that very tightly woven OptiMesh containers are capable of retaining bone cement during vertebroplasty.

A Description of the OptiMesh Vertebroplasty

Procedure

The procedure begins by gaining access to the central-anterior portion of the vertebral body. This may be accomplished through the transpedicle or the posterolateral approach. The surgeon begins by puncturing the cortex of the vertebra at the appropriate spot and then advances a guide pin, under fluoroscopic control, into the central-anterior part of the vertebral body. A cannulated drill prepares the entrance channel, into which a guide tube of approximately 5 mm internal diameter is passed to the desired depth within the entrance portal. A small-diameter expandable reamer is passed through the guide tube to the appropriate depth, and it is sequentially expanded while it is rotated, producing a cavity of about 12 to 14 mm in diameter.

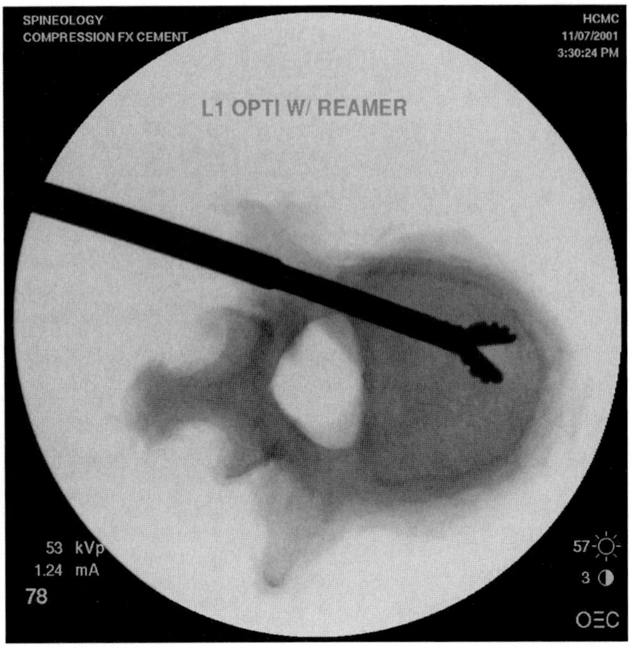

FIG. 25.9. The Spineology Research Group developed a miniaturized expandable reamer (5 mm in diameter) that can be inserted through the pedicle to create a small cavity within the vertebral body.

A porous fabric balloon is passed through the tube and into the cavity. Bone graft or bone cement is then injected into the balloon, also under fluoroscopic control, until the cavity is slightly overfilled, causing elevation of the compressed vertebral body and stabilization of the construct. Figures 25.9 and 25.10 illustrate the tools and devices developed.

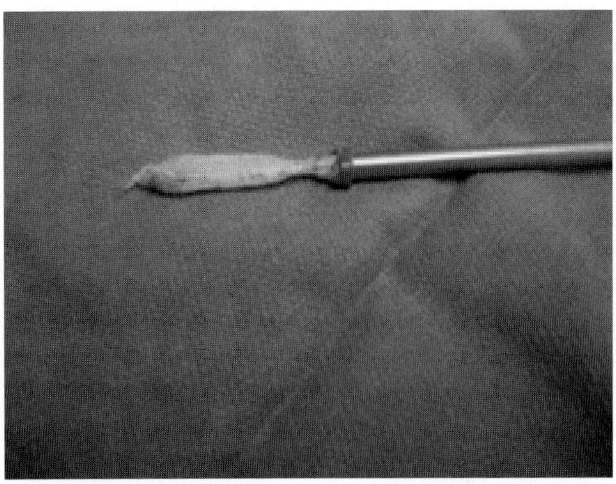

FIG. 25.10. A small OptiMesh container with a tight weave that is intended for retaining the flow of bone cement during vertebroplasty.

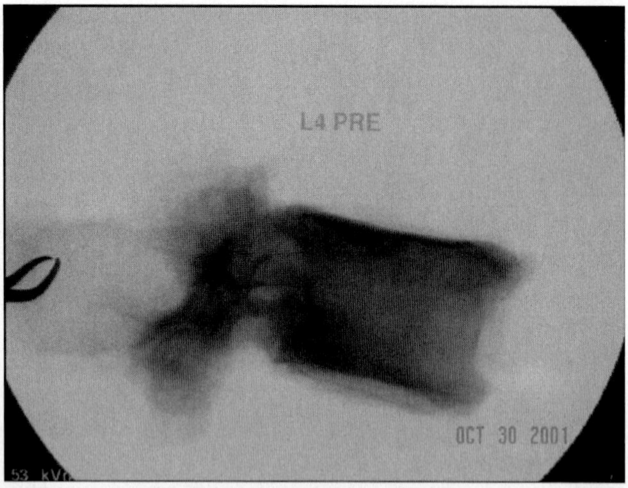

FIG. 25.11. A vertebral element removed from an elderly osteoporotic woman, before fracture and fixation.

Figures 25.11 to 25.16 illustrate the steps in the procedure. At the end of the injection cycle, a small amount of cement exudes through the tight weave of the fabric. These small "fingers" of cement lock the cement bolus in position.

The Spineology Research Group experimented with a variety of porosities until the one ideal for appropriately restraining and/or containing the injected materials was determined. The intention, in the case of bone cement, was to contain the cement sufficiently

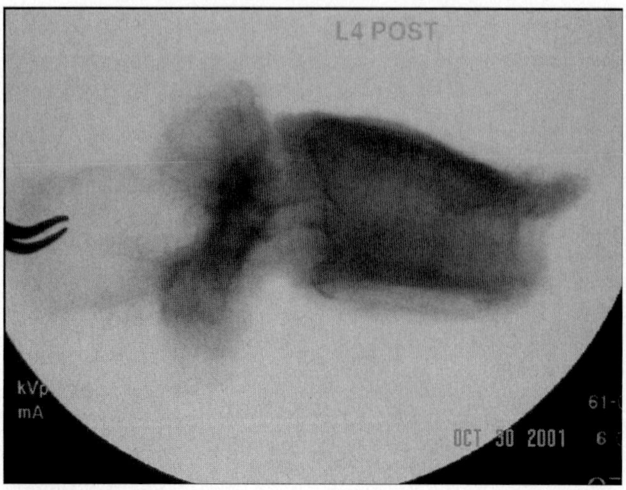

FIG. 25.12. The vertebral body of Fig. 25.11 has been compressed to 50% of its preinjury height with the use of a force plate.

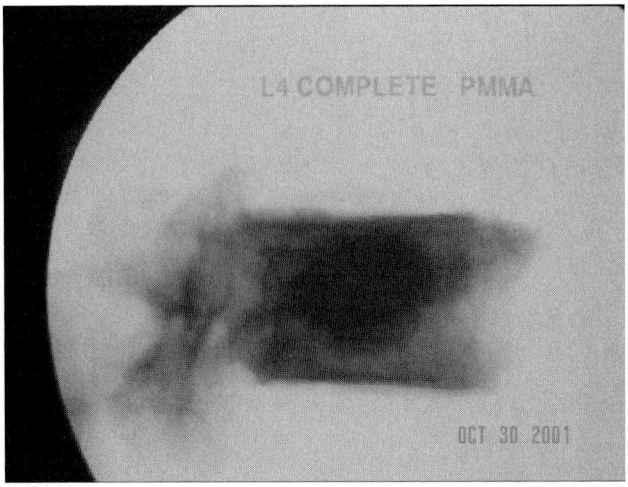

FIG. 25.13. The vertebral body of Fig. 25.12 after expansion and stabilization of the fracture through the use of the OptiMesh container of Fig. 25.9 and bone cement. Note the complete restoration of height and the absence of cement into the spinal canal.

to allow for complete expansion of the balloon, and some degree of overfilling, so that a certain amount of cement would extrude through the mesh of the balloon. The group did this so that the balloon would be bonded securely and intimately to the cancellous bone of the vertebral body. The group chose a tight weave, to prevent gross leakage of the cement.

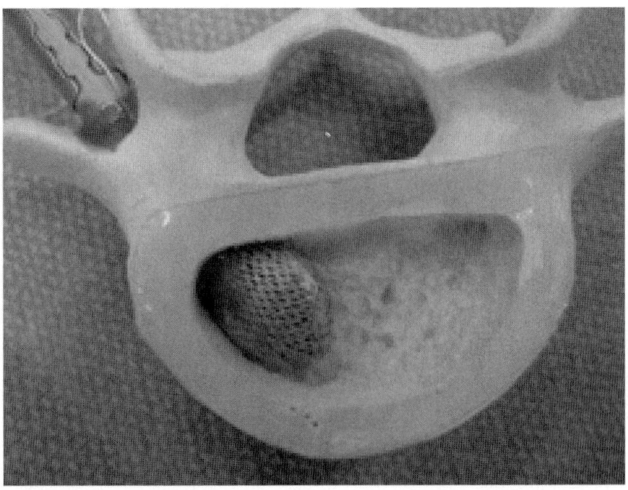

FIG. 25.14. If morselized bone graft is used, the container fills without any extrusion of bone graft.

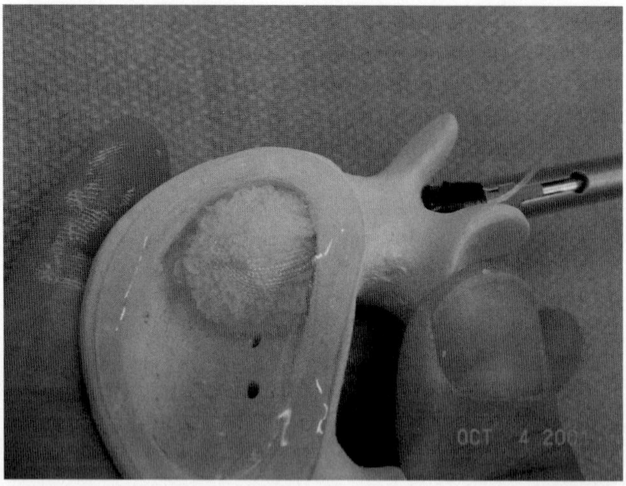

FIG. 25.15. If bone cement is used, small "fingers" of cement extrude during the last phase of the filling. These fingers lock to the bolus of cement into the surrounding cancellous bone. Gross leakage of cement is prevented as long as the weave is tight enough and the volume of injected cement is carefully controlled.

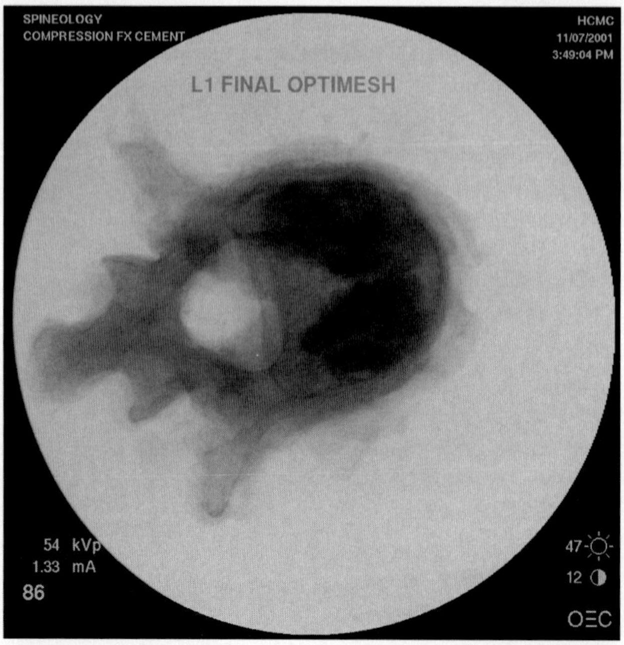

FIG. 25.16. Two tightly woven OptiMesh containers have been filled by OptiMesh System tools with bone cement. Note the absence of cement flow into the triangular space anterior to the spinal canal.

TABLE 25.1. *Comparison of OptiMesh vertebroplasty with standard vertebroplasty*

Outcome	Anterior OptiMesh	Vertebroplasty
Percentage of initial height restoration	98	86
Average height restored (mm)	5.05	1.22
Average volume of cement injected (mL)	8.75	12.2

Ten vertebral specimens in each group were compressed to 50% of their original height. Each was then treated by injection of bone cement until height was restored or until cement leakage was seen.

Laboratory Experiments and Results

Using fresh human cadaver vertebral bodies derived from elderly osteoporotic people, the group performed the following sequence of maneuvers:

1. Obtained radiographs of the specimens in three planes.
2. Compressed the specimen to 50% of its original anterior body height by using a pneumatic ram.
3. Obtained new radiographs of the specimens in three planes.
4. Inserted injection tubes into the vertebral bodies by using commonly two recommended techniques: standard vertebroplasty or optimesh vertebroplasty.
5. Filled the cavity with bone polymethylmethacrylate (PMMA) bone cement.
6. Measured vertebral height.
7. Obtained new radiographs of all specimens.

Table 25.1 illustrates the results of the experiment on ten specimens. These results suggest that containing bone cement with minimally porous mesh containers can effectively expand vertebral compression fractures as effectively as standard vertebroplasty, with less volume of cement and less likelihood for leakage.

SUMMARY AND CONCLUSIONS

Our initial experiments demonstrate that slightly porous, implantable mesh containers may effectively reduce and stabilize osteoporotic vertebral compression fractures in a modified vertebroplasty procedure. Furthermore, the system appears to provide a greater degree of reduction with less cement volume and, qualitatively at least, less tendency to leak cement outside of the intended location. More sophisticated and more extensive testing is underway.

REFERENCES

1. Arnold W. [Early surgical treatment of traumatic paraplegia with an external fixation device and diagonal vertebroplasty] *Unfallchirurg* 1985;88(7):293–298.
2. Barr JD, Barr MS, Lemley TJ, et al. Percutaneous vertebroplasty for pain relief and spinal stabilization. *Spine* 2000;25:923–928.
3. Deramond H, Depriester C, Toussaint P, et al. Percutaneous vertebroplasty. *Semin Musculoskelet Radiol* 1997; 1(2):285–296.
4. Dudeney S, Lieberman I. Percutaneous vertebroplasty in the treatment of osteoporotic vertebral compression fractures: an open prospective study. *J Rheumatol* 2000;27:2526.
5. Einhorn TA. Vertebroplasty: an opportunity to do something really good for patients. *Spine* 2000;25:1051–1052.
6. Galibert P, Deramond H, Rosat P, et al. [Preliminary note on the treatment of vertebral angioma by percutaneous acrylic vertebroplasty.] *Neurochirurgie* 1987;33:166–168.
7. Galibert P, Deramond H. [Percutaneous acrylic vertebroplasty as a treatment of vertebral angioma as well as painful and debilitating diseases.] *Chirurgie* 1990;116:326–334; discussion, 1990;116:335.

8. Garfin SR, Yuan HA, Reiley MA. New technologies in spine: kyphoplasty and vertebroplasty for the treatment of painful osteoporotic compression fractures. *Spine* 2001;26:1511–1515.
9. Grados F, Depriester C, Cayrolle G, et al. Long-term observations of vertebral osteoporotic fractures treated by percutaneous vertebroplasty. *Rheumatology (Oxford)* 2000;39:1410–1414.
10. Heini PF, Wälchli B, Berlemann U. Percutaneous transpedicular vertebroplasty with PMMA: operative technique and early results. A prospective study for the treatment of osteoporotic compression fractures. *Eur Spine J* 2000;9:445–450.
11. Jensen ME, Evans AJ, Mathis JM, et al. Percutaneous polymethylmethacrylate vertebroplasty in the treatment of osteoporotic vertebral body compression fractures: technical aspects. *AJNR Am J Neuroradiol* 1997;18: 1897–1904.
12. Kaufmann TJ, Jensen ME, Schweickert PA, et al. Age of fracture and clinical outcomes of percutaneous vertebroplasty. *AJNR Am J Neuroradiol* 2001;22:1860–1863.
13. Lieberman IH, Dudeney S, Reinhardt MK, et al. Initial outcome and efficacy of "kyphoplasty" in the treatment of painful osteoporotic vertebral compression fractures. *Spine* 2001;26:1631–1638.
14. Mathis JM, Barr JD, Belkoff SM, et al. Percutaneous vertebroplasty: a developing standard of care for vertebral compression fractures. [Review.] *AJNR Am J Neuroradiol* 2001;22:373–381.
15. Murphy KJ, Lin DD. Vertebroplasty: a simple solution to a difficult problem. *J Clin Densitom* 2001;4:189–197.
16. Watts NB, Harris ST, Genant HK. Treatment of painful osteoporotic vertebral fractures with percutaneous vertebroplasty or kyphoplasty. [Review.] *Osteoporos Int* 2001;12:429–437.
17. Wenger M, Markwalder TM. Surgically controlled, transpedicular methyl methacrylate vertebroplasty with fluoroscopic guidance. *Acta Neurochir (Wien)* 1999;141:625–631.
18. Bostrom MP, Lane JM. Future directions. Augmentation of osteoporotic vertebral bodies. [Review.] *Spine* 1997; 22(24 Suppl):38S–42S.
19. Jarvik JG, Deyo RA. Cementing the evidence: time for a randomized trial of vertebroplasty. *AJNR Am J Neuroradiol* 2000;21:1373–1374.
20. Levine SA, Perin LA, Hayes D, et al. An evidence-based evaluation of percutaneous vertebroplasty. *Manag Care* 2000;9(3):56–60,63.
21. Belkoff SM, Mathis JM, Jasper LE, et al. The biomechanics of vertebroplasty. The effect of cement volume on mechanical behavior. *Spine* 2001;26:1537–1541.
22. Heini PF, Berlemann U, Kaufmann M, et al. Augmentation of mechanical properties in osteoporotic vertebral bones—a biomechanical investigation of vertebroplasty efficacy with different bone cements. *Eur Spine J* 2001;10:164–171.
23. Heini PF, Berlemann U. Bone substitutes in vertebroplasty. *Eur Spine J* 2001;10(Suppl 2):S205–S213.
24. Hitchon PW, Goel V, Drake J, et al. Comparison of the biomechanics of hydroxyapatite and polymethylmethacrylate vertebroplasty in a cadaveric spinal compression fracture model. *J Neurosurg* 2001;95(2 Suppl): 215–220.
25. Liebschner MA, Rosenberg WS, Keaveny TM. Effects of bone cement volume and distribution on vertebral stiffness after vertebroplasty. *Spine* 2001;26:1547–1554.
26. Tohmeh AG, Mathis JM, Fenton DC, et al. Biomechanical efficacy of unipedicular versus bipedicular vertebroplasty for the management of osteoporotic compression fractures. *Spine* 1999;24:1772–1776.
27. Harrington KD. Major neurological complications following percutaneous vertebroplasty with polymethylmethacrylate: a case report. *J Bone Joint Surg Am* 2001;83:1070–1073.
28. Ratliff J, Nguyen T, Heiss J. Root and spinal cord compression from methylmethacrylate vertebroplasty. *Spine* 2001;26(13):E300–E302.
29. Castel E, Lazennec JY, Chiras J, et al. Acute spinal cord compression due to intraspinal bleeding from a vertebral hemangioma: two case-reports. *Eur Spine J* 1999;8:244–248.
30. Padovani B, Kasriel O, Brunner P, et al. Pulmonary embolism caused by acrylic cement: a rare complication of percutaneous vertebroplasty. *AJNR Am J Neuroradiol* 1999;20:375–377.
31. Perrin C, Jullien V, Padovani B, et al. [Percutaneous vertebroplasty complicated by pulmonary embolus of acrylic cement.] *Rev Mal Respir* 1999;16:215–217.
32. Encarta® World English Dictionary © 1999 Microsoft Corporation. Developed for Microsoft by Bloomsbury Publishing Plc.
33. Spineology Company: Internal documents. Stillwater, MN: Spineology Research Group, 2000–2001.

26

Vertebroplasty: The Value of Prophylactic Augmentation

Paul F. Heini

Department for Orthopaedic Surgery, University of Berne, Berne, Switzerland

Epidemiological data indicates that the number of elderly people in all Western countries will increase during the next century. Accordingly, the number of people suffering from osteoporosis will grow. Osteoporosis-related fractures represent an enormous medical and socioeconomic problem (1). Approximately 1.5 million fractures annually are attributable to osteoporosis. These include 700,000 vertebral fractures, 250,000 distal forearm Colles fractures, 250,000 hip fractures, and 300,000 fractures of other limb sites (2). Melton estimated the costs of spinal fractures in 1995 to reach about 1 billion CHF (700 million US$) for the United States (3), and Lippuner et al. calculated the costs for the acute treatment of osteoporotic fractures in Switzerland (mainly caused by vertebral fractures) to exceed 600 million CHF (400 million US$), which is more than 2% of the whole health care budget (4). In Canada, the costs due to hip fractures alone are estimated to nearly quadruple from $650 million to $2.4 billion until 2040 (5).

The already high number of fractures attributable to osteoporosis is expected to double by 2030 and will challenge the health care system of every country. The spine is the most common site of osteoporotic fractures (6). The risk that a white woman over the age of 50 will sustain a vertebral fracture in her remaining lifetime is approximately 32% (7). In the United States, 25% of the women over the age of 70 and 50% of the women over the age of 80 years show evidence of vertebral fractures, the majority of which occur in the midthoracic region and the thoracolumbar junction (8,9).

However, osteoporosis is not only an epidemiological and socioeconomic problem but also a catastrophe for the individual patient. Spontaneous and fast collapse of multiple vertebrae is often observed in daily clinical practice (Fig. 26.1A–C). The consequences are loss of physiological spinal alignment and, in rare cases, potential neurological impairment (10,11). Declines in physical function and changes in appearance contribute to social isolation, loss of self-esteem, and impaired quality of life (12).

Despite encouraging results regarding medical treatment, its effect is slow (13,14). In an advanced stage of the disease, local fractures cannot be prevented. Furthermore, there exist considerable problems of compliance with treatment and a certain degree of intolerance to oral bisphosphonates (15).

Percutaneous reinforcement of fractured osteoporotic vertebral bodies with acrylic bone cement has become a widely used technique with reportedly significant and rapid pain relief in as many as 80% to 90% of the patients (16–20).

A

B

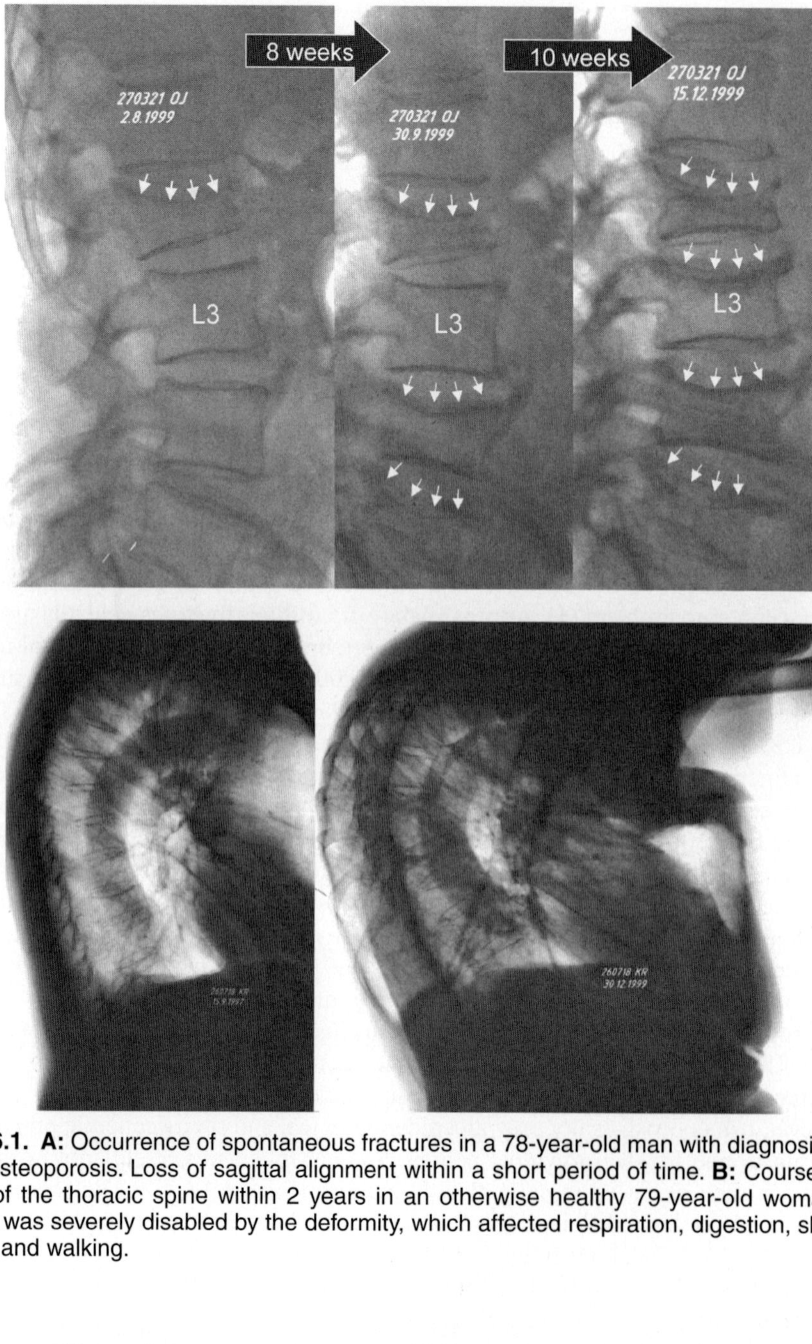

FIG. 26.1. **A:** Occurrence of spontaneous fractures in a 78-year-old man with diagnosis of primary osteoporosis. Loss of sagittal alignment within a short period of time. **B:** Course of collapse of the thoracic spine within 2 years in an otherwise healthy 79-year-old woman. The patient was severely disabled by the deformity, which affected respiration, digestion, sleeping, sitting, and walking.

Adverse effects of the treatment are complications of the cement extravasation and an increased fracture risk for adjacent vertebrae, as shown in a survey of 25 patients in a long-term follow-up study (21). An *in vitro* study on whole motion segments instead of single vertebrae revealed a lower failure load and a lower stiffness after reinforcement, in contrast to the native state (22).

The indications for the treatment and the extent of reinforcement remain open questions at this time. The treatment of painful fractures refractory to conservative measures

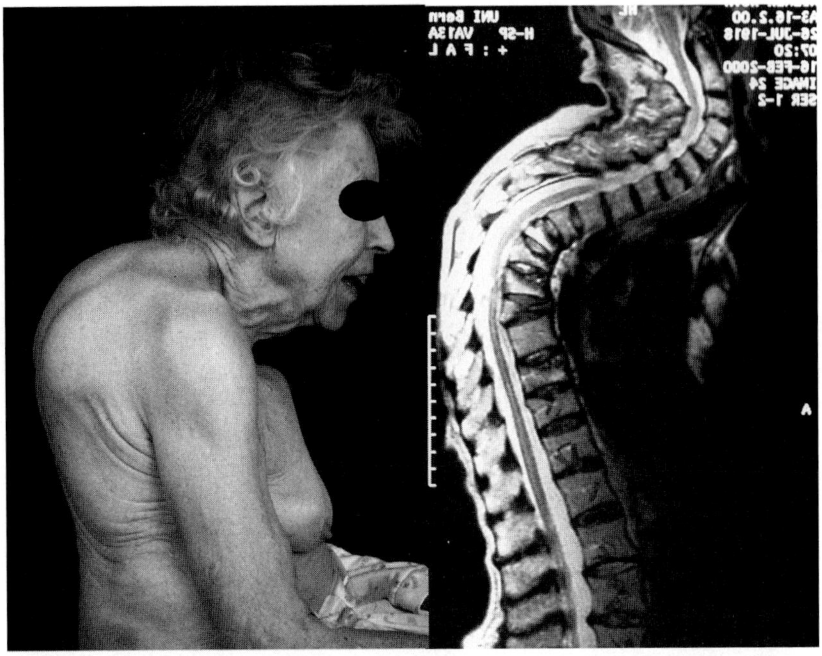

C

FIG. 26.1. *Continued.* **C:** The clinical picture shows the deformed spine and sternum. In the magnetic resonance image, the spinal cord is not seen to be affected; the deformity is caused by the collapse of the four vertebral bodies T-4 to T-7.

for 3 weeks is a generally accepted indication (23). However, there are no data and no reports regarding the rationale of prophylactic reinforcement and its technical feasibility.

As mentioned before, the spontaneous and fast collapse of multiple vertebrae with loss of posture is a clinical problem. Multiple studies have tried to define the fracture risk on the basis of multiregression analysis of many parameters (24–27). However, it is not possible from these parameters to reliably draw consequences for an individual patient that provide a rationale for the prophylactic treatment of nonfractured vertebrae. The data for vertebral fractures are not as predictive as the data for hip fractures (26). Despite this lack of basic data, physicians are forced in their clinical daily life to decide to what extent a reinforcement should be performed. Addressing the problem of failure of adjacent vertebrae, surgeons changed their attitude regarding the extent of augmentation: In cases of severe osteoporosis, they perform augmentation very extensively.

SURGICAL TECHNIQUE FOR MULTISEGMENTAL REINFORCEMENT

The operative technique is very efficient and allows six to eight injections in a 1-hour session; that is, it allows the reinforcement of six to eight vertebrae unilateral or three to four bilateral. The procedure is performed with local anesthesia; an anesthesiologist on standby continuously monitors the vital signs. After fluoroscopic localization of the levels to be augmented, the skin and soft tissues over the pedicles are anesthetized with mepivacaine hydrochloride 1%, with deep injections down to the periosteum (Fig. 26.2A). Under fluoroscopic p-a control, a skin stab incision is established, and a 2.0-mm K-wire is guided into the pedicle of each vertebra to be reinforced. In severe osteoporo-

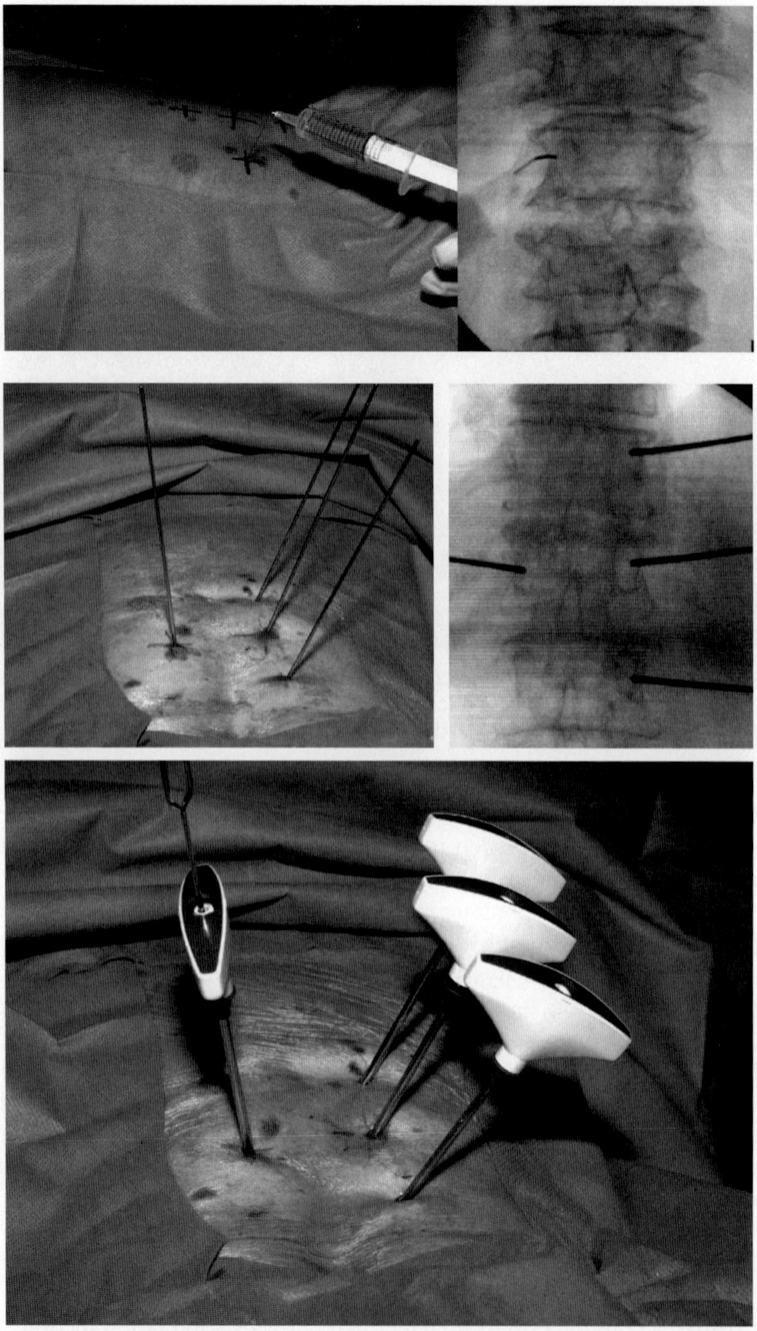

A

B

FIG. 26.2. Surgical technique. **A:** Local anesthesia is administered over the pedicles to be injected. **B:** A stab incision is made, and K-wires 2 mm in diameter and 20 cm in length are inserted under C-arm control; 8-gauge filling cannulas are guided over the K-wires into the vertebral body. The depth is controlled by the C-arm. The cannulas are set into the center of the vertebral body.

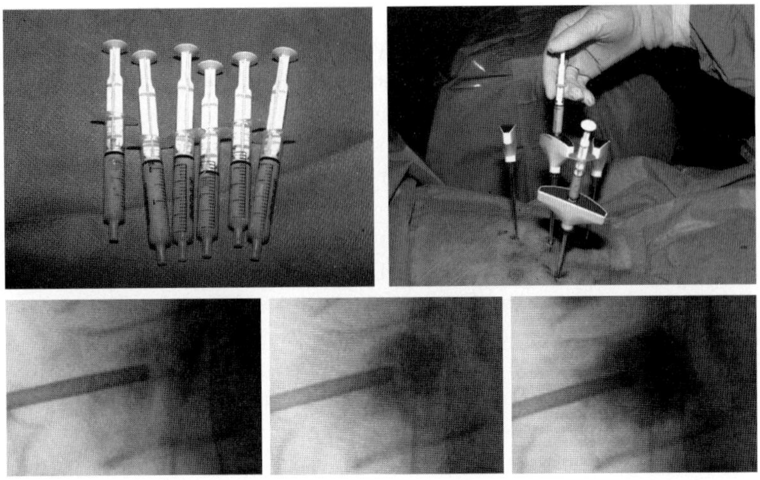

C

FIG. 26.2. *Continued.* **C:** Polymethylmethacrylate (PMMA) with contrast dye added is aspirated into 2-mL syringes. After at least 2 minutes into curing in order to achieve optimal viscosity, the cement is injected under continuous C-arm control. The cement should behave like a growing cloud. The example shows a bilateral injection into an L-1 fracture with augmentation of the adjacent vertebrae unilaterally.

sis, the wire can be advanced by hand; otherwise, some gentle hammer blows may be necessary. Under lateral projection control, the wires are adjusted to the appropriate depth-that is, the center of the vertebral body. For the cement injection, disposable bone marrow biopsy cannulas of 7- or 8-gauge diameter and 10 to 15 cm of length are used. The cannulas are guided over the K-wires, which are then removed (see Fig. 26.2B). The free passage in front of the cannula is checked by a blunt probe.

The augmentation material consists of a low-viscosity bone cement (Palacos® LV-40, manufactured by Essex Chemie). In order to enhance the radiographic visibility, a nonionic liquid contrast dye is added to the cement during the mixing procedure (Iopamiro 300®, manufactured by Bracco) in the ratio of 10 mL of contrast dye per one portion of polymethylmethacrylate (PMMA). Alternatively, a special formula designed for vertebroplasty is used (Vertebroplastic™ Cement, manufactured by De Puy AcroMed). The material is filled into 2-mL standard syringes. At least 2 minutes into the cement curing, filling of the vertebral bodies is commenced under continuous fluoroscopic control in the lateral view. The cement remains injectable for the following 3 or 4 minutes. The simultaneous filling of two vertebral bodies is possible. The flow of the cement must be monitored very carefully and should look like a growing cloud (Fig. 26.2C). Leakages of cement posteriorly into the spinal canal and anteriorly through the nutritional vessels must be avoided. The maximum amount of cement to be injected is determined by the procedure. In cases of normal filling ("growing cloud"), the augmentation is stopped as soon as the filling of the entire vertebral frame is visible. If cement extrudes, the filling is stopped immediately. However, in such cases, the position of the needle can be slightly altered, which may allow further filling with less liquid cement. Before the withdrawal of the needles, the material should be allowed to fully cure, to avoid dragging cement into the soft tissues. Experience with the Vertebroplastic Cement reveals optimal radiopacity and a long time for application. However, the cement in its initial state is very liquid, and up to 5 minutes into curing is needed before injection is started. The use of the cement in the early liquid state increases the risk of extravasation and embolization.

Additional analgesia may be needed either during placement of the K-wires and cannulas or, in particular, during the injection of cement, which sometimes is felt as regional low back pain. In these cases, intravenous administration of alfentanil hydrochloride (Rapifen) also helps patients keep the prone position for the required 45 to 60 minutes of the entire procedure.

The viscosity and visibility of the cement are of utmost importance during the procedure. Supplementation of contrast dye or the use of an adapted formula is indispensable. The viscosity of the cement immediately after mixing is far too low to perform a safe procedure because of the risk of extravasation or embolization. Therefore, curing of the cement until an adapted viscosity is achieved is important. The resistance for injection is determined mainly by the dimension of the cannula. A large cannula allows injection of the cement at a higher viscosity and contributes to the safety of the procedure. The use of 2-mL syringes provides optimal relation between force and feeling and provides direct flow control.

A prototype cannnula with a side opening that can be used with a guide wire as well has been shown *in vitro,* to provide a more symmetrical filling pattern and to carry a decreased risk for extravasation (28).

CLINICAL EXPERIENCE WITH MULTIPLE-LEVEL REINFORCEMENT

Primary Outcome

Since the late 1990s, percutaneous reinforcement of osteoporotic vertebrae has been performed in 183 patients. Overall, 200 procedures were performed; 15 patients underwent two procedures, and one underwent three. In these 183 patients, 566 vertebral bodies were reinforced: on average, three vertebrae per patient. The number of levels treated per patient is shown in Fig. 26.3A.

In 35% of the patients, four or more levels were reinforced. The average amount of cement injected was 7 mL (Fig. 26.3B), and the distribution of levels treated is shown in Fig. 26.3C.

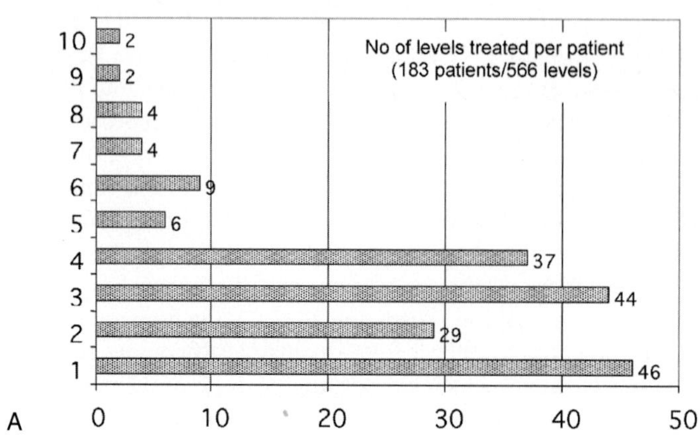

FIG. 26.3. A: The number of levels treated per patient is displayed: 25% received a single-level injection, 60% received injections at two to four levels, and 15% received injections at five or more levels.

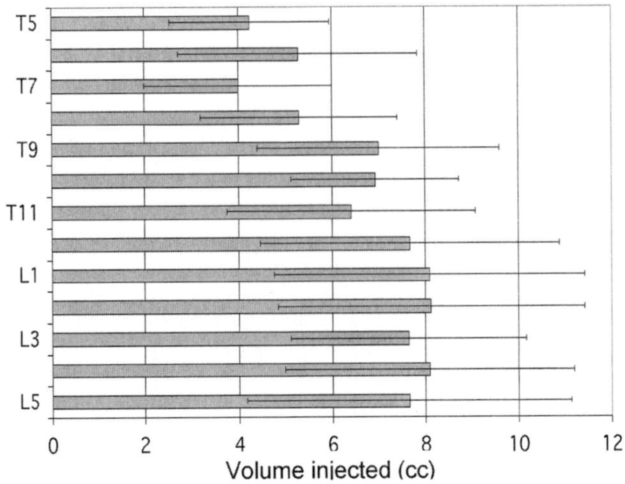

B

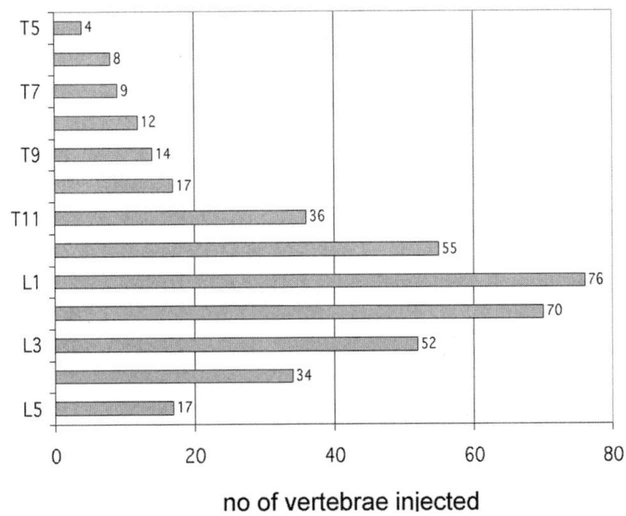

C

FIG. 26.3. *Continued.* **B:** Amount of polymethylmethacrylate (PMMA) injected, depending on the level treated. On average, 7 mL were injected. (In a subgroup of 144 patients, 404 levels were treated.) **C:** Distribution of levels (404) treated of a subgroup of patients (*n* = 144). The main part of fractures is located at the thoracolumbar junction.

In these patients, 95% (190) of the 200 interventions could be performed with local anesthesia. Extravasation of bone cement into the intervertebral disc or adjacent soft tissue was observed in about 20% of the cases. However, there was a single case with clinical sequelae of L-2 nerve root irritation that subsided after a periradicular infiltration of 40 mg of a crystalline steroid. The average operating time was 40 minutes.

Two-Year Follow-Up

A subgroup of 54 patients with a minimal follow-up period of at least 2 years was surveyed. The pain decrease observed in this group was 4.8 points (from 7.6 to 2.8) measured with a visual analogue scale. The intervention ameliorated the pain in 87% of the patients. In eight patients, new fractures were encountered: two caused by new falls, three that appeared 6 months and 1.5 years after the procedure, and three shortly after the first intervention.

Multilevel Reinforcement

Sixty-four patients had four or more vertebrae reinforced; these patients had severe osteoporosis and most suffered from multiple fractures, the age of which could not be defined. The indication for this multilevel treatment was based on the presence of severe osteoporosis as it was estimated from the radiographic pattern and from the intraoperative findings. Few patients had fractures extending from the thoracic spine to the lumbar spine. In these cases, the location of the predominant pain was reinforced first and the effect was observed. If afterwards the patients felt improvement at that location and presented new pain at another site, this pain was then consecutively treated, too. In cases in which nonfractured vertebrae were surrounded by fractured ones, the so-called sandwich vertebrae were reinforced as well. From a technical point of view, the filling of intact, nonfractured vertebrae is easier because the filling pattern appears more regular and extravasations are less frequent (Fig. 26.4A–C).

A

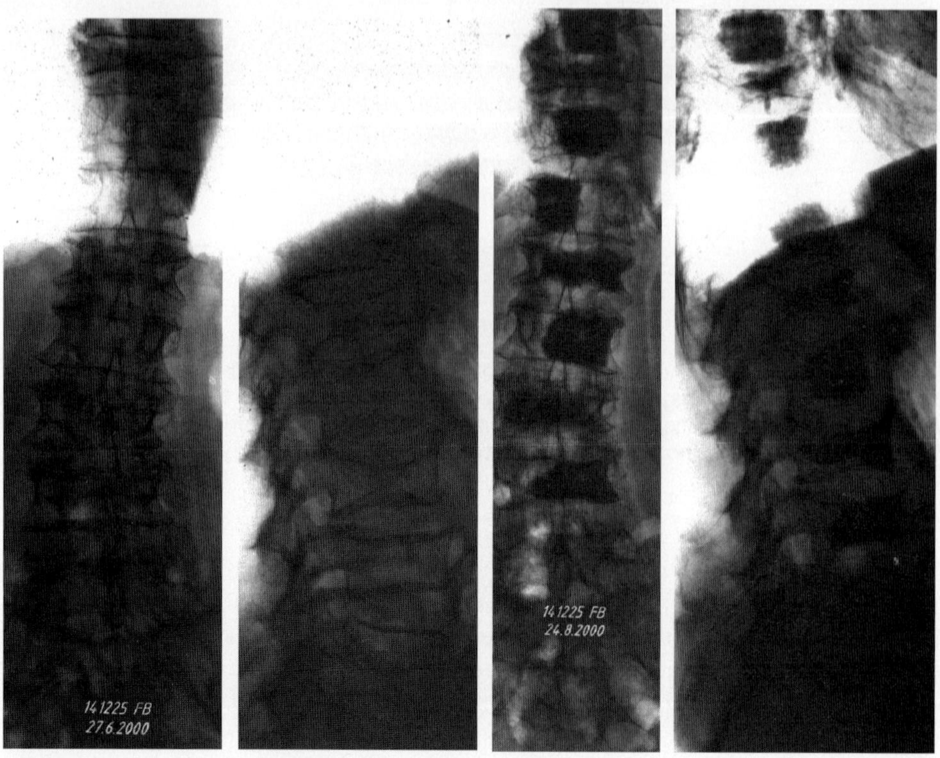

FIG. 26.4. A: Example of severe osteoporosis (T-score for the lumbar spine, –2.8) in a 75-year-old women with disabling back pain. Multiple fractures from L-1 to L-4 and in T-10 were present. Eight-level reinforcement from T-9 to L-4 was performed and yielded immediate important pain relief.

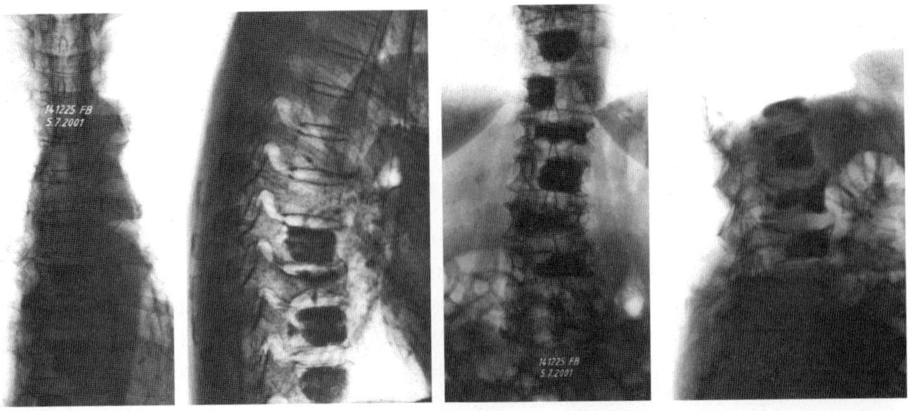

B

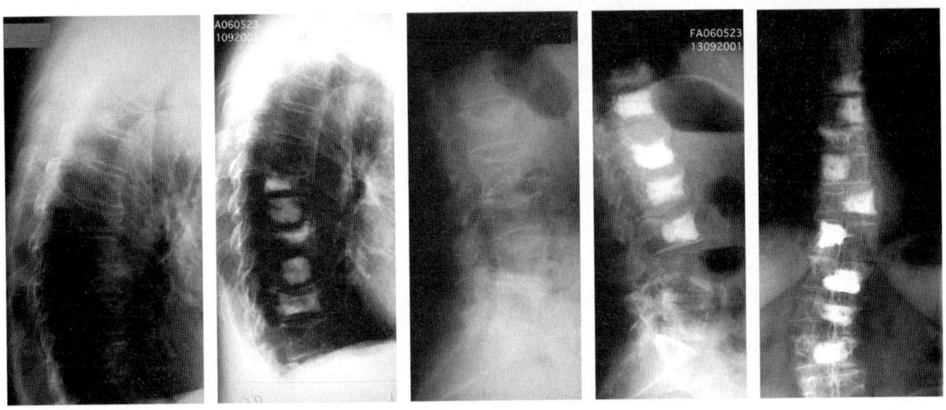

C

FIG. 26.4. *Continued.* **B:** Follow-up assessment after 1 year reveals lasting pain relief and a stable situation in the radiograph without further collapse of the reinforced vertebrae or the adjacent ones. Because of the severity of the osteoporosis, all vertebrae between T-10 and L-4 (those at highest risk for failure) were treated, and the adjacent superior vertebrae were reinforced as well. The patient was furthermore treated with alendronate. **C:** Fractures of T-7, T-9, and T-11 in a 78-year-old women with pain at her midthoracic region for 5 months and no history of trauma. Cement injection from T-7 to T-11, including the "sandwich" vertebrae, provided prompt pain relief. At follow-up 4 months later, the patient mentioned low back pain to be her main problem after the other pain had disappeared, and because of the fractures in L-1, L-2, and L-3, reinforcement was performed from T-12 to L-3. This procedure was also successful, providing a decrease of back pain (Visual Analogue Scale score decreased from 9 to 2).For the second procedure, Vertebroplastic Cement was used; that material has much higher radiopacity in contrast to the author's custom-made formula.

Preoperative Workup

Patients to undergo reinforcement should have a good quality radiographic examination, preferably standing radiographs in two planes of the area of interest. It can be helpful to compare earlier radiographs because the age of a fracture is sometimes hard to determine. The author and colleagues perform additional investigations (magnetic resonance imaging, computed tomography, bone scanning) only if there are other pathological processes to be assessed or if the fracture pattern cannot be judged by the conventional radiographs. The clinical findings are important: In the initial phase of a fracture, there is sharp, radiating, sometimes breathtaking pain. After a week or more, pain starts to be localized, with tension and fatigue going up and down. Fractures at the thoracolumbar junction are quite often accompanied by an extension of the pain toward the lumbar spine and the buttocks. Pain localization and tenderness on knocking the spine helps the surgeon decide on the levels to be reinforced.

CONCLUSIONS

Vertebroplasty bears an enormous potential. The described technique allows reinforcement of multiple levels within a short intervention time at reasonable cost. It is possible to reinforce 12 vertebrae within two sessions of about 45 minutes each. That means that a reinforcement from T-6 to L-4 can be performed in patients with severe osteoporosis and multiple fractures, the age and the tendency for further collapse of which cannot be foreseen. From the perspective of the clinician, there is better information (bone density, risk profiles) that allows the surgeon to select and characterize patients at high risk for imminent fractures. These patients should be treated prophylactically in order to prevent collapse and loss of spinal alignment. Current experience has shown the feasibility and safety of this procedure.

REFERENCES

1. Barrett-Conner E. The economics and human costs of osteoporotic fractures. *Am J Med* 1995;98:3–8.
2. Riggs BL, Melton LJ. The worldwide problem of osteoporosis: insights afforded by epidemiology. *Bone* 1995;17(5 Suppl):505S–511S.
3. Melton LJ 3rd: (1995) How many women have osteoporosis now? *J Bone Miner Res* 1995;10:175–177.
4. Lippuner K, von Overbeck J, Perrelet R, et al. Incidence and direct medical costs of hospitalizations due to osteoporotic fractures in Switzerland. *Osteoporos Int* 1997;7(5):414–425.
5. Wiktorowicz ME, Goeree R, Papaioannou A, et al. Economic implications of hip fracture: health service use, institutional care and cost in Canada. *Osteoporos Int* 2001;12(4):271–278.
6. Melton LJ 3rd, Kan SH, Frye MA, et al. Epidemiology of vertebral fractures in woman. *Am J Epidemiol* 1989; 129:1000–1011.
7. Cummings SR, Black DM, Rubin SM. Lifetime risks of hip, Colles', or vertebral fracture and coronary heart disease among white postmenopausal women. *Arch Intern Med* 1989;149(11):2445–2448.
8. Kanis JA, McCloskey EV. Epidemiology of vertebral osteoporosis. *Bone* 1992;13(Suppl 2):S1–S10.
9. Lee YL, Yip KM. The osteoporotic spine. [Review.] *Clin Orthop* 1996;(323):91–97.
10. Heggeness MH. Spine fracture with neurological deficit in osteoporosis. *Osteoporos Int* 1993;3:215–221.
11. Korovessis P, Maraziotis T, Piperos G, et al. Spontaneous burst fracture of the thoracolumbar spine in osteoporosis associated with neurological impairment: a report of seven cases and review of the literature. [Review.] *Eur Spine J* 1994;3:286–288.
12. Ryan PJ, Blake G, Herd R, et al. A clinical profile of back pain and disability in patients with spinal osteoporosis. *Bone* 1994;15:27–30.
13. Watts NB, Becker P. Alendronate increases spine and hip bone mineral density in women with postmenopausal osteoporosis who failed to respond to intermittent cyclical etidronate. *Bone* 1999;24(1):65–68.
14. Riggs BL, Melton LJ 3rd. The prevention and treatment of osteoporosis. [Review.] *N Engl J Med* 1992;327: 620–627.
15. Ettinger B, Pressman A, Schein J. Clinic visits and hospital admissions for care of acid-related upper gastrointestinal disorders in women using alendronate for osteoporosis. *Am J Manag Care* 1998;4:1377–1382.
16. Watts NB, Harris ST, Genant HK. Treatment of painful osteoporotic vertebral fractures with percutaneous vertebroplasty or kyphoplasty. *Osteoporos Int* 2001;12:429–437.
17. Cotten A, Boutry N, Cortet B, et al. Percutaneous vertebroplasty: state of the art. *Radiographics* 1998;18: 311–320; discussion, 1998;18:320–323.
18. Galibert P, Deramond H, Roast P, et al. [Preliminary note on the treatment of vertebral angioma by percutaneous acrylic vertebroplasty]. *Neurochirurgie* 1987;33:166–168.
19. Heini PF, Wälchli B, Berlemann U. Percutaneous transpedicular vertebroplasty with PMMA: operative technique and early results. A prospective study for the treatment of osteoporotic compression fractures. *Eur Spine J* 2000;9:445–450.
20. Jensen ME, Evans AJ, Mathis JM, et al. Percutaneous polymethylmethacrylate vertebroplasty in the treatment of osteoporotic vertebral body compression fractures: technical aspects. *AJNR Am J Neuroradiol* 1997;18: 1897–1904.

21. Grados F, Depriester C, Cayrolle G, et al. Long-term observations of vertebral osteoporotic fractures treated by percutaneous vertebroplasty. *Rheumatology (Oxford)* 2000;39:1410–1414.
22. Berlemann U, Ferguson S, Nolte LP, et al. Adjacent vertebral failure following vertebroplasty: a biomechanical investigation. *J Bone Joint Surg (in press).*
23. Watts NB, Harris ST, Genant HK, et al. Treatment of painful osteoporotic vertebral fractures with percutaneous vertebroplasty or kyphoplasty. *Osteoporos Int* 2001;12:429–437.
24. Nakaoka D, Sugimoto T, Kaji H, et al. Determinants of bone mineral density and spinal fracture risk in postmenopausal Japanese women. *Osteoporos Int* 2001;12:548–554.
25. Black DM, Steinbuch M, Palermo L, et al. An assessment tool for predicting fracture risk in postmenopausal women. *Osteoporos Int* 2001;12:519–528.
26. Cummings SR, Nevitt MC, Browner WS, et al. Risk factors for hip fracture in white women. Study of Osteoporotic Fractures Research Group. *N Engl J Med* 1995;332:767–773.
27. van der Voort DJ, Geusens PP, Dinant GJ. Risk factors for osteoporosis related to their outcome: fractures. *Osteoporos Int* 2001;12:630–638.
28. Heini PF, Dain Allred D: The use of a side-opening cannula in vertebroplasty. A technical note. *Spine* 2002;27:105–109.

27

When to Operate?

Stephen Eisenstein

Centre for Spinal Studies, Robert Jones & Agnes Hunt Orthopaedic Hospital, Oswestry, Shropshire, United Kingdom

The answer is: very seldom. Osteoporosis is a generalized condition of bone, and the surgery required for vertebral fracture requires good quality adjacent bone for grafting and fixation. These ingredients are not available in patients with osteoporosis that is sufficiently severe t result in fracture in the first place. The kind of surgery considered feasible for these patients, if indications could be found, is the kind of surgery usually associated with trauma to normal bone: namely, anterior excision of the crushed vertebra with replacement grafting and fixation, to achieve correction of the kyphosis and a solid fusion across both adjacent disc spaces. In common experience, this surgery is fraught with complications related to major surgery in frail patients, further vertebral collapse, loss of fixation, and recurrent deformity in adjacent vertebrae, with pain.

Nevertheless, there is at least one report of success with this type of surgery, involving 22 patients (1). This is not the common experience, but the author has attended two of these procedures with Professor Kaneda and noted the meticulous technique applied. More recently, there has been widespread enthusiasm for vertebroplasty, the restitution of vertebral body strength by means of pushing one or other form of cement in soft form through the relevant pedicles into the collapsed body (2–7). The great benefit of this procedure is the dramatic (95%) reduction in pain (8), but no claims are made for correction of deformity. Daunting complications are possible with vertebroplasty, but they are rare (9).

Kyphoplasty is vertebroplasty in which a balloon or bag is expanded inside the vertebral body with force sufficient to restore some vertebral body height before the cement is pumped into the bag (10). The average corection of kyphosis is 50% (8).

To the extent that these procedures are now being performed percutaneously by radiologists and with local anesthetics, they may possibly not count as surgical operations (11).

The indications for major open surgery for decompression, bone grafting, or both must be sought among the consequences of osteoporotic kyphotic deformity: namely, pain, cosmesis, neurological deficit, and further fracture. Of these, neurological deficit is the most pressing indication. It is also the least common and the one for which open surgery is most likely to do some good; hence, the nature of the initial response earlier to the question of when to operate.

Surgery is not a solution to the problem; it is a confession of failure of prevention. This reasoning must also apply to vertebroplasty and kyphoplasty, but these new procedures at least achieve great benefits for very little intervention.

REFERENCES

1. Kaneda K, Asano S, Hashimoto T, et al. The treatment of osteoporotic-posttraumatic vertebral collapse using the Kaneda device and a bioactive ceramic vertebral prosthesis. *Spine* 1992;17:S295–S303.
2. Barr JD, Barr MS, Lemley TJ, et al. Percutaneous vertebroplasty for pain relief and spinal stabilisation. *Spine* 2000;25:923–928.
3. Campbell DG. Percutaneous vertebroplasty: a novel treatment for acute vertebral fractures. *Med J Aust* 2001; 175:55–56.
4. Gangi A, Kastler BA, Dietemann JL. Percutaneous vertebroplasty guided by a combination of CT and fluoroscopy. *AJNR Am J Neuroradiol* 1994;15:83–86.
5. Grados F, Depriester C, Cayrolle G, et al. Long-term observations of vertebral osteoporotic fractures treated by percutaneous vertebroplasty. *Rheumatology (Oxford)* 2000;39:1410–1414.
6. Heini PF, Wälchli B, Berlemann U. Percutaneous transpedicular vertebroplasty with PMMA: operative technique and early results. A prospective study for the treatment of osteoporotic compression fractures. *Eur Spine J* 2000; 9:445–450.
7. Ikeuchi M, Yamamoto H, Shibata T, et al. Mechanical augmentation of the vertebral body by calcium phosphate cement injection. *J Orthop Sci* 2001;6:39–45.
8. Garfin SR, Yuan HA, Reiley MA. New technologies in spine: kyphoplasty and vertebroplasty for the treatment of painful osteoporotic compression fractures. *Spine* 2001;26:1511–1515.
9. Harrington KD. Major neurological complications following percutaneous vertebroplasty with polymethylmethacrylate: a case report. *J Bone Joint Surg Am* 2001;83:1070–1073.
10. Lieberman IH, Dudeney S, Reinhardt MK, et al. Initial outcome and efficacy of "kyphoplasty" in the treatment of painful osteoporotic vertebral compression fractures. *Spine* 2000;26:1631–1638.
11. Jensen ME, Dion JE. Percutaneous vertebroplasty in the treatment of osteoporotic compression fractures. *Neuroimag Clin North Am* 2000;10:547–568.

28

Osteoporotic Thoracolumbar Fractures: When Is Surgery Indicated?

Luc Vanden Berghe

Department of Orthopaedic Surgery, St. Lucas Ziekenhuis, Brugge, Belgium

Lumbar osteoporotic fractures are increasing because of the aging of the population; the risk of osteoporotic fractures increases dramatically with age. The lifetime risk of sustaining an osteoporotic fracture is 16%, and although it seems to occur more frequently in women, studies have shown that the prevalence of vertebral fractures is as great in men as in women (1).

Reductions in bone density and the thinning and loss of trabecular bone result in corresponding reductions in strength of the vertebrae. This can lead to inability to support loads and to compression fractures, even after minor stress such as lifting objects or minor injuries such as falls. Half of the fractures, however, are not attributed to a known loading activity. Such spontaneous fractures may be the result of fatigue damage from loading during normal activities (1,6).

Most osteoporotic compression fractures become asymptomatic, but sometimes compression fractures can cause progressive kyphosis, increasing pain, increasing disability, and neurological lesions. Spinal canal compromise, however, is seldom seen (2,5,7).

Burst fractures are less common in the elderly population but can cause spinal canal compromise and neurological deficits.

TYPES OF LUMBAR OSTEOPOROTIC FRACTURES

The most common types are the wedge compression fracture and the burst fracture

The *wedge compression fracture* is often a low injury fracture; it may be the result of a hyperflexion force and a compression force on the lumbar spine. It affects only the anterior column, and in most cases, less than 50% of the vertebral body height is reduced. It is most common at the thoracic spine and the thoracolumbar junction. It is less common in the lower lumbar spine. In most cases, the spinal canal and the posterior structures are not affected. Most compression fractures are considered stable without the potential for progressive deformity or neural compression (2).

The *lateral wedge compression fracture* is less common. It is also usually a low injury fracture and the result of fatigue damage caused by asymmetrical loading of the lumbar vertebra. It may cause laterolithesis or scoliosis of the lumbar spine. It too is usually considered a stable fracture and does usually not affect the spinal canal (5).

The *burst fracture* is the result of a combined axial and flexion force on the lumbar spine. The force is greater than that causing the wedge compression fracture, and this type of fracture is often unstable with the potential for progressive deformity, spinal canal compromise, and neurological injuries (2).

The *stability of the spinal fracture* determines treatment. Stable fractures can be treated conservatively; in unstable fractures, surgical treatment has to be considered.

A spinal fracture can be considered stable if the vertebra is able to withstand physiological loads without the development of unacceptable deformity, neurological damage, or intolerable pain from abnormal motion (7).

CONSERVATIVE TREATMENT OF OSTEOPOROTIC FRACTURES

Because most osteoporotic fractures are stable, become asymptomatic, and do not affect the spinal canal, the conservative treatment of osteoporotic fractures is still the optimal. Immediate surgery is considered only if the fracture is severely unstable or if there is neurological damage or risk for neurological damage (2,5,7).

The traditional conservative treatment consists of bed rest during a short period in the acute phase, followed by casting or bracing, if tolerated, and early ambulation. Most osteoporotic fractures become asymptomatic and necessitate no further treatment. Treating the underlying cause can prevent new osteoporotic fractures.

There is growing interest in fortification of the vertebral bodies with bone cement or other materials.

Patients with a kyphotic deformity caused by a single or multiple compression fractures may experience increasing back pain, increasing disability, or deformity and may become candidates for surgery.

SURGICAL TREATMENT OF OSTEOPOROTIC FRACTURES

Operative treatment may be indicated for lesions that are considered unstable, especially if there is spinal canal compromise with neurological deficits.

If there is spinal canal compromise by bone or soft tissue fragments, a decompression of the spinal column, through an anterior, posterior, or posterolateral approach, may be indicated. When the spinal canal is decompressed, the spinal column is usually further destabilized, and fusion with instrumentation is often necessary.

Instrumentation and fusion may also be indicated for the treatment of painful deformities.

Evolution of Instrumentation

Before 1960, patients with osteoporotic fractures were usually treated conservatively with bed rest and casting. In cases with spinal canal compromise, a posterior decompression, combined in rare cases with posterior fusion, was sometimes performed.

In the last quarter of the twentieth century, there was a revolution in spinal surgery with the introduction of spinal instrumentation by Harrington and others (3).

The *Harrington instrumentation* was developed for the surgical treatment of deformities of the spine but was adapted for the surgical stabilization of thoracolumbar fractures in the early 1960s. Because of the limitation in fixation points, however, the surgical complication and pseudarthrosis rates were high. These high complication rates motivated spinal surgeons to improve the instrumentation to more stable constructs.

Edwardo Luque improved the Harrington system by adding multilevel sublaminar wire fixation combined with the use of two rods or a rectangle. But there were disadvantages to the use of sublaminar wires: the wires could not be used at the levels where a laminectomy was performed, and, if they were used at the upper end of a construct, there was often a tendency for junctional kyphosis and wire cutout to occur. The passage of wires under the lamina carried the risk for neurological damage.

In the early 1980s, *Yves Cotrel and Jean Dubousset* developed a new system that combined the use of two rods with multiple hooks in order to achieve segmental fixation. The rods could easily be contoured to achieve a good sagittal balance. The system was developed for the treatment of spinal deformities and lower lumbar disease but was soon adapted for the treatment of fractures of the thoracolumbar spine. Pedicle screws were designed to improve the fixation in the lumbar spine and to allow the use of the system in special circumstances. The two rods were crosslinked to improve the stability of the construct. Higher fusion rates and lower complication rates were reported.

The *VSPISOLA system* was also developed for the treatment of spinal deformities and lower lumbar disease but became commonly used in the treatment of spinal fractures. It allowed the combination of hooks, sublaminar wires, and pedicle screws with smooth rods and became a very versatile system. The combination of pedicle screws and plates offered a very rigid screw-plate fixation system (4).

With the development of the spinal instrumentation, the treatment of unstable thoracic and lumbar fractures evolved from bed rest, body casting, and bracing to early internal fixation and mobilization, a similar evolution as in the treatment of hip fractures and other fractures.

However, because of the weakness of the osteoporotic bone, achieving a stable fixation in an osteoporotic spine was a major challenge. Hardware pullout, during or after surgery, became a major concern when spinal instrumentation was used in osteoporotic patients. Because of the stiffness of instrumented segments, the development of a symptomatic junctional kyphosis proximal to the cephalad extent of the instrumentation was not uncommon and often led to further surgery. The increased stress to the adjacent, unfused levels sometimes resulted in painful degenerative changes at this levels. Because of the high complication rate in osteoporotic patients, the initial enthusiasm was quickly tempered.

Some of the complications can be prevented by using multiple fixation points, attempting less deformity correction, and addressing coronal and sagittal balance. Approaching the anterior spinal column with structural grafting increases the fusion rate and decreases hardware failure.

Today, it is realized that in every patient, the possible advantages and disadvantages of surgery have to be carefully weighed. Often, not operating on the patient proves to be the best solution, inasmuch as a surgical intervention carries a high complication rate in osteoporotic patients, especially if there are multiple compression fractures and kyphosis.

Surgical Treatment: Types of Instrumentation

Posterior Instrumentation

Selection of the appropriate instrumentation is important. The instrumentation should allow segmental fixation to decrease the stress at any site and should allow the combination of pedicle screws, hooks, and sublaminar wires. Usually, two rods or plates are used, often connected with two or more transverse connections to form a rectangular, stable construct.

Sublaminar wires are ideal for use in the osteoporotic spine because they allow multiple fixation points and have high pullout strength. They are used most frequently in the thoracic spine because the use of pedicle screws is not widely accepted at the thoracic level. Sublaminar wires should not be used to end the construct and cannot be used at levels where decompression or laminectomy is performed. There is an increased risk of neurological complications when the wires are inserted under the lamina (5).

Pedicle screws have become the standard fixation tool in the lumbar spine. The pedicle is the strongest site accessible posteriorly to obtain a three-dimensional fixation on the vertebra. The screws can be inserted safely in the majority of patients, especially if a laminectomy or laminotomy has been performed. The fixation with pedicle screws is less strong in the osteoporotic spine, and they should be applied at several levels or combined with sublaminar hooks to share the loads. In the osteoporotic spine, the pedicles often have a large diameter, and larger screws may be used to achieve stronger fixation. The fixation can also be augmented with bone cement or injectable carbonated apatite.

Sublaminar or pedicle hooks can be used at the thoracic spine, but their pullout strength is less than the pullout strength of sublaminar wires, unless used in a bilateral claw configuration. They are most commonly used to end the construction at the upper end, in a claw configuration.

Proper selection of the *cephalad level of instrumentation* is important. The construct should not end at the apex of a sagittal curve or at the thoracolumbar junction. All pathological levels, especially the kyphotic segments, should be included.

The most effective superior anchors at the thoracic level are bilateral hooks in a claw configuration. To decrease stress on the proximal anchor, the proximal ends of the rods should be bent in enough kyphosis, and, if possible, the levels below the proximal anchor should be instrumented with sublaminar wires or hooks (3).

The posterior ligamentous complex above the superior anchors should be preserved to prevent the development of junctional kyphosis.

For the *distal fixation,* the use of pedicle screws has gained acceptance, especially at the lumbar level. In osteopenic bone, distal fixation can be improved by inserting pedicle screws at more than one level. Instrumentation to the sacrum should be avoided because the complication rate (hardware pullout, pseudarthrosis) increases.

Anterior Instrumentation

Anterior instrumentation can be used in burst fractures. Two screws are inserted in the vertebral body above and two in the vertebral body below the fractured vertebra. The screws are connected with rods (Kaneda system) or a plate (Z-plate).

Osteoporotic Vertebral Fractures: When Is Surgery Indicated?

Immediate Operative Treatment

Immediate operative treatment of thoracic lumbar injuries is indicated for lesions that are considered unstable or have the potential for further neurological compromise.

*Flexion-compression injuries (T-11 to L-4)*affect the anterior column and are usually the result of a hyperflexion or compression force. As a rule, fractures with greater than 50% loss of the anterior column are an indication for surgical treatment because they have the potential for continued kyphotic decompensation. In the osteoporotic patient, however surgical treatment is rarely indicated for this type of fracture. Trying to correct the kyphosis with internal fixation often leads to hardware failure and recurrence of the kyphosis. If the kyphosis necessitates surgical correction, anterior column support with structural grafts or shortening procedures are indicated. The anterior column support should be combined with a segmental posterior fixation with hooks and sublaminar wires at the thoracic level and pedicle screws at the lumbar level. It should be remembered that most of the compression fractures are stable fractures and that the complication rate of internal fixation is high in osteoporotic patients with hardware pullout, junctional kyphosis, and general medical problems.

Burst fractures of the thoracolumbar spine are usually the result of combined axial and flexion force. This force is greater than the force that causes wedge compression fracture. This type of fracture may compromise the spinal canal and lead to neurological injuries. Burst fractures are mechanically unstable and are associated with a 20% incidence of neurological compromise. These fractures must be considered for surgical intervention. Decompression and stabilization should be performed in the first three days after injury, for the best result.

Considerable controversy still exists concerning the treatment of retropulsed bone in the canal and its role in the cause of posttraumatic stenosis and neurological injury.

In cases of significant canal compromise and incomplete or complete neurological injury, anterior decompression is preferred. The vertebral body is removed, the spinal canal is decompressed, and the vertebral body should be replaced with a structural cage or graft. It is important to preserve the endplates of the level above and below the affected vertebral body. The anterior decompression and reconstruction can be combined with anterior internal fixation or posterior internal fixation with vertebral or pedicle screws.

Flexion distraction fractures are uncommon in elderly people. If they are unstable, internal stabilization should be considered.

Late Surgical Treatment

Late surgical treatment may be considered if progressive kyphosis develops, causing increasing pain and disability. Usually, a posterior approach is preferred with segmental instrumentation and limited correction. If greater correction is indicated, a shortening procedure or a combined anterior and posterior approach may be necessary. Decortication and grafting technique should be adequate, because the pseudarthrosis rate is higher in osteoporotic patients.

The type of treatment also depends on the *general condition of the patient.* Spinal surgery is major surgery and may not be tolerated by patients in poor general condition, such as those with nutritional deficiencies. The risk/benefit ratio has to be calculated for every patient.

SUMMARY

The majority of patients with osteoporotic thoracolumbar fractures are still treated nonoperatively with brace immobilization and early ambulation. Medical treatment can help prevent further fractures.

Immediate or urgent surgery is indicated for unstable fractures with a neurological deficit or with the risk of a neurological deficit as a result of compression of the spinal cord or the cauda equina. In most cases, a combined anterior and posterior approach with anterior decompression, vertebral body replacement, and posterior segmental fixation is the treatment of choice.

Delayed surgery can be considered in cases of progressive kyphosis, increasing pain, or increasing disability. In the planning of surgical treatment in these cases, the challenges of internal fixation in an osteoporotic spine with hardware pullout should always be considered. In osteoporotic patients, the pseudarthrosis rates are high, and there is the risk of junctional kyphosis, especially when stiff implants are used and the kyphosis is corrected. Painful degenerative changes at the cephalad level are not unusual.

Failures can be avoided by using multiple sites of fixation, attempting a lesser degree of deformity correction, avoiding ending the instrumentation in kyphotic segments, and combining anterior support and posterior instrumentation.

Because of their inherent challenges, surgical intervention and internal fixation should be avoided if possible in the treatment of osteoporotic fractures.

REFERENCES

1. Andersson GB, Bostrom MP, Eyre DR, et al. Consensus summary on the diagnosis and treatment of osteoporosis. *Spine* 1997;22(24 Suppl):63S–65S.
2. Bridwell KH, DeWald RL: *The textbook of spinal surgery.* Philadelphia: JB Lippincott, 1991:857–1000.
3. Devlin VJ, Asher MA: Long fusions from the thoracic spine to the sacrum: problems, principles, and techniques. In: Margulies JY, Floman Y, Farcy JP, et al., eds. Lumbosacral and spinopelvic fixation. Philadelphia: Lippincott-Raven, 1996:805–814.
4. Fellrath RF, Chewning SJ: ISOLA instrumentation in the stabilization of thoracolumbar fractures. *Semin Spine Surg* 1995;2;109–115.
5. Hu SS: Internal fixation in the osteoporotic spine. *Spine* 1997;22:43S–48S.
6. Myers ER, Wilson SE: Biomechanics of osteoporosis and vertebral fracture. *Spine* 1997;22:25S–31S.
7. Spivak JM, Vaccaro AR, Cotler JM: Thoracolumbar spine trauma: principles of management. *J Am Acad Orthopaed Surg* 1995;6:353–360.

29

Augmentation of Pedicle Screws with Calcium Apatite Cement

Paul I.J.M. Wuisman

Department of Orthopaedic Surgery, Academisch Ziekenhuis, Vrije Universiteit, De Boelelaan, Amsterdam, The Netherlands

To attain rigid spinal stabilization, spinal instrumentation with screw-rod fixation anteriorly, posteriorly, or both is now widely used. The instrumentation is usually used to correct a progressive spinal deformity, to stabilize a mechanical instable spinal segment, or both. The advantage of screws as a part of the constructs is that they provide a rigid bony fixation upon which internal fixation devices can be mounted. Rapid graft incorporation and successful spinal fusion have been shown to be more likely to occur with rigid internal fixation (1–3). Rigid internal fixation reflects the strength of screw attachment to the spine, which in turn is directly related to the quality of bone into which the pedicle screw is placed (2,4,5). Consequently, dense, good-quality trabecular bone enhances solid fixation, whereas osteoporotic and poor-quality bone, as in osteogenesis imperfecta, carries an increased risk of screw loosening and postoperative pullout (2,4–8). Extreme poor bone quality may even preclude the use of screw fixation (4–6,8,9). Experimental studies with human cadaver vertebrae have demonstrated the suitability of *in situ* setting calcium apatite cement (CAC) in augmenting initial fixation of pedicle screws in senile (osteoporotic) trabecular bone (10,11). This chapter reports operative strategies and outcome with the use of CAC [Norian Skeletal Repair System (SRS); Norian Corporation] for the augmentation of pedicle screws in 14 patients with severe progressive osteoporotic spinal deformities.

MATERIAL AND METHODS

Fourteen patients with a symptomatic progressive spinal deformity associated with severe osteoporosis were surgically treated by correction and stabilization of the deformity. The patients' ages ranged between 8 and 78 years; the average was 46.2 years. There were 10 female and 4 male patients. All patients had clinical symptoms caused by a severe osteoporotic spinal deformity: Six patients had progressive neurological symptoms associated with a spinal stenosis, spondylolisthesis, or a degenerative scoliosis; five patients suffered from osteogenesis imperfecta, all with a progressive spinal deformity; and three patients had an idiopathic osteoporosis of the spine (of these three, two developed kyphosis and one developed kyphoscoliosis at the thoracolumbar junction). Routine radiographs, magnetic resonance imaging scans, and or computed tomographic scans were obtained to analyze the deformity. In addition, for all patients, a dual energy x-ray absorptiometry (DEXA) scan of the lumbar spine and the trochanteric region was obtained to estimate the bone mineral density. All patients showed decreased bone mineral density measurements at twice the standard deviation below the expected mean value. Fifty-eight spinal segments were fused: 102 transpedicle screws were augmented, 24 anteriorly and 78 posteriorly. In every patient, bone graft substitution was performed to obtain segmental or multisegmental fusion.

Surgical Procedure

In total, 58 spinal segments were fixed with a screw-rod system posteriorly and a double rod-screw system anteriorly. Each screw was augmented with in situ setting CAC. CAC is a poorly crystalline material similar in structure to the mineral phase of bone that allows ingrowth of adjoining blood vessels and subsequent development of bone into the artificial scaffold provided (12,13). It can be applied in paste form, and it hardens at physiological temperatures. In a canine metaphyseal defect model, it has been shown to be osteoconductive and completely biocompatible; resorption of the CAC appears to be a result of normal cell-mediated processes (13).

Posterior Approach

In eight cases, bilateral posterior transpedicle screw augmentation (with 78 screws) was performed. The patients were positioned on a radiolucent Wilson frame. A posterior midline incision was made, followed by detachment of the paraspinal musculature laterally up to the outer margins of the transverse processes. Once the vertebral levels were confirmed fluoroscopically, a hemilaminectomy was performed bilaterally at all levels where augmentation of the pedicles was planned. The pedicles of each vertebra were identified and prepared under direct visualization and fluoroscopically. A small awl was used to ream a canal into the vertebral body through its pedicle. The depth of the hole was measured to determine the screw length; at the same time, the wall of the canal was controlled to ensure that the cortex had not been breached. Under fluoroscopic control, the pedicle screw was inserted. Upon manual testing of the rigidity of this initial screw placement, and under fluoroscopy, the author and colleagues observed that several screws were clinically loose. The screws were then removed, and a second (direct) control of the canal was examined with a probe to ensure that the cortex had not been breached. The CAC was then prepared and injected (about 2.0 to 3.0 mL per screw hole) into the screw hole, in a nonpressurized, retrograde manner, and the screw was reinserted under direct view and image intensification. Throughout the process of screw hole preparation, augmentation, and screw insertion, the dura and the nerve root were deviated medially for protection and also to enable direct visualization of cortical defect or cement leakage. Whenever leakage occurred, the cement was immediately removed. After cement hardening, all screws were tested manually and confirmed to be rigid. The connecting rods (or plates) were then mounted, and stabilization or correction of the spinal deformity was finally performed. The procedure was finished with a posterolateral bone grafting; the grafts were retrieved from the posterior iliac crest.

Anterior Approach

For anterior stabilization, a thoracolumbar approach (for four patients) and a lumbar retroperitoneal approach (for two patients) had been chosen to for the anterior correction-stabilization and fusion (Fig. 29.1). The patients were given general endotracheal anes-

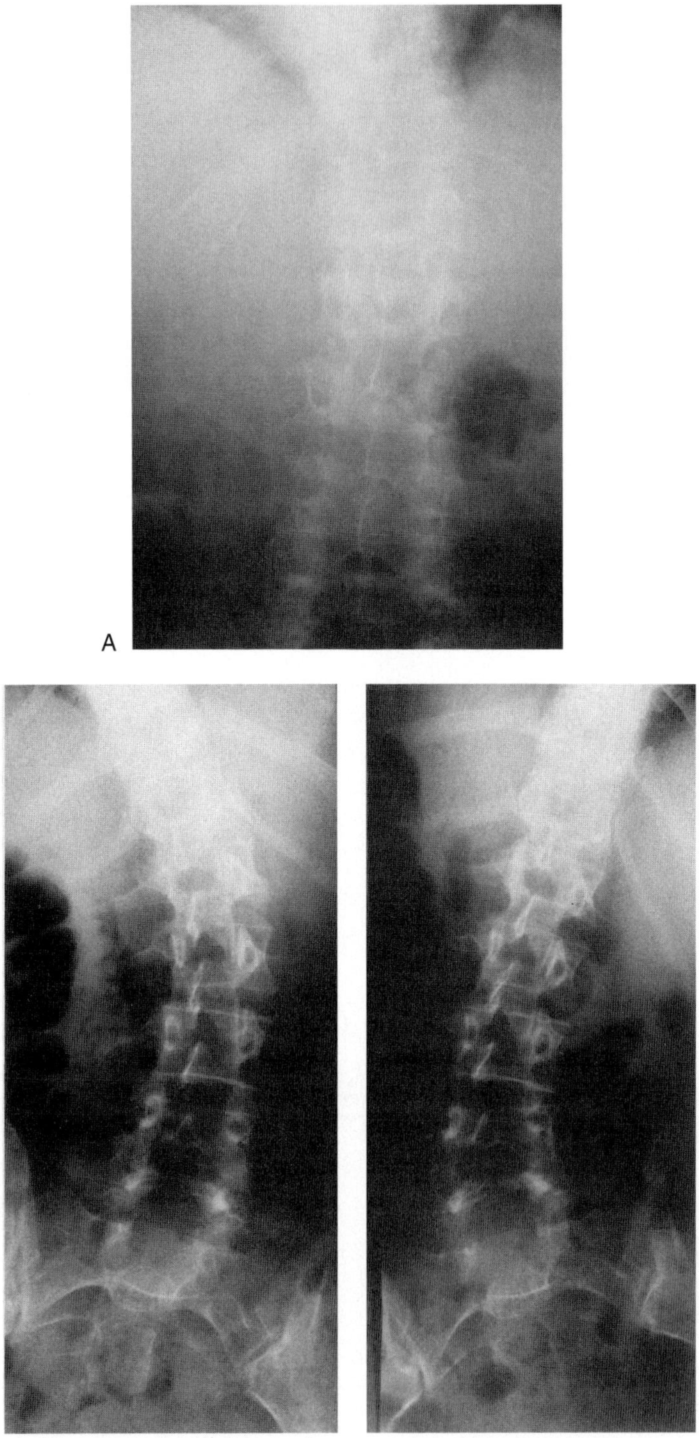

FIG. 29.1 **A:** Anteroposterior radiograph of a 19-year-old woman known with osteogenesis imperfecta and severe osteoporosis, showing a right convex lumbar scoliotic deformation. **B:** Anteroposterior bending radiographs, showing the multilevel instability.

(continued on next page)

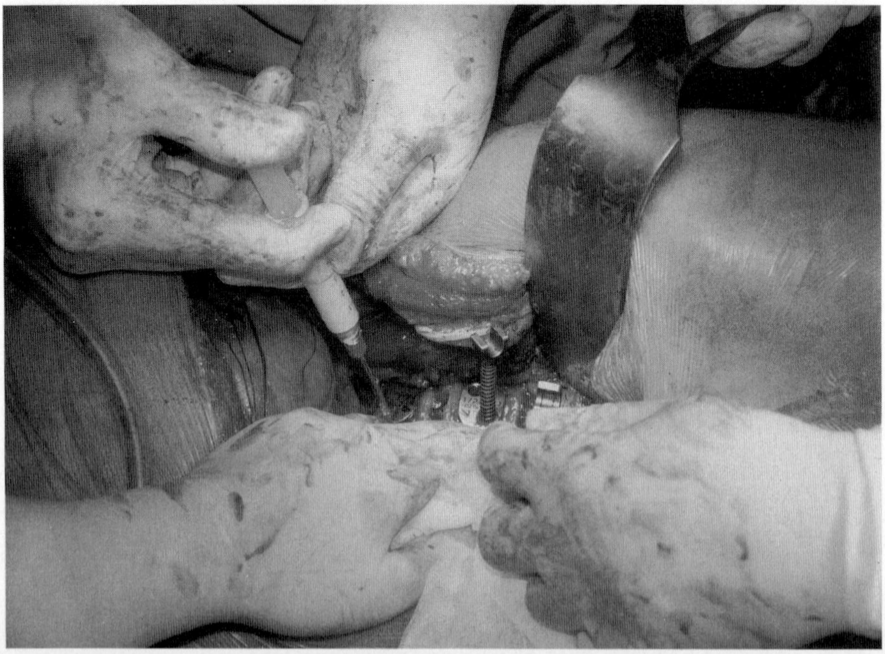

C

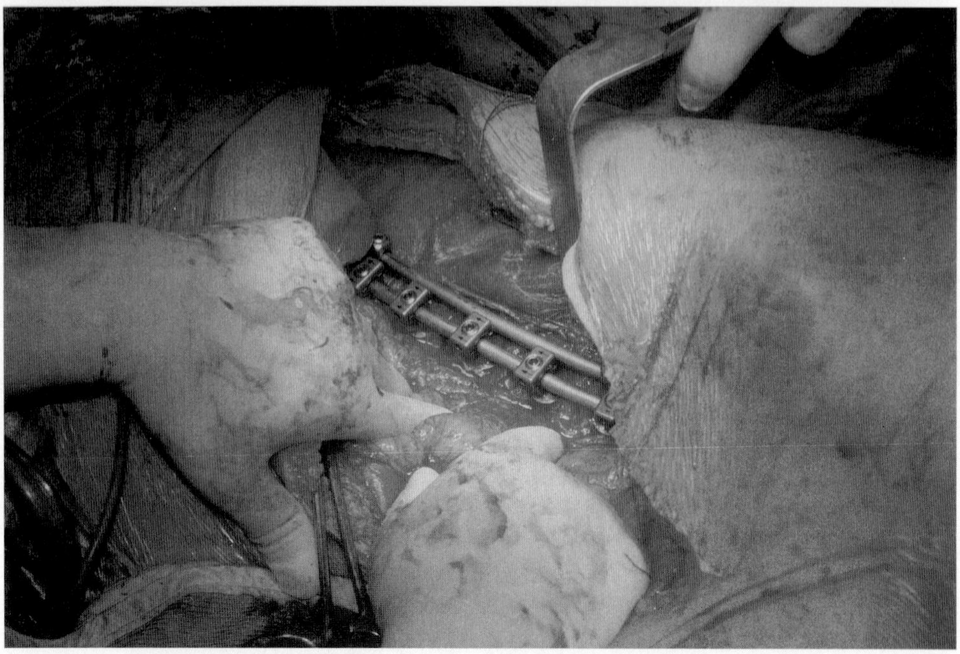

D

FIG. 29.1 *Continued.* **C:** Intraoperative picture, showing the injection of the calcium apatite cement into the prepared screw hole. **D:** Intraoperative picture, showing stabilization of the thoracolumbar spine with a double rod-screw system.

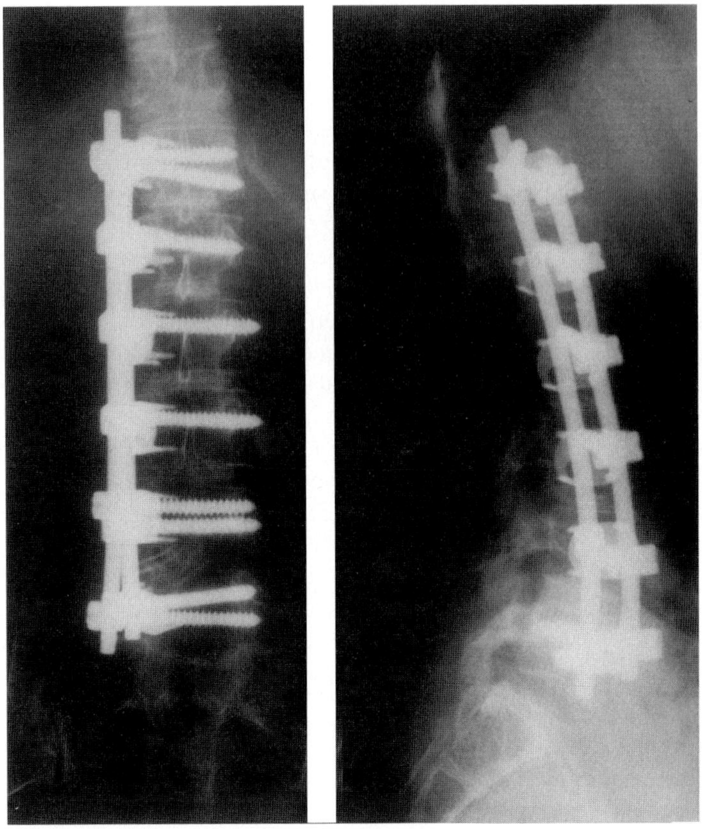

E

FIG. 29.1 *Continued.* **E:** Postoperative anteroposterior and lateral radiographs, showing successful fusion of T-12 to L-5.

thetic and then turned in the lateral decubitus position on a radiolucent table. Once the vertebral levels were confirmed fluoroscopically, the lumbar segmental vessels were divided and ligated, and the psoas major muscle was retracted off the spine in a posterior direction to expose the vertebral bodies. Thereafter, the segmental intervertebral discs were reamed. To prepare the ventral screws, an awl was used to prepare the screw hole in the vertebral body, after which a self-tapping screw was inserted. The opposing cortical wall of the vertebral body was not perforated, in order to prevent leakage of the CAC. The positions of the screws were monitored with anteroposterior and lateral fluoroscopy. Upon manual testing of the rigidity of this initial screw placement, the author and colleagues observed that several screws were clinically loose. Subsequently, all screws were removed, and the CAC was prepared and injected into the screw hole. The injection was performed in a nonpressurized, retrograde manner with a 10-mL syringe and a 12-gauge needle. Per screw hole, 2.0 to 3.0 mL of CAC was injected. The screws were then reinserted in pairs and held in place until the CAC hardened (about 10 to 15 minutes). After hardening, bone grafting was performed (a free vascularized fibula graft in two patients, iliac crest grafts in four patients) Subsequently, a double-rod system was mounted to stabilize or correct the deformity. Closure of the wound was performed with aspiration tubes (in the pleural cavity) and or Redon drains (in the retroperitoneal bed).

SURGICAL RESULTS

The mean length of the postoperative follow-up period was 24 months (range, 14 to 66 months). The average duration of surgery was 8 hours and 13 minutes (range, 5 to 12 hours). two to three ventral screws and four pedicle screws (two spinal segments) could be augmented in one step with 2.0 to 3.0 mL of CAC per screw hole. Thereafter, a new portion of cement was prepared, and another set of screws was placed. During cement injection and screw reinsertion, cement leakage was observed out of the entrance of the screw hole in a retrograde manner. After augmentation, definitive screw reinsertion, and cement hardening, all screws revealed to be clinically rigid with the exception of one (0.3%) ventral screw. Cement leakage occurred at the base of the pedicle of the corpus vertebrae in seven (9%) of 78 screw augmentation procedures. The cement was promptly removed before touching the medial deviated dura or nerve root and before hardening. With the technique described, no cement-related or device-related complications occurred. Bone fusion of the spine was achieved in all cases (100% fusion rate). However, radiographic evaluation of the screw-cement-bone interface was difficult because of overprojection of the metal devices and the variable quality of the radiographs in time. All patients with neurological symptoms experienced complete relief of those symptoms; however, two patients still complained about back pain after the procedure. In four patients, an almost complete correction of the deformity was achieved, and in one patient, a partial correction was performed. In three other patients, an *in situ* fusion was accepted and achieved (all patients with osteogenesis imperfecta and severe osteoporosis).

ILLUSTRATIVE CASE REPORT

A 19-year-old woman, known to have osteogenesis imperfecta type I according to the Sillence classification, presented with severe lumbar and sacroiliac pain to such a degree that she had been bedridden 50% of the time during the few years before presentation. Physical examination revealed no deformities of her extremities but a painful right convex thoracolumbar scoliosis. The deformity was easily corrected by lateral bending. Radiographs showed a right convex scoliosis of T-12 to -L-5 (45 degrees; see Fig. 29.1A), with severe spinal instability (T-12 to -L-5) as seen on anteroposterior bending (see Fig. 29.1B) and flexion-extension lateral radiographs. Magnetic resonance imaging studies of the lumbar spine showed normal bone, discs, and soft tissues and no spinal cord or nerve root compression. DEXA studies showed decreased lumbar spine values (0.62 g per square centimeter; the normal value for age-matched women is about 1.21 g per square centimeter). Before surgery, the patient was pain free only in a thoracolumbar orthosis; she was also treated with calcium, vitamin D, and pamidronate. Six months after initial treatment, an anterior fusion (T-12 to L-4) with CAC augmented screws and a double-rod system was performed (see Fig. 29.1C,D). Fusion was established by reaming the intervertebral discs, followed by iliac crest grafting. After surgery, the patient complained about a temporary genitofemoral nerve palsy, which resolved spontaneously within 6 months. Regular follow-up radiographs showed a maintained, complete correction of the scoliotic deformity, unchanged position of the ventral screws, and solid fusion (see Fig. 29.1E). Twenty-four months after the operation, the patient gave birth to healthy twins. During the pregnancy, she complained only about mild back pain.

DISCUSSION

Progressive spinal deformity caused by osteoporosis is usually a disease of the elderly. Surgical intervention may be considered in severely osteoporotic patients with one or more vertebral fractures and spinal canal compromise or worsening of a preexisting deformity (a degenerative scoliosis) and neurological deficits. Reconstruction of such a spine poses technical challenges: The benefit of improvement in the quality of life (as demanded by many patients) by a surgical intervention should outweigh the potential technical and medical risks.

Experimental and clinical studies have demonstrated that graft incorporation and successful bone fusion is more likely to occur when rigid internal fixation is achieved (2,3). In patients suffering from severe osteoporosis or other diseases that adversely affect the quality of bone (of which osteogenesis imperfecta is a unique group) in whom degenerative (osteoporotic) scoliotic spinal deformities develop, attainment of a rigid internal fixation can be extremely difficult and, in very severe cases, may be precluded (4,6,7,8,14). Although most of the literature reports about surgical intervention in severe osteoporotic cases are anecdotal, results of several studies about surgical interventions in aged patients tend to be supportive and have shown improved function and pain relief after surgery (15,16). In an outcome study of 84 patients aged 40 years or older who underwent spinal reconstructive surgery for a spinal deformity, overall satisfaction with the functional was 81%, and there was significant improvement in most of the functional measures (15). However, surgical intervention in the elderly may have increased perioperative and postoperative complications. In a cohort study of patients treated for degenerative spondylolisthesis (mean age, 57.8 years) or spinal fractures (mean age, 35.7 years) with pedicle screw fixation and rods/plates, the spondylolisthesis cohort showed significantly higher rates of intraoperative loss of fixation (1.7% versus 0.2%) and postoperative loosening and pullout (3.8% versus 2.3%) (16). These findings are supported by laboratory experiments demonstrating that osteopenia compromises pedicle screw fixation (4,6,17,18). When pedicle screw devices are applied in (elderly) osteoporotic patients, the screw-bone interface is easily disrupted, which leads to an increased risk of postoperative loosening or pullout (4,8,16,18). To improve pedicle screw fixation, several strategies have been used: alteration of the point of screw purchase, the use of screws with a larger diameter, and transfer of the loads on the screws to nearby anatomical structures. In addition, manipulation of the screw-bone interface by augmentation of the screws is another logical step for facilitating a rigid screw fixation. In this regard, several studies have demonstrated the effectiveness of polymethylmethacrylate (PMMA) and CAC in the augmentation of pedicle screws in cadaver specimens (8,10,11,18,19). CAC is a composite of monocalcium phosphate monohydrate [$Ca(H_2PO_4)_2H_2O$], α-tricalcium phosphate [$Ca_3(PO_4)_2$], and calcium carbonate [$CaCO_3$] dry mixed; a sodium phosphate solution is subsequently added and converts it into a paste. Within 10 minutes of delivery, the paste hardens at physiological pH as a result of the crystallization of dahllite (carbonated hydroxyapatite) (12,13). It attains 50% of its maximum strength 1 hour after its implantation, 90% 4 hours after, and maximum strength 24 hours after. In comparison with PMMA, it has both the advantage of being nonexothermic during solidification and the potential for being resorbed and replaced in time by normal bone (12,13). Encouraging clinical experiences have been gathered in the application of CAC in upper and lower limb fractures (20–23). However, no reports of the clinical use of CAC as an screw augmentation technique in spinal surgery are available. Experimentally, CAC compares favorably with PMMA in the enhancement of initial fixation of pedicle screws (11).

Although the postaugmentation pullout strengths seen with PMMA and CAC augmentation are similar, the failure modes of the two types of augmentation are quite different. CAC-augmented screws tend to pull out without causing any bone fracture, stripping the cement at the restored bone screw interface (11). In contrast, the pedicle often fractures at or near its junction with the vertebral body during pullout of PMMA-augmented screws; with the cement remains intact, whereas the bone around it fails (11). Preferential failure of the screw-bone interface with CAC augmentation may have some advantages: revision after screw fixation failure is simplified by removal of the screw, débridement, re-augmentation, and screw reinsertion. In addition, the failure at the screw-bone interface does, in fact, reduce the risk of pedicle fracture, and therefore reduces the risk of injury to the nerve roots.

There are several potential disadvantages of augmentation of screws with CAC. In particular, preparation and injection of the CAC was time consuming, limiting the number of injections into two to three (ventral) and four (posterior) prepared screw holes with the existing technique. The whole procedure lengthened the operation time considerably: per set of two to four screws, about 10 minutes extra. A part of this problem may be explained by inexperience with the procedure, the technique employed to prepare the CAC, and the injection technique. In addition, to perform the CAC injection safely posteriorly, a hemilaminectomy was necessary to exclude leakage of the CAC and remove the CAC if leakage happened. Preparation of the pedicle, therefore, is important: in the author's opinion, a disruption of the wall of the pedicle precludes injection. In this regard, computer-assisted preparation and insertion of pedicle screws may reduce the number of incorrectly placed screws (24), but leakage of CAC needs to be considered constantly, especially in transpedicle screw augmentation. More recently, the CAC preparation and injection technique has been improved, shortening this part of the procedure considerably. Another drawback in the author's series is the difficulty in detecting the cement margins on radiographs. It was almost impossible to clearly define the cement-screw and the cement-bone interfaces. Therefore, the cement filling along the length of the screw was difficult to assess. In addition, cement dislodgment and cement fracture could not be clearly defined on radiographs. The difficulties in assessment were attributable partly to the different qualities of the radiographs (different angles, different exposure times) in time and partly to the overprojection of the screws and rods. In this regard, there are no comparable data from *in vitro* studies: These studies focused on biomechanical parameters by comparing the pullout resistance of different screws with or without augmentation (8,10,11,18,19). The amount of injected CAC (2 to 3 mL per screw hole), however, was comparable with those in the *in vitro* studies (10,11). Lucency in the cement-bone interface or around the screw, although difficult to assess, was not observed on any of the radiographs throughout the follow-up period. Bone fusion was attained in 100% of cases; only one lumbar screw was loose during and after surgery. No further screw loosening or screw migration was observed postoperatively.

This study has all the shortcomings of a nonprospective, nonrandomized study. The procedure described, however, appeared safe and helped establish fixation of the pedicle screws. Nevertheless, indications for spinal fusion in severe osteoporosis and the criteria for augmentation of pedicle screws in the surgical treatment of osteoporotic spinal deformities have not been clearly defined yet. Although the author's results with the surgical technique employed for cement augmentation of ventral and pedicle screws is promising and showed no serious complications, there are still many questions to be addressed. The method of screw hole preparation, cement characteristics (e.g., viscosity, composition, porosity) injection (pressurized, nonpressurized, the use of a seal), screw types (self-tapping or non—self-tapping) and sizes still need further study. The authors and colleagues opted to inject the cement in a nonpressurized manner in order to decrease the risk of cement leakage out of the bone through the already weakened trabecular structure of the osteoporotic vertebrae. However, cement leakage was still seen despite this precautionary measure. The author therefore advocates that hemilaminectomy should be performed at all levels that require fusion, in order to visualize and promptly remove leaked cement.

REFERENCES

1. Bernhardt M, Swarzt DE, Clothiaux PL, et al. Posterolateral lumbar and lumbosacral fusion with and without pedicle screw internal fixation. *Clin Orthop* 1992;284:109–115.
2. Kornblatt MD, Casey MP, Jacobs RR. Internal fixation in lumbosacral spine fusion: a biomechanical and clinical study. *Clin Orthop* 1986;203:141.
3. Schwab FJ, Nazarian DG, Mahmud F, et al. Effects of spinal instrumentation on fusion of the lumbosacral spine. *Spine* 1995;20(18):2023–2028.
4. Halvorson TL, Kelley LA, Thomas KA, et al. Effects of bone mineral density on pedicle screw fixation. *Spine* 1994;19:2415–2420.
5. Hasegawa K, Takahashi HE, Uchiyama S, et al. An experimental study of a combination method using a pedicle screw and a laminar hook for the osteoporotic spine. *Spine* 1997;22:958–963.
6. Hanscom DA, Winter RB, Lutter L, et al. Osteogenesis imperfecta. Radiographic classification, natural history, and treatment of spinal deformities. *J Bone Joint Surg Am* 1992;74:598–616.
7. Ishikawa S, Kumar SJ, Takahashi HE, et al. Vertebral body shape as a predictor of spinal deformity in osteogenesis imperfecta. *J Bone Joint Surg Am* 1996;78:212–219.
8. Law M, Tencer AF, Anderson PA. Caudo-cephalad loading of pedicle screws: mechanisms of loosening and methods of augmentation. *Spine* 1993;18:2438–2443.
9. West JL, Bradford DS, Ogilvie JW. Results of spinal arthrodesis with pedicle screw-plate fixation. *J Bone Joint Surg Am* 1991;73:1179–1184.
10. Lotz JC, Hu SS, Chiu DFM, et al. Carbonated apatite cement augmentation of pedicle screw fixation in the lumbar spine. *Spine* 1997;22:2716–2723.
11. Moore DC, Maitra RS, Farjo LA, et al. Restoration of pedicle screw fixation with an *in situ* setting calcium phosphate cement. *Spine* 1997;22:1696–1705.
12. Constantz BR, Ison IC, Fulmer MT, et al. Skeletal repair by *in situ* formation of the mineral phase of bone. *Science* 1995;267:796–799.
13. Frankenberg EP, Bauer TW, Jiang M, et al. Mechanical integrity of calcium phosphate cement in *in vivo* metaphyseal defect models over time. Transactions of the 42nd Annual Meeting of the Orthopaedic Research Society, Atlanta, Georgia, 1996;21:224–228.
14. Weinstein JN, Rydevik BL, Rauschning W. Anatomic and technical considerations of pedicle screw fixation. *Clin Orthop* 1992;284:34–46.
15. Hu SS, Holly EA, Lele C, et al. Patient outcomes after spinal reconstructive surgery in patients > or = 40 years of age. *J Spinal Disord* 1996;9:460–469.
16. Yuan HA, Garfin SR, Dickman CA, et al. A historical cohort study of pedicle screw fixation in thoracic, lumbar and sacral spinal fusions. *Spine* 1994;19(Suppl):S2279–S2296.
17. Soshi S, Shiba R, Kondo H, et al. An experimental study on transpedicular screw fixation in relation to osteoporosis of the lumbar spine. *Spine* 1991;16:1335–1341.
18. Zindrick MR, Wiltse LL, Widel EH, et al. A biomechanical study of intrapeduncular screw fixation in the lumbosacral spine. *Clin Orthop* 1986;203:99–112.
19. Wittenberg RH, Lee KS, Shea M, et al. Effect of screw diameter, insertion technique and bone cement augmentation of pedicular screw fixation strength. *Clin Orthop* 1993;296:278–287.
20. Jupiter JB, Winter S, Sigman S, et al. Repair of five distal radius fractures with an investigational cancellous bone cement: a preliminary report. *J Orthop Trauma* 1997;11:110–116.
21. Kopylov P, Jonsson K, Thorngren KG, et al. Injectable calcium phosphate in the treatment of distal radial fractures. *J Hand Surg [Br]* 1996;21:768–777.
22. Leutenegger A. Integration and resorption of calcium phosphate ceramics in defect filling of fractures of the tibial head. Radiologic long-term results. [In German.] Helv Chir Acta 1994;60:1061–1066.
23. Stankewich CJ, Swiontkowski MF, Tencer AF, et al. Augmentation of femoral neck fracture fixation with an injectable calcium-phosphate bone mineral cement. *J Orthop Res* 1996;14:786–793.
24. Laine T, Schlenzka D, Makitalo K, et al. Improved accuracy of pedicle screw insertion with computer-assisted surgery. A prospective trial of 30 patients. *Spine* 1997;22:1254–1258.

30

Vertebrectomy and Vertebral Reconstruction

Everard A. Munting

Department of Orthopedic Surgery, Cliniques Saint Pierre, 134O Ottignies, Louvain-la-Neuve, Belgium

The management of vertebral osteoporotic compression fractures by open surgical procedures involving osteosynthesis, decompression, or balance correction is very seldom indicated. Most often, osteoporotic vertebral compression fractures are rather well tolerated. Vertebroplasty by injection of acrylic cement in the fractured vertebra has shown rather remarkable results regarding pain control in patients with significant symptoms. The so-called kyphoplasty technique even seems able to correct sagittal deformity in selected cases.

In cases in which conservative management has failed and percutaneous procedures are not indicated, the goals and potential benefits of major surgery must be weighed against the significant risks of local and general complications in a group of patients that are often elderly and frail, presenting with associated pathological processes. Potential local complications include mechanical failure of the osteosynthesis, further vertebral collapse, skin slough, and wound infection, all of which would necessitate repeated surgery. General complications of all kinds, from minor to severe, are to be expected in most cases and result in prolonged hospital stays. Fortunately, in this author's experience, this did not result in significant sequelae. In view of the frequent occurrence of postoperative complications, these matters must be thoroughly discussed with the patient and family before any surgical decision is made.

SURGICAL INDICATIONS

Surgery for vertebral compression fractures should be discussed when significant pain and loss of function, nonresponsive to conservative means, is attributable to one or several of the following conditions:

1. Sagittal or frontal imbalance.
2. Spinal stenosis with neurological deficit or nerve root impingement.
3. Instability related to vertebral body pseudarthrosis or adjacent disc degeneration.

The general status of the patient must be carefully assessed. Nutritional and hydration status are of paramount importance and must be corrected before surgery. Respiratory therapy, when necessary, should be started before the procedure.

THERAPEUTIC GOALS

If the surgical option is discussed, all aspects of the problem—neural compromise, spinal balance, and stability—must be considered jointly. The goals of the surgical procedure must be precisely defined along with careful preoperative planning.

Neural compromise is an uncommon complication of isolated osteoporotic vertebral compression fractures. When it occurs, it is often related to a combination of posterior wall recession or angular kyphosis and preexisting degenerative spinal stenosis. Even when asymptomatic, it must be considered in cases of sagittal balance correction because the straightening of the spine may increase the stenosis.

Altered sagittal balance precludes a straight standing position without muscular effort and severely affects the walking capacity. The induced passive tension in the paraspinal muscles, as well as on the nerve roots and the dural sac, is a significant nociceptive feature. Besides the lasting pain, severe loss of a straight standing and sitting position is associated with the loss of a straight vision and normal horizon line. This has a major negative impact on global life quality of the affected patient and contributes to social exclusion. Correction of severely compromised sagittal balance, if achieved, consistently results in a major and spectacular improvement in the well-being of the patient.

Instability, with its consequences in terms of pain and neurological compromise, is a frequent observation in these patients. It is often the result of a combination of several factors, including degenerative disc and facet disease, muscular insufficiency, and, sometimes, pseudarthrosis. If a surgical treatment is chosen, instability must be addressed despite the technical difficulties. After decompression of encroached neural structures, iatrogenic instability must also be assessed and, if present, treated by appropriate osteosynthesis.

SURGICAL PLANNING

Approach and Sequences

The choice of the surgical approach—posterior, anterior or both—is of crucial importance. In case of long-standing, significant kyphosis, a posterior approach is, in any case, mandatory. Indeed, kyphosis correction by a single anterior approach is probably impossible, but if it is feasible, it results in significant stretching of the dural sac, which carries a very high risk of neurological complications.

A posterior approach can be combined with an anterior approach, either simultaneously or as a two-staged procedure, in case of severe spinal canal compromise of anterior origin. The author and colleague usually prefer a single posterior approach, but in selected cases, simultaneous anterior and posterior approaches are the best option.

Correction of Deformity

The planning of deformity correction includes the precise assessment of the extent, if any, of reducibility and the site or sites where this reduction occurs: within the intervertebral disc or discs or within the fractured vertebral body. These observations influence the choice of the type and eventual sequences of surgical approach. Quite often, in elderly patients, major deformity is the result of a combination of vertebral collapse and disc degeneration. This may result in surprisingly reducible deformity, associated with major intervertebral instability with its related dynamic neural impingement.

A rigid deformity must be corrected only after careful and extensive release of all structures surrounding the involved area (1). Kyphosis correction must be obtained mostly by gentle external maneuvers, either by pushing on the back if the patient is in the lateral decubitus position or by modifying the position of the operating table if the patient is in the prone position. Acting simultaneously on the rods can be done only if they are secured to the spine by multiple anchoring points. Again, if significant force is necessary to corrected the deformity, the structures around the area of correction must be freed more extensively before further attempts of correction. This is probably the most important technical point in this type of surgery. Interbody distraction with a spreader is contraindicated because it always results in the migration of the tool through the osteoporotic vertebral bodies.

Neural Release

The decompression and release of adhesions of the neural structures in the spinal canal and the intervertebral foramina must be carried out carefully. The author and colleagues prefer canal calibration and partial laminotomy for decompression, in order to keep as many bone structures available for the arthrodesis.

Undercutting of the bone structures in the spinal canal at the osteotomy site must be done to avoid an induced, potentially severe stenosis when the osteotomy is closed. However, laminectomy involving one or two levels about the osteotomy site should also be performed, if necessary, in order to achieve a good decompression.

Osteosynthesis

All modalities and maneuvers should be used to obtain strong and stable fixation of the spine. The author and colleagues prefer titanium instrumentation to facilitate postoperative imaging of the spinal canal. They always try to combine different types of anchoring means to improve the stability of the construct. Pedicle screws proximal to the osteotomy site are always combined with hooks, sublaminar wires, or both. To improve the purchase of the pedicle screws in the bone, they usually inject 1 to 3 mL of high-viscosity acrylic cement in each pedicle. They use a 1-mL syringe, whose size allows its introduction in the pedicle. The tip of the syringe is cut off, which allows the injection of the cement that, because its high viscosity, will be pressurized between the bone trabeculae when the screw is inserted .

Reconstruction Means

In most cases in which sagittal balance correction is intended, the author and colleagues try to perform a subtraction osteotomy with no need for anterior implants. Furthermore, this provides abundant autograft from the osteotomy site. When anterior reconstruction is needed, they use exclusively freeze-dried, gamma ray—irradiated, cortical allografts (usually a segment of femoral shaft) supplemented with autograft, if locally available (2).

Infrastructure

This type of procedure should be carried out only by an experienced team, with the use of a cell saver and somatosensory or motor evoked potentials when working at the thoracic level.

SURGICAL TECHNIQUES

Four basic surgical techniques are used to correct sagittal deformities. Three basic principles have been used, and not always published, for many years by several well-known French authors and authors from the english-speaking world. Technical details regarding osteosynthesis, bone substitutes, or bone reinforcement have been associated or modified over the years by several teams.

The *single posterior approach with subtraction osteotomy* includes pedicles and posterior wall resection with posterior fixation (Fig. 30.1) (3,4) [developed by René Louis and Jacques Sénégas, cited by Argenson (1)]. This technique is best indicated in cases of significant, rigid deformity or if a posterior fusion is present. It is the technique of choice in the low lumbar spine (L-4 or L-5) and in high thoracic fractures with or without neurological compromise. Extensive release of the structures near the osteotomy is the key factor for success. The center of rotation of the single, large corrective movement is located about the anterior longitudinal ligament. This procedure may be associated with significant bleeding and can be technically challenging.

Multiple posterior subtraction osteotomies about the facet joints with long segmental posterior fixation, which are less aggressive for the patient, allow only minor sagittal correction. Careful canal calibration with removal of the ligamentum flavum must be carried out at each involved level to prevent iatrogenic spinal canal stenosis. In this procedure, the corrective movement involves multiple centers of rotation located about the posterior longitudinal ligament. It is indicated in patients with multilevel compression fractures with rather minor sagittal imbalance and in which have some disc height still remains.

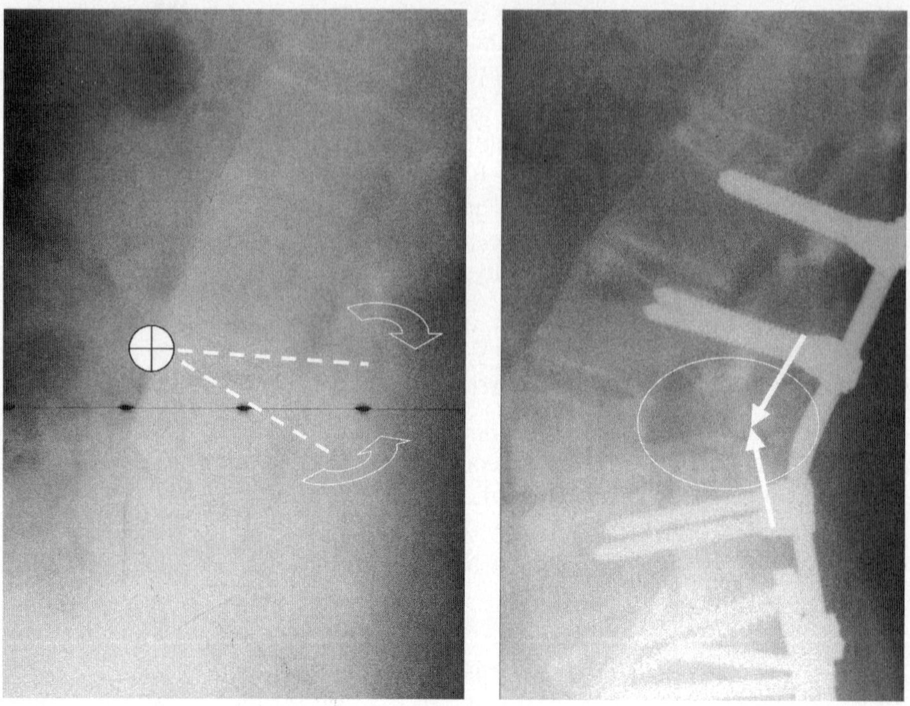

FIG. 30.1. Preoperative and postoperative radiographs of a patient with ankylosing spondylitis. A posterior subtraction osteotomy was carried out. Notice the complete resection of the L-4 pedicle.

Anterior corpectomy and reconstruction with autograft, allograft, or an artificial implant is another option (Fig. 30.2) (5–7). This is indicated particularly in cases of vertebral pseudarthrosis or in severe, acute, or subacute compression fracture with spinal canal compromise. The procedure is rather easy if only an anterior approach is needed and if the posterior wall can be left in place. If spinal canal decompression must be carried out along with posterior release, the bleeding can be significant. The procedure is also technically challenging because one of two procedures is needed: either a simultaneous anterior and posterior approach with the patient in the lateral decubitus position or a three-staged procedure that includes posterior release, anterior release and vertebral reconstruction, and a posterior segmental fixation. This is, in any case, major surgery whose indications must be thoroughly weighed in this group of fragile patients.

Posterior calibration, subtraction about the facets, and posterior fixation in compression, associated with *anterior discectomy and fusion in distraction* with ring allograft or cages (Fig. 30.3) derived from the technique described by Robertson and Whitesides (8), is best indicated in cases of severe but reducible deformity related to a combination of vertebral compression fracture and unstable degenerative disc disease. Because the center of rotation of the corrective movement is located about the posterior longitudinal ligament, there is little risk of stretching of the neural structures or of inducing spinal canal stenosis when the osteotomy is closed. This procedure can be performed by either a simultaneous approach or a two-staged approach. The technique allows significant cor-

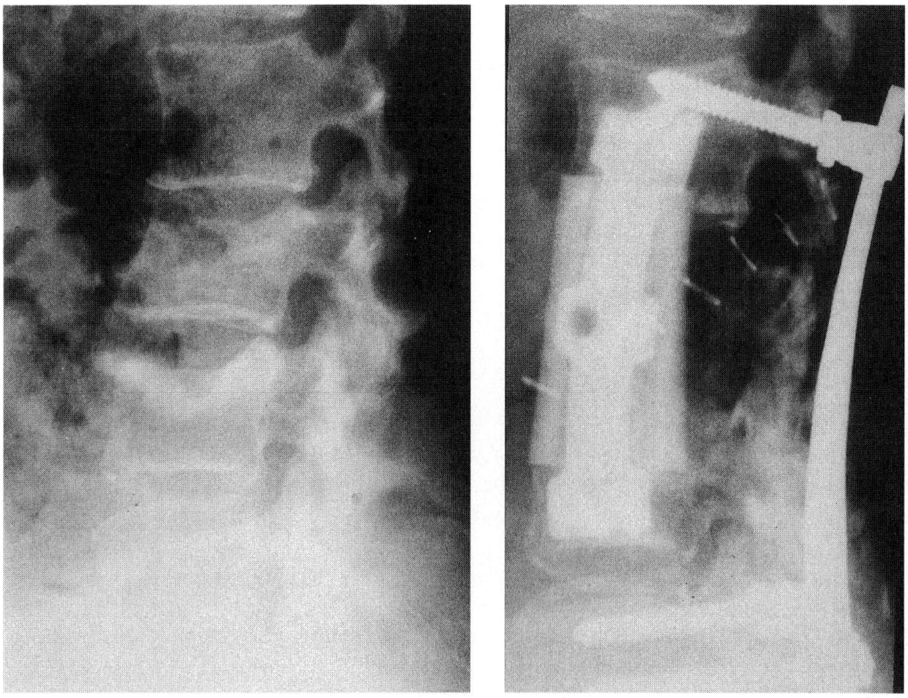

FIG. 30.2. Preoperative and postoperative radiographs of a patient with intractable pain and osteoporotic compression fractures after radiotherapy for lymphoma. There was no significant imbalance. Posterior osteosynthesis and arthrodesis were followed by anterior reconstruction with a cortical allograft. The graft was trimmed to the correct size and shape and provides large bearing surfaces, with the adjacent endplates favoring bone healing.

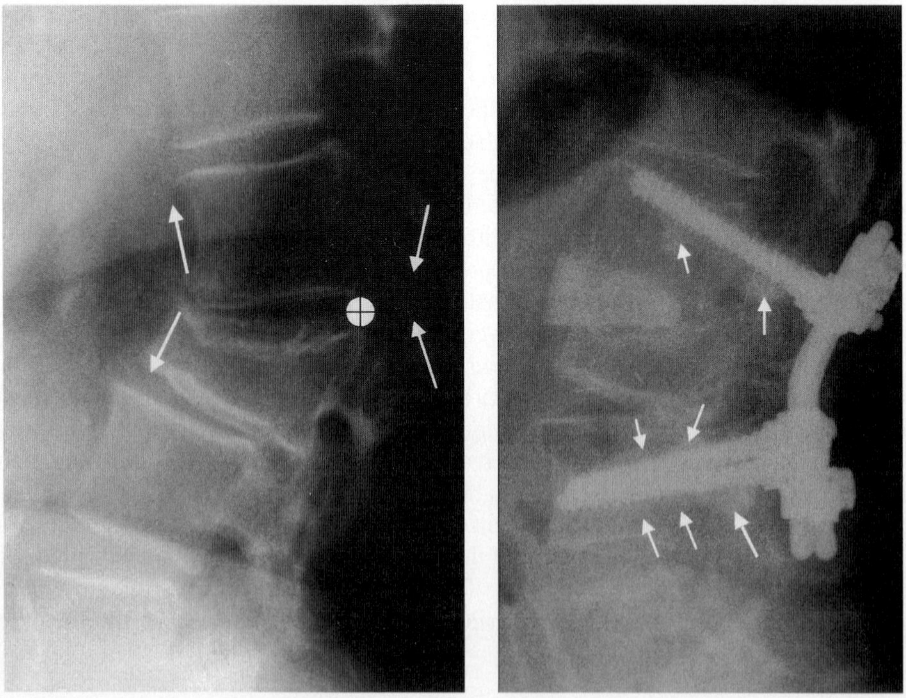

FIG. 30.3. L-2 compression fracture with associated disc disease, causing retrolisthesis of L-3 on L-4 with spinal canal stenosis. The case was managed by a simultaneous anterior and posterior approach. The sagittal imbalance was corrected with a cortical ring allograft inserted between L-2 and L-3. Posterior spinal canal calibration was carried out for neural release along with osteosynthesis, providing good stability. Notice the acrylic cement around the pedicle screws (*small arrows, right*).

rection and is associated with excellent and reliable fusion. The vertebral body fracture must, however, be consolidated.

CONCLUSIONS

Surgical management of osteoporotic vertebral compression fractures remains seldom indicated. The objectives must be well defined and followed by careful surgical planning, taking into account all particulars of the patient. Preoperative workup includes assessment of the patient's nutritional and hydration status, the severity of the osteoporosis, and the extent of spinal canal compromise.

If by the time of surgical planning the impression is that not all goals can be achieved, it is often preferable to renounce surgery altogether, because partial fulfillment of the preoperative goals often, if not always, results in total failure of the surgery. Indeed, in view of the poor bone quality, no osteosynthesis, no matter how many anchoring points are obtained, will support the stresses induced by a persisting sagittal imbalance. Conversely, appropriate correction by means of an osteotomy must be stabilized by a strong osteosynthesis. If it is not, pseudarthrosis, hardware loosening, and loss of correction will occur and lead to the necessity of repeated surgery with an increasing toll of complications.

Despite all these drawbacks, when meticulous surgery is performed in very selected cases after careful planning and preparation, the results are surprisingly good and appreciated by the patient, despite the often very difficult postoperative period.

REFERENCES

1. Argenson C. In: *Cahiers d'enseignement de la SOFCOT. Conférences d'enseignement.* Paris: Expansion Scientifique Française, 1990:205–234.
2. Munting E, Manche E, Faundez A. Vertebral reconstruction with cortical allograft: long-term evaluation. *Eur Spine J* 2001;10:S153–S157.
3. Roy-Camille R, Lelièvre JP Pseudarthroses des corps vertébraux du rachis dorso-lombaire. *Rev Chir Orthop* 1975;61:249–257.
4. Thomasen E. Vertebral osteotomy for correction of kyphosis in ankylosing spondylitis. *Clin Orthop* 1985; 194:142–151.
5. Bradford DS, Winter RB, Lonstein JE, et al. Techniques of anterior spinal surgery for the management of kyphosis. *Clin Orthop* 1977;128:129–139.
6. Kostuik JP. Anterior fixation for fractures of the thoracic and lumbar spine with or without neurologic involvement. *Clin Orthop* 1984;189:103–115.
7. Louis R. Ostéotomies vertébrales par voie antérieure. *Rev Chir Orthop* 1971;57(Suppl 1):163–174.
8. Robertson JM, Whitesides TE. Surgical reconstruction of late posttraumatic thoracolumbar kyphosis. *Spine* 1985;10:307–312.

31

Principles of Cost/Benefit Ratios

Christian Mélot

Faculty of Medicine, Free University of Brussels, and Department of Intensive Care, Erasme University Hospital, Brussels, Belgium

EFFICACY, EFFECTIVENESS, AND EFFICIENCY

Physicians can predict that the third millennium will be an era of health care cost containment and outcomes assessment, in which they will measure and obtain the greatest value possible from health care services and products to achieve the highest satisfaction of the patients.

To reach this target, the major challenge of this century will be to ensure the transfer of the research results with proven benefits (efficacy) to the daily clinical practice for the advantage of the individual patient (effectiveness) at the lowest cost for the benefit of the society (efficiency) (Table 31.1).

Efficacy studies answer the question: can it work? Does a procedure, service, or program do more good than harm to people who fully comply with the associated recommendations or treatments? Such studies pertain to an ideal world in which patients are carefully chosen to participate to a trial.

Effectiveness studies answer the question: does it work in the real world? Does the procedure, service, or program do more good than harm to those people to whom it is offered? This form of health care evaluation, in which both the efficacy of a service and its acceptance by those to whom it is offered are considered, is the evaluation of effectiveness or usefulness.

The efficiency evaluation answers the question of whether a certain health procedure, service, or program is worth undertaking in comparison with other things that could be done with the same resources. Should the health care resources necessary to make the procedure, service, or program available to those who could benefit from it be spent in this way rather than some other way? Although efficiency evaluation provides important information to decision makers, it addresses only one dimension of health care program decisions. It must be preceded by efficacy and effectiveness evaluations.

If an ethical dimension is added by taking into account the distributive justice, then two other questions must be asked: Is the procedure, service, or program accessible to all people who could benefit from it? Is it reaching those who need it?

The terms "*efficiency evaluation*" and "*economic evaluation*" are often used interchangeably. In these evaluations, the outcomes or benefits are defined differently for each type of analysis, but costs are uniformly defined in monetary terms.

TABLE 31.1. *Efficacy, effectiveness and efficiency evaluations*

Ideal world	Real world	
Efficacy evaluation	Effectiveness evaluation	Efficiency evaluation
Outcomes in research studies (e.g., randomized clinical trials with selected group of patients)	Risk-adjusted outcomes in a clinical setting (e.g., applying the research results to most of the patients)	Risk-adjusted costs in an economic world (e.g., economic evaluation using cost-minimization analysis, cost-effectiveness analysis, cost-utility analysis, and cost-benefit analysis)

NOMENCLATURE FOR COSTS

Economists are more concerned with how society chooses to allocate limited resources rather than what something costs per se. Cost may be used to sum resource use of several types, allowing an economic comparison of services with a common scale. Accounting methods are used to develop costs from resource use (Table 31.2).

Costs can be considered from several possible perspectives. For hospitals, costs are their expenses related to providing a service. For payers, the cost is what the providers charge, plus their administrative expenses. In principle, cost studies often seek to determine societal costs, which can be used in cost-effectiveness analyses to gain the widest perspective. However, societal costs are never directly measurable; thus, combinations of costs proxies from one or several sources are often used as estimates.

Costs can be classified as direct or indirect. Varying definitions of indirect costs may lead to uncertainty in categorizing a particular cost. Direct costs relate to the provision of medical care, and indirect costs are other societal costs. An example of direct costs structure in osteoporosis is shown in Fig. 31.1 (1). Direct medical costs can also be divided into two components: in-hospital direct costs and follow-up direct costs. Inpatient costs comprise hospital costs (e.g., room, laboratory testing, pharmacy) and physicians' or surgeons' professional billing. Follow-up direct costs include physician office visits, outpatient testing, medications, home health providers, and additional hospitalizations.

Indirect costs reflect lost patient or business opportunity and may be referred to as *productivity costs* (2). Productivity costs represent true costs to society and should not be ignored in a cost-effectiveness or cost-utility analysis. Some health economists argue for inclusion of productivity costs in the denominator of the cost-utility ratio, measured in quality-adjusted life-years. Others argue that productivity costs should be included in the

TABLE 31.2. *Nomenclature for costs*

Cost perspective	Provider (e.g., hospital, health professional) Payer (e.g., insurance, Social Security) Patient
Cost category	Direct costs Indirect costs
Cost per service	Average costs Marginal costs Incremental costs
Accounting method	Top-down costing Bottom-up costing

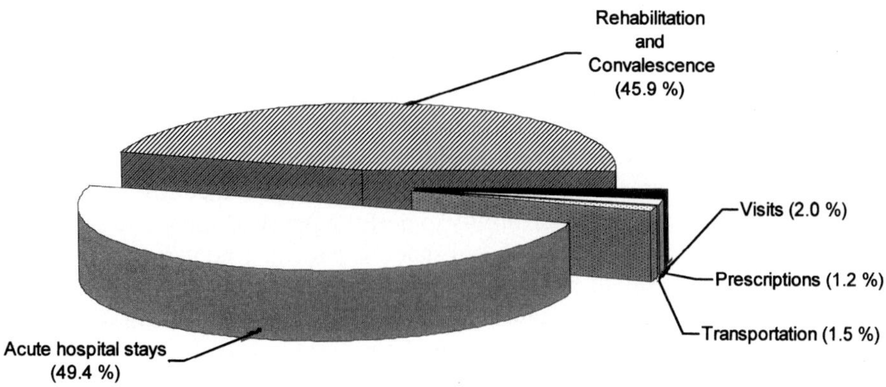

FIG. 31.1. Structure of direct costs in osteoporosis [drawn with the figures of Levy P, et al. (1)].

numerator of the cost-utility or cost-effectiveness ratio, measured in monetary units by the human-capital method or the friction-cost method.

The human-capital approach views a person as a capital investment, valued by his or her economic contribution to society. Therefore, the value of a human life is considered the discounted current value of future earnings that can be expected over the person's lifetime. The friction-cost method estimates the short-term effects of illness by studying consequences at the level of the company. Its basic premise is that loss of productivity as a result of disease depends on time needed to restore the original productivity level. The friction-cost approach assumes that sick employees are replaceable and that production losses are confined to the friction period, which is the time needed to replace a sick worker.

Costs can be also evaluated per service by measuring average, marginal, or incremental costs of two or more procedures, services, or programs (3,4). Average cost is calculated by dividing all costs for a therapy or test by the number of uses of that therapy or test. The marginal cost is the cost of producing one extra unit of outcome. The incremental cost is the difference in the cost between two treatments. Average costs include all resources used, including overhead, whose costs would not be decreased if those resources were not used. Marginal costing accepts fixed costs as a given and focuses only on variable costs or those additional resources consumed by each additional patient. Incremental costing focuses only on difference in costs between two treatments or procedures.

What a hospital charges for a service is not its costs (5). Measuring hospital costs is difficult and has been approached with either top-down or bottom-up accounting (6). Top-down accounting involves dividing all the money spent on a hospitalization or procedures by the number of episodes of care involving hospitalization or those procedures. In contrast, a bottom-up approach involves individual costs of all resources used for a service (e.g., supplies, equipment depreciation, facilities, salaries).

Finally, inflation and discounting must be introduced in evaluating costs in the future. Costs in the future must be deflated by multiplication with a constant to convert from any one year to another, on the basis of the medical inflation rate. Future costs must also be discounted to reflect the opportunity costs of current money units, or future costs must be expressed at their present value. Costs are generally discounted at a rate of 3% to 5% per year.

OUTCOMES EVALUATION

Figure 31.2 is a diagram of the range of outcomes—disease progression and health status—associated with osteoporosis. Disease progression outcomes refer to progressive bone structure alteration with fractures of long bones and of the axial skeleton, resulting in hospitalization, disability, and death. Health status outcomes refer to the way in which the underlying disease process manifests itself to patients. Symptoms such as fatigue, stiffness, and pain often decrease the ability to perform physical and social functions and result in a decline in the patient's emotional state. As patients find that they are unable to function as well as they would like, the perceived quality of life decreases. In quantifying health status, general health status measures represent overall health-related functioning, whereas disease-specific measures for osteoporosis describe more clinically relevant domains and can be more sensitive to changes in clinical status.

The integration of mortality and quality-of-life end points can be accomplished with health utility analyses (see Fig. 31.2). Health state utilities reflect patient preferences for a particular health state under conditions of uncertainty. Utility scores integrate all aspects of a patient's health status characteristics into a single number between 0 and 1, in which 0 represents death and 1 represents perfect health. Utilities can be estimated directly through either the use of the standard gamble or the time trade-off techniques (7). By multiplying utilities (the quality of life) by survival (the duration of life), quality-adjusted life-years (QALYs) may be calculated and used in cost-utility analyses. Dividing an estimate of the difference in costs between a treatment and its alternative by an estimate of the difference in QALYs yields an estimate of the incremental cost-utility analysis (or the incremental cost-effectiveness analysis, if the denominator is the difference in natural units, i.e., life-years gained) (4).

The "Quality-adjusted Time Without Symptoms of disease and Toxicity of treatment" (Q-TWiST) method focuses on the integration of both quality and quantity of life into a single analysis to be used for treatment comparisons (8). The Q-TWiST method makes treatment comparisons in terms of survival time without symptoms of disease or toxicity

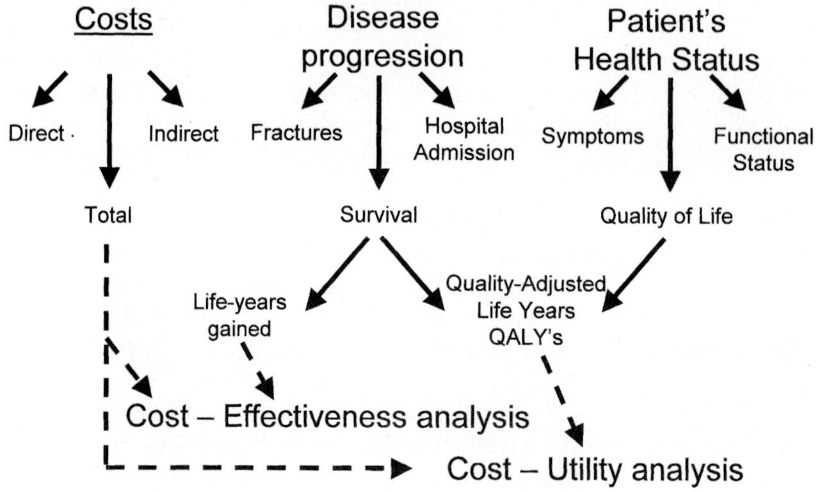

FIG. 31.2. Clinical outcomes associated with disease progression and patient's health status in osteoporosis. Principles of cost-effectiveness and cost-utility analyses.

of treatment (i.e., the survival time remaining after subtracting periods of time with symptoms or toxicity from the overall survival time). The Q-TWiST method allows a portion of the time spent with toxicity, relapse, or other clinical health states to be included in the comparison, inasmuch as these health states often have some health-related quality-of-life value for patients.

EFFICIENCY EVALUATION METHODOLOGIES

In efficiency evaluation—that is, assessing the financial impact of a new drug, technique, or procedure—four methods are commonly used: (a) cost-minimization analysis, (b) cost-effectiveness analysis, (c) cost-utility analysis, and (d) cost-benefit analyses. Whatever the type of analysis used, all costs are measured in monetary terms.

Cost-Minimization Analysis

Cost-minimization analysis focuses on the differences in direct costs associated with the study treatments. In this type of analysis, the treatments to be compared are considered equally efficacious according to previous research; thus, only treatment costs are compared. The objective of cost-minimization analysis is to identify the most efficient treatment method. Cost-minimization analysis is an appropriate form of evaluation to use when there is reason to believe that the outcomes of the procedures or treatments under consideration are the same. When there is strong evidence to suggest that there are no great differences in clinical outcomes, the analysis can concentrate on identifying the lowest cost option (9).

Cost-Effectiveness Analysis

Cost-effectiveness analysis is perhaps the most widely used method of evaluating new treatments or procedures. It compares total (direct and indirect) costs of a given clinical outcome measure for different therapeutic options. Benefits are expressed in terms of nonmonetary outcomes; thus, this type of analysis can be used only to compare interventions that produce similar outcomes. Cost-effectiveness analysis may also compare resource use associated with different therapies. The objective of this type of analysis is to determine the least costly method of achieving a given outcome.

To carry out a cost-effectiveness analysis, it is necessary to have suitable measures of effectiveness. The choice of these depends on the objectives of the particular interventions under review. In all cost-effectiveness analysis, however, measures of effectiveness should be defined in appropriate natural units and, ideally, expressed in a single dimension.

Common measures used in several studies have been "lives saved" and "life years gained" (10–12). Other measures of effectiveness have included the number of symptom-free days after treatment (13), the number of patients with a successful diagnosis in the case of alternative diagnostic strategies (14), the number of complications avoided by the treatment (15), and the numbers of episodes of fever cured and deaths prevented by the treatment (16). Most of the studies just cited expressed effectiveness in terms of a single dimension and thereby permitted direct comparison between alternative procedures in terms of their marginal cost per unit of outcome (4).

Cost-Utility Analysis

Information provided by cost-effectiveness analysis can be extremely useful in clarifying choices between different treatments for particular diseases or disabilities. It is, however, limited in its ability to assist decision makers in choosing between programs, because the units of outcome often vary—for example, reductions in blood pressure in comparison with cases of cancer of the cervix diagnosed. Moreover, cost-effectiveness analysis is not able to combine reductions in morbidity and reductions in mortality into a single index; thus, direct comparison is not possible between treatments that vary on these two dimensions.

Cost-utility analysis is therefore a variation of cost-effectiveness analysis that considers patient preferences for the effects of the therapy. In the concept of QALYs, 1 year of life in perfect health is set at 1.0 (1 QALY). Years with less than optimal health are scored as less than 1.0. The basic assumption is that 2 years scored 0.5 add up to the equivalent of 1 year of complete wellness ($2 \times 0.5 = 1$ QALY).

In this approach, the problem is the assignment of values (utilities) to health states. Utilities can be measured through one of several techniques based on decision theory, such as the rating scale, the standard gambling, or the time trade-off (7,17,18).

The first technique, referred as the *categorical or rating scale,* is to use a line with end points marking the best and worst possible health states at the top and bottom of the scale, respectively. The subject is asked to place the health state for which the utility is being measured (the intermediate state) somewhere between these two extremes.

The second method is the *standard gamble* or *reference lottery* technique. The subject is presented with a hypothetical choice between the actual health state being assessed and a lottery. The lottery provides a chance with a variable probability p of best outcome (perfect health) and the complementary chance ($1 - p$) of the worst outcome (death). The value of p for which the subject is indifferent to the choice is equal to the utility of the actual health state of the patient. The standard gamble is analogous to asking, "What probability of dying from surgery would you accept if the surgery would be guaranteed to restore perfect health if you survived?" The worse the health state is, the higher is the probability of dying from surgery that would be acceptable in order to restore health.

In the *time trade-off,* the subject is presented with a choice between the intermediate health state with a fixed survival time and the best possible health for a shorter survival time t, which is varied. As in the standard gamble, there is a value of t for which the subject would be indifferent to the choice. The percentage of life expectancy represented by t is equal to the utility for the intermediate state. The time trade-off is analogous to asking the subject, "How much of your remaining life expectancy would you be willing to give up if you could be restored to perfect health?" The worst the actual health status is, the more time a patient would be willing to forgo.

The rating scale is the simplest to understand but, paradoxically, has been shown in some studies to be more difficult for patients, probably because the units on the scale are relatively meaningless (19). Another major shortcoming is that comparisons between different measurements are hard to interpret. The time trade-off appears to be the easiest for patients to understand and perform (19). By definition, the standard gamble is the gold standard for utility measurement but is more difficult to understand than time trade-off because the concept of probability is difficult for many patients to grasp. Comparisons of the three approaches have shown that the standard gamble yields the highest expected utilities and the rating scale yields the lowest (20). The standard gamble and the time trade-off have shown acceptable reproducibility with repeated measurements, and the time trade-off shows acceptable validity in comparison with the reference technique standard gamble.

Cost-Benefit Analysis

Cost-benefit analysis is sometimes used loosely as a general term covering all types of economic evaluation, but among health economists, the term is usually restricted to the forms of evaluations that are used to place a monetary value on benefits and outcomes. Cost-benefit analysis defines both benefits and costs in monetary terms. Benefits are typically defined as costs avoided by the use of the intervention. Such costs may include hospitalization, days of disability, or loss of productivity as a result of premature death. The objective is to determine whether the cost savings realized outweighs the costs incurred from the therapy. Because therapeutic benefits are translated into monetary units, this type of analysis is ideal for comparing the value of treatments that have different therapeutic outcomes. For example, the cost and benefit of diverse medical therapies and surgical techniques can be compared. Although cost-benefit analysis provides a mechanism for such decisions, its usefulness is limited by the reluctance of many people to accept the assignment of a monetary value to patient health outcomes.

An alternative is to establish what people are willing to pay for health services if they were required to pay for them. This approach was used by Thompson (21), who sought to establish how much people would be willing to pay for a hypothetical cure for rheumatoid arthritis. Specially trained interviewers posed the following question to 247 patients: "What percentage of your family's total monthly income would you be willing to pay regularly for a complete cure for arthritis?" Of the patients questioned, 84% gave what were considered plausible responses; they indicated a willingness to pay a mean of 22% of the household income.

SENSITIVITY ANALYSIS

Estimates of the benefits of health practices, in terms of mortality and morbidity probabilities, are rarely known with certainty. The most easily applied method available to deal with uncertainty is sensitivity analysis. In this method, the most uncertain features and assumptions in the cost-effectiveness calculation are varied one at a time over the range of possible values. This permits the robustness of the results to be tested in light of variations in the values of key variables. Different forms of sensitivity analysis exist (22): (a) *Simple sensitivity analysis* entails varying one or more of the components of an evaluation to see how it affects the results; (b) in *extreme scenarios,* if two treatments are being compared, the extreme estimates of cost and effectiveness would be identified so that the two options can be compared under pessimistic (high-cost and low-effectiveness) and optimistic (low-cost and high-effectiveness) assumptions; and (c) *probabilistic sensitivity analysis* assigns ranges and distributions to variables, and computer programs are used to select values at random, from each range and to record the results. The advantage of the probabilistic approach is that it can simultaneously deal with a large number of variables and indicate the degree of confidence that can be attached to each option.

CONCLUSIONS

The appropriate choice of method of economic evaluation depends on the context in which choices need to be made. When outcomes are identical, the most straightforward form of cost minimization can be applied. When this condition does not apply, other forms of evaluation that require the more difficult task of outcome or benefit measurement should be applied. For many years, cost-effectiveness analysis has been the most widely used form of economic evaluation. It offers a powerful approach that may be used to help guide clinical decision and policy making. However, its limitations have meant that considerable research effort has been devoted to the development of cost-utility analysis. Beyond this, cost-benefit analysis offers the most comprehensive and theoretical form of economic evaluation, but its application in the context of health care is sometimes difficult because of the reluctance of many people to assign a monetary value to patient health outcomes. With the current changes in health care, accountability and costs are increasingly important, and physicians can expect to see more studies with these methods and greater incorporation of economic evaluation into the medical care delivery system.

REFERENCES

1. Levy P, Levy E, Audran M, et al. The cost of osteoporosis in men: the French situation. *Bone* 2002;30:631–636.
2. Rothermich EA, Pathak DS. Productivity-cost controversies in cost-effectiveness analysis: review and research agenda. *Clin Ther* 1999;21:255–267.
3. Mélot C. Economic evaluation in health care. In: Gunzburg R, Szpalski M, eds. *Lumbar spinal stenosis.* Philadelphia: Lippincott Williams & Wilkins, 2000:357–365.
4. Mélot C. Methodology for economic evaluation. In: Szpalski M, Gunzburg R, eds. *The degenerative cervical spine.* Philadelphia: Lippincott Williams & Wilkins, 2001:287–295.
5. Finkler SA. The distinction between costs and charges. *Ann Intern Med* 1982;96:102–109.
6. Finkler SA, Ward DM. *Essentials of costs accounting for health care organizations,* 2nd ed. New York: Aspen, 1999:11–43.
7. Mélot C. Principles of cost-benefit analysis. In: Szpalski M, Gunzburg R, Pope MH, eds. *Lumbar segmental instability.* Philadelphia: Lippincott Williams & Wilkins, 1999:259–273.
8. Mélot C. Principles of quality assessment. In: Gunzburg R, Szpalski M, eds. *Lumbar disk herniation.* Philadelphia: Lippincott Williams & Wilkins, 2002:243–254.
9. Robinson R. Economic evaluation and health care: costs and cost-minimization. *BMJ* 1993;307:726–728.
10. Churchill DN, Lemon BC, Torrance GW. Cost-effectiveness analysis comparing continuous ambulatory peritoneal dialysis to hospital haemodialysis. *Med Decis Making* 1984;4:489–500.
11. Ludbrook A. A cost-effectiveness analysis of the treatment of chronic renal failure. *Appl Econ* 1981;13:337–350.
12. Oster G, Epstein AM. Cost-effectiveness of antihyperlipemic therapy in the prevention of coronary heart disease. The cost of cholestyramine. *JAMA* 1987;258:2381–2387.
13. Sintonen H, Alander V. Comparing the cost-effectiveness of drug regimens in the treatment of duodenal ulcers. *J Health Econ* 1990;9:85–101.
14. Hull R, Hirsh J, Sackett DL, et al. Cost-effectiveness of clinical diagnosis, venography, and noninvasive testing in patients with symptomatic deep-vein thrombosis. *N Engl J Med* 1981;304:1561–1567.
15. Magid D, Schwartz B, Craft J, et al. Prevention of Lyme disease after tick bites. A cost-effectiveness analysis. *N Engl J Med* 1992;327:534–541.
16. Sudre P, Breman JC, McFarland D, et al. Treatment of chloroquine-resistant malaria in African children: a cost-effectiveness analysis. *Int J Epidemiol* 1992;21:146–154.
17. Kaplan RM, Bush JW. Health-related quality of life measurement for evaluation research and policy analysis. *Health Psychol* 1982;1:61–80.
18. Sonnenberg FA. Introduction to decision theory and utilities. In: Staquet MJ, Hays RD, Fayers PM, eds. *Quality of life assessment in clinical trials.* Oxford, UK: Oxford University Press, 1998:93–117.
19. Torrance GW. Social preferences for health states. An empirical evaluation of three measurement techniques. *Soc Econ Plan Sci* 1976;10:129–136.
20. Read JL, Quinn RJ, Berwick DM, et al. Preferences for health outcomes: comparison of assessment methods. *Med Decis Making* 1984;4:315–329.
21. Thompson MS. Willingness to pay and accept risks to cure chronic disease. *Am J Public Health* 1986;76: 392–396.
22. Robinson R. Economic evaluation and health care: cost-effectiveness analysis. *BMJ* 1993;307:793–795.

32

Cost Analysis of Medical and Surgical Treatment of Vertebral Fractures

Angelo A. Licata

Department of Endocrinology, Metabolic Bone Center, The Cleveland Clinic Foundation, Cleveland, Ohio

The treatment of osteoporosis has advanced dramatically since 1990, and the development of better therapies is expected. New medical and diagnostic modalities have made this disease a treatable one, no longer constrained by the untreatable process of aging. Reconstructive surgery of acute vertebral fractures may change the approach for the future and complement the medical approach.

Both vertebroplasty and kyphoplasty have changed the approach to treating acute fracture and pain. Each procedure has its own unique advantages and disadvantages. The short-term economic costs of the procedures are ultimately among the determinants for implementation. These alone, however, are not sufficient, because the impact of other issues, such as effects on quality of life and long-term savings in extended care costs, must be fully assessed as well. As yet, no trials have evaluated these surgical interventions and their relative costs in comparison with routine medical care. This chapter presents preliminary observations of costs in the medical and surgical treatment of acute fractures in patients treated at three centers in the United States.

The study is a retrospective analysis of extant data at two surgical sites and one medical site. Both surgical sites are affiliated with large academic institutions and, as such, would skew data toward higher costs. The medical site is a large health maintenance organization (HMO) with no expressed academic affiliation. Cost drivers in the initial acute management of vertebral fractures were obtained from the institutional data base. Data beyond the initial year of treatment were severely limited. Long-term cost drivers were sought but not obtained in all cases.

STUDY SITES

The medical facility was Group Health Cooperative of Seattle, Washington, the largest HMO in the northwestern United States. This is a consumer-governed organization in which a consumer-elected board of directors appoints the president, who in turn selects the medical director. It has an enrollment of 592,000 members. The HMO has its own medical staff and contracts with clinicians in areas not served by the HMO medical staff. The cost structure is about 92% of the national average.

The vertebroplasty site was at an academic institution affiliated with the University of San Diego School of Medicine. Patient data ($n = 9$) were abstracted from the practice of one physician during the period 1999 to 2000. The cost structure in this geographic region is about 115% the national average.

The kyphoplasty site was an orthopedic surgeon's practice at the Cleveland Clinic Foundation, a private nonprofit foundation with a 1000-bed hospital, an outpatient clinic facility, a research institute, and an education foundation. It has about 1000 full-time salaried physicians. Its spine center treats more than 4000 patients yearly, primarily with a nonsurgical approach involving medical and physical therapy modalities. The cost structure is 90% of the national average.

The demographics of all patients enrolled in the study are noted in Table 32.1 along with the average cost per case. The costs of care are those accrued during the first year of therapy at all sites. The cost for kyphoplasty is the average for three treatment levels. Of patients undergoing kyphoplasty, 30% had multiple myeloma; 44% underwent treatment for one vertebra ($8540), 41% for two vertebrae ($10,150), and 15% for three vertebrae ($11,300).

Table 32.2 lists the direct cost drivers for treatment of the initial vertebral fracture during the first year. Long-term cost drivers are not known; these would include the 5-year costs associated with, but not limited to, increased risk of further fractures, long-term care, home health care, and hospitalizations for complications such as ileus, decreased pulmonary function, management of depression and pain, and sleep disorders. Over 4.4 years, medical costs rose an additional $7000 for these long-term costs drivers, thereby increasing the average costs to about $9500 for this time period. The long-term costs beyond the initial surgical procedures are not well established. An additional $1100 is estimated for vertebroplasty costs because of home health care and treatment of ileus, pulmonary problems, depression, and sleep disturbance. The time frame involved is unclear but less than 5 years. However, these charges are limited to a small number of cases, as noted in Table 32.1, and at best are approximations of what would be the "universe" of vertebroplasty cases. It is unclear what fraction of the surgical costs are attributable to the "academic mission" that may be part of institutional overhead and hidden in these surgical charges. More detailed breakdown of charges is listed below.

Nonoperative medical care costs are distributed over several areas, as noted in Table 32.3. The average cost, excluding drugs, is $2150 per year. Pharmacy charges for outpatient drugs increase the average by $350.

The average annual cost can increase substantially, depending on treatment for complications such as recurring vertebral or nonvertebral fractures (especially those of the hip), decubitus ulcers from long-term immobility, gait disturbance, deconditioning of the musculature, and weight loss. Aging and frailty increase the complication rate. Data show a doubling and tripling of the baseline average costs for some patients. About 20% of patients with a prevalent vertebral fracture sustain a new one within the following year. These patients have an increased incidence of complications in comparison with a control population (i.e., same age but no diagnosis of osteoporosis). The incidences of decreased pulmonary function and hip fractures are 20.7% and 12.3% higher, respectively; the incidences of urinary tract infection, depression, and decubitus ulcers are 2% to 4% higher.

Vertebroplasty cost analysis results are listed in Table 32.4. The average cost per case was $3900 for nine patients. Certain charges are not included in this average value; these include technical and professional fees for anteroposterior and lateral radiography and lumbar/thoracic magnetic resonance imaging performed at other institutions. Pharmacy costs for the procedure are also not listed.

Kyphoplasty cost analysis is noted in Table 32.5. The total professional fees account for 16% of the total; the technical fees, 84%.

TABLE 32.1. *Demographic and average cost data*

Site	Number	Average age (years)	Gender % (women/men)	Costs/year (US $)
1. Medical	75	77	81/19	2500
2. Vertebroplasty	9	Not available	Not available	3900
3. Kyphoplasaty	54	68	60/40	9600

TABLE 32.2. *Direct cost drivers for treatment during the first year*

Medical therapy	Vertebroplasty	Kyphoplasty
Specialists' fees	Angio-suite	Operating room costs
Home health care	Physicians' fees	Surgeons' fees
Pharmacy	Imaging costs	Hospital stay
Hospitalization costs	Instruments	Instruments
		Imaging costs

TABLE 32.3. *Medical care costs*

Cost driver	% Total charge
Hospital outpatient	5
Hospital inpatient	14
Unallocated (no specific data)	15
Other (home health care, laboratory, ambulance)	15
Medical specialist	10
Primary care provider	11
Pharmacy	16
Long-term care	14

TABLE 32.4. *Vertebroplasty cost breakdown*

Cost driver	Cost per case (avg. US $)	% Total
Equipment and supplies	1740	41
Physician fees	1310	31
Angio-suite	76	2
Imaging	135	3
Other, laboratory administration	287	7
Postanesthetic care unit	352	8

TABLE 32.5. *Kyphoplasty cost analysis*

Cost driver	Cost per case (avg. US $)	% Total
Operating room	4400	47
Physicians'/nurses' fees	2600	28
Laboratory/pharmacy tests	18	<1
Durable medical	57	1
Physical therapy	50	1
Imaging	520	6
Hospital	1690	18

COMMENTS

These data are a first approximation for analyzing medical and surgical treatment costs of vertebral fractures. The data show a substantially higher cost for the kyphoplasty in the initial patient encounter, but the costs of both surgical procedures were greater than the initial cost outlay for medical treatment. The unresolved issue is whether there are long-term benefits from surgery that would control costs to a greater degree than would medical therapy. Some of the long-term benefit is intangible and difficult to quantitate. These are the issues subsumed under the notion of quality of life. Pain relief is certainly one of these and is the major cost driver for treatment in all cases. If the surgical procedures continue to display improvement in this parameter, they will be favored over conventional medical therapy and its use of analgesic drugs that cause central nervous system side effects and increase susceptibility to falls and fractures. The immediacy of pain control with kyphoplasty and vertebroplasty is certainly an important advance. The reconstruction of collapsed vertebrae from kyphoplasty is an added benefit that has significant long-term implications. Maintaining correct anatomical alignment may be a major ameliorating factor for long-term costs. Control of pain, curtailment of medical costs, and increased daily productivity are a few of the potential long-term benefits. Long-term costs drivers have not yet been evaluated adequately. Quite clearly, the very limited nature of this study cannot provide such an evaluation; more study sites are required. How surgical therapy may affect long-term cost drivers is clearly speculative. One area that has not been fully explored is the relationship between prevalent fractures and future fractures. Data show clearly that patients with prevalent fractures are at risk for future fractures. In one study, data showed progressive increases in new fractures in the year after the incident vertebral fracture (1). Almost 20% of patients sustain a new vertebral fracture within the year. Drug therapy can control further fractures within a year of initiation (2–4). Long-term costs may be curtailed because of this effect. What would surgery accomplish in this situation? Would it curtail or increase further fractures? Is a blend of medical and pharmaceutical therapy the optimal approach? These notions must be critically evaluated with a larger data base and a greater dispersion of sites in academic and nonacademic centers.

REFERENCES

1. Lindsay R, Silverman SL, Cooper C, et al. Risk of new vertebral fractures in the year following a fracture. *JAMA* 2001;285:320–323.
2. Harris ST, Watts NH, Genant HK, et al. Effects of risedronate treatment on vertebral and nonvertebral fractures in women with postmenopausal osteoporosis. *JAMA* 1999;282:1344–1352.
3. Liberman UA, Weiss SR, Broll J, et al. Effect of oral alendronate on bone mineral density and the incidence of fractures in postmenopausal osteoporosis. *N Engl J Med* 1995;333:1437–1443.
4. Ettweger B, Block DM, Mitlate BH, et al. Reduction of vertebral fracture risk in postmenopausal women treated with raloxifene. *JAMA* 1999;282:637–645.

Subject Index

Note: Page numbers followed by f indicate figures; page numbers followed by t refer to tables.